Ambulatory Surgery and Office Procedures In Head and Neck Surgery

Ambulatory Surgery and Office Procedures in Head and Neck Surgery

Edited by

K.J. Lee, M.D., F.A.C.S.
*Chief of Otolaryngology,
Hospital of Saint Raphael;
Director, Hospital of Saint Raphael
Ear Research and Educational Center;
Director, Hospital of Saint Raphael
Laser Surgery Center,
New Haven, Connecticut*

Carol H. Stewart
Branford, Connecticut

Grune & Stratton, Inc.
Harcourt Brace Jovanovich, Publishers
Orlando   New York   San Diego   Boston   London
San Francisco   Tokyo   Sydney   Toronto

Copyright © 1986 by Grune & Stratton, Inc.

All rights reserved. No part of this publication may be reproduced or transmitted in any form or by any means, electronic or mechanical, including photocopy, recording, or any information storage and retrieval system, without permission in writing from the publisher.

Grune & Stratton, Inc.
Orlando, Florida 32887

Distributed in the United Kingdom by
Grune & Stratton, Ltd.
24/28 Oval Road, London NW 1

Library of Congress Catalog Number 86-19487
International Standard Book Number 0-8089-1803-6
Printed in the United States of America
86 87 88 89   10 9 8 7 6 5 4 3 2 1

Dedication

This book is dedicated to Linda Lee and Ryan Stewart.

CONTENTS

Preface   *xi*
Contributors   *xiii*

1. Otolaryngology—Head and Neck Physical Diagnosis
   K.J. Lee and Thomas Vris   1

2. Office Photography
   Stewart D. Fordham and Robert P. Rowe   19

3. Fiberoptic Nasopharyngolaryngoscopy
   Eiji Yanagisawa and Koichi Yamashita   31

4. Fiberoptic Bronchoscopy
   Jacob Loke and S.Y. So   41

5. Fiberoptic Esophagoscopy
   Myron H. Brand and Frank J. Troncale   49

6. Videolaryngoscopy
   Eiji Yanagisawa   63

7. Instrumentation and Techniques of Office Removal of Foreign Bodies
   K.J. Lee and Raymond A. Gaito, Jr.   73

8. Chemical Peel and Dermabrasion
   Emil P. Liebman   79

9. Scar Revision and Facial Flaps
   Ronald H. Hirokawa and Richard C. Bryarly   93

10. Hair Transplant
    Ronald C. Savin   103

11. Collagen Injection
    Douglas D. Dedo   119

12. Otoplasty
    K.J. Lee and Nathan E. Nachlas   125

13. Blepharoplasty
    Ronald H. Hirokawa and Richard C. Bryarly   135

14. Cervical-Facial Liposuction
    Julius Newman and Abram Nguyen   149

15. Voice Restoration
    Vijay K. Anand and Kenneth E. Lee   185

16. The Carbon Dioxide Laser in Outpatient Surgery
    James H. Kelly and Marvin P. Fried   191

17. Cryosurgery in Outpatient Surgery
    Richard L. Fabian   199

18. Allergy Skin Testing
    Denise Metz and June Bubier   207

19. The Modified RAST—An Aid in Diagnosis and Management of Allergic Patients
    Donald J. Nalebuff   215

20. The Clinical and Practical Aspects of Auditory Brainstem Response
    Lori Wills   229

21. The Clinical and Practical Aspects of Electronystagmography
    Kenneth H. Brookler   247

22. The Principles and Practicality of Hearing Aid Dispensing
    Mary S. MacDonald — 267

23. Rhinomanometry
    Thomas V. McCaffrey and Eugene B. Kern — 277

24. The Clinical and Practical Aspects of Office Pulmonary Function Tests
    Frederick L. Sachs — 285

25. Development and Management of an Outpatient Surgical Facility in the Office of an Otolaryngological Group Practice
    James J. Pappas and Sharon S. Graham — 295

26. Designing the Facility
    Howard A. Tobin — 303

27. The Computer for Business
    John V. Barto and Carol H. Stewart — 315

    Index — 321

Preface

It has been estimated that 60 percent or more of all Otolaryngology/Head and Neck surgery can be performed in an ambulatory surgical environment. We have put forth in this book not only descriptions of surgical procedures that can be performed on an ambulatory surgery basis, but also examples of free-standing ambulatory surgery centers. Common procedures that can be performed in an ambulatory surgical environment, such as tonsillectomy and septal reconstruction, have not been included; it is assumed that such techniques have been mastered during residency. Other procedures, such as mastoidectomy–tympanoplasty, can also be performed in an ambulatory surgery center, provided the patient is ASA Class I.

It is our hope that this book will stimulate more innovative use of out-patient surgery facilities.

K. J. Lee, M.D., F.A.C.S.
Carol Stewart

Contributors

Vijay K. Anand, M.D. Chief of Voice Restoration Clinic, and Attending Surgeon, Department of Otolaryngology, Manhattan Eye, Ear and Throat Hospital, New York, New York

John V. Barto Datatek Computer Services, Inc., Guilford, Connecticut

Myron H. Brand, M.D., F.A.C.P., F.A.C.G. Attending Gastroenterologist, Hospital of Saint Raphael; Assistant Clinical Professor of Medicine, Yale University School of Medicine, New Haven, Connecticut; Consultant in Gastroenterology, Milford Hospital, Milford, Connecticut

Kenneth H. Brookler, M.D., M.S., FRCS(C), F.A.C.S. Otology & Neurotology & Facial Nerve Surgery, New York, New York

Richard C. Bryarly, M.D. Assistant Professor, Department of Otolaryngology, LSU Medical Center, Shreveport, Louisiana

June Bubier, R.N. Providence, Rhode Island

Douglas Dedo, M.D., F.A.C.S. Clinical Assistant Professor of Otolaryngology—Head and Neck Surgery, University of Miami School of Medicine, Miami, Florida; Attending Physician, Good Samaritan Hospital and Saint Mary's Hospital, West Palm Beach, Florida

Richard L. Fabian, M.D., F.A.C.S. Attending Physician, New England Deaconess Hospital and Dana Farber Institute; Assistant Clinical Professor, Massachusetts Eye and Ear Infirmary, Boston, Massachusetts

Marvin P. Fried, M.D., F.A.C.S. Associate Professor of Otolaryngology, Harvard Medical School; Surgeon, Brigham and Women's Hospital; Associate Surgeon in Otolaryngology, Beth Israel Hospital; Assistant in Otolaryngology, Children's Hospital Medical Center; Assistant Surgeon, Massachusetts Eye and Ear Infirmary, Boston, Massachusetts

Stewart D. Fordham, M.D., M.A. Staff Physician, California Hospital Medical Center, Los Angeles, California

Raymond A. Gaito, Jr., M.D.   Resident in Otolaryngology, Yale School of Medicine, New Haven, Connecticut

Sharon S. Graham, M.A.   The Ear & Nose-Throat Clinic, P.A., Little Rock, Arkansas

Ronald H. Hirokawa, M.D., F.A.C.S.   Attending Physician, Hospital of Saint Raphael and Yale New Haven Hospital, New Haven, Connecticut

James H. Kelly, M.D., F.A.C.S.   Chief of Otolaryngology, Sinai Hospital of Baltimore; Attending Physician Johns Hopkins Hospital, Baltimore, Maryland

Eugene B. Kern, M.D.   Department of Otorhinolaryngology, Mayo Clinic, Rochester, Minnesota

K. J. Lee, M.D., F.A.C.S.   Chief of Otolaryngology, Hospital of Saint Raphael; Director, Hospital of Saint Raphael Ear Research and Educational Center; Director, Hospital of Saint Raphael Laser Surgery Center, New Haven, Connecticut

Kenneth E. Lee   Harvard University, Cambridge, Massachusetts

Emil P. Liebman, M.D., F.A.C.S.   Clinical Professor, Department of Otorhinolaryngology and Bronchoesophagology; Chief Section of Facial Plastic and Reconstructive Surgery Temple School of Medicine, Philadelphia, Pennsylvania

Jacob Loke, M.D., F.A.C.P.   Associate Professor of Medicine; Attending Physician, Yale School of Medicine, New Haven, Connecticut

Thomas V. McCaffrey, M.D.   Department of Otorhinolaryngology, Mayo Clinic, Rochester, Minnesota

Mary McDonald, M.A., C.C.C.-A.   Clinical Audiologist, New Haven Ear, Nose, Throat & Cosmetic Facial Plastic Surgery Center, New Haven, Connecticut

Denise Metz, R.N., B.A.   Providence, Rhode Island

Nathan Nachlas, M.D.   Instructor, Department of Otolaryngology, Head and Neck Surgery, Johns Hopkins Hospital, Baltimore, Maryland

Donald J. Nalebuff, M.D.   Chief, Department of Immunology, Holy Name Hospital, Teaneck, New Jersey

Julius Newman, M.D.   Chairman, Department of Cosmetic Surgery, The Graduate Hospital, Philadelphia, Pennsylvania

Abram Nguyen, M.D.   Senior Fellow, Department of Cosmetic Surgery, The Graduate Hospital, Philadelphia, Pennsylvania

James J. Pappas, M.D.   The Ear & Nose-Throat Clinic, P.A., Little Rock, Arkansas

Robert P. Rowe, M.D.   Associate Professor of Head and Neck Surgery, Loma Linda University School of Medicine, Loma Linda, California

Frederick L. Sachs, M.D.   Associate Clinical Professor of Medicine, Yale University School of Medicine; Associate Chief, Department of Medicine, Yale New Haven Hospital; Attending Physician at Yale New Haven Hospital and The Hospital of Saint Raphael, New Haven, Connecticut

Ronald Savin, M.D.   Clinical Professor of Dermatology, Yale School of Medicine; Attending Physician, Yale New Haven Hospital; Attending Physician, Hospital of Saint Raphael, New Haven, Connecticut

S.Y. So, M.B.B.S., M.R.C.P.   Senior Lecturer in Medicine, University of Hong Kong, Hong Kong

Carol H. Stewart   Branford, Connecticut

Howard A. Tobin, M.D., F.A.C.S.   Director, Facial Plastic and Cosmetic Surgical Center, Abilene, Texas

Frank J. Troncale, M.D.   Chief of Gastroenterology, Hospital of St. Raphael; Assistant Clinical Professor of Medicine, Yale University School of Medicine, New Haven, Connecticut; Consultant in Gastroenterology, Milford Hospital, Milford, Connecticut

Thomas Vris, M.D.   Attending Surgeon, Norwalk Hospital, Norwalk, Connecticut

Lori Wills, M.S., C.C.C.-A.   Audiologist, New Haven Ear, Nose, Throat and Facial Plastic Surgery Center, New Haven, Connecticut

Koichi Yamashita, M.D.   Professor and Chairman, Department of Otolaryngology, Kanazawa Medical University, Uchinada, Ishikawa, Japan

Eiji Yanagisawa, M.D., F.A.C.S.   Clinical Professor of Otolaryngology, Yale School of Medicine; Attending Physician, Yale New Haven Hospital; Attending Physician, Hospital of Saint Raphael, New Haven, Connecticut; Attending Physician, Milford Hospital, Milford, Connecticut; Consultant, Meriden-Wallingford Hospital, Meriden, Connecticut; Consultant, Waterbury Hospital, Waterbury, Connecticut

LEGENDS CHAPTER 3, FIGURES 7A–P

Fig. 3-7. Examples of normal and abnormal fiberscopic findings. (A) Nasopharynx showing torus tubaris, lateral nasopharyngeal wall, and soft palate. (B) Enlarged torus tubaris. Note mucus coming out of the eustachian tube orifice in a patient with acute otitis media. (C) Markedly enlarged adenoids. This patient has no otitis media with effusion because the tubal orifice is not blocked by the adenoid mass. (D) An abscess obstructing the pharyngeal tubal orifice. (E) Enlarged adenoids with mildly enlarged torus tubaris. (F) Marked hypertrophy of adenoids with closure of eustachian tube orifice. This patient had mucous otitis media. (G) Carcinoma of nasopharynx. (H) Nasopharynx of cleft palate patient with patent eustachian tube orifice. (I) Panoramic view of the base of tongue, larynx, and hypopharynx. (J) Enlarged faucial tonsils. (K) Normal larynx at rest. (L) Edematous vocal cords. (M) Laryngeal nodules. (N) Large sessile polyp. (O) Epiglottic carcinoma. (P) Extensive carcinoma involving epiglottis, false and true cords, aryepiglottic folds, and arytenoids.

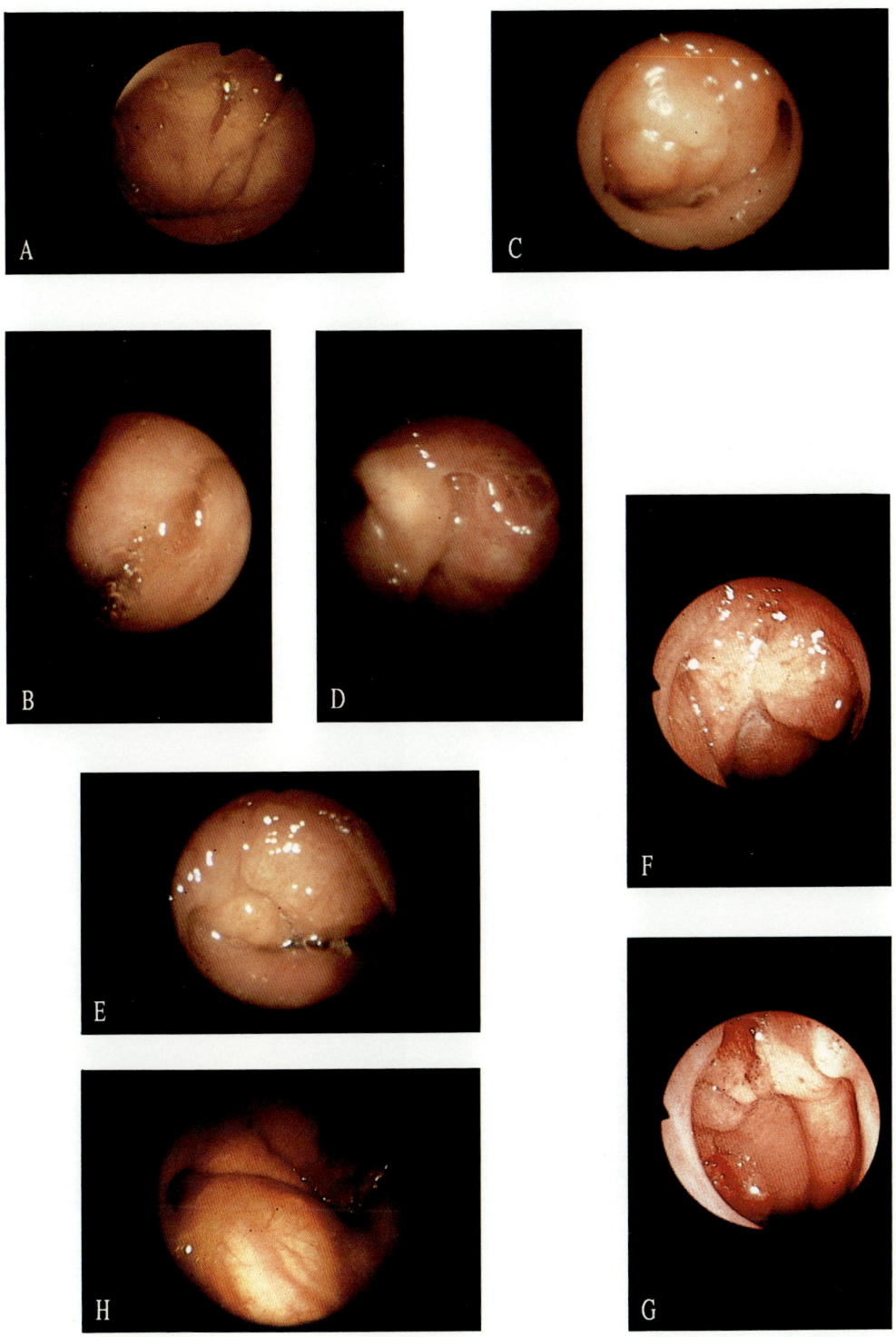

Chapter 3, Figure 7A–H

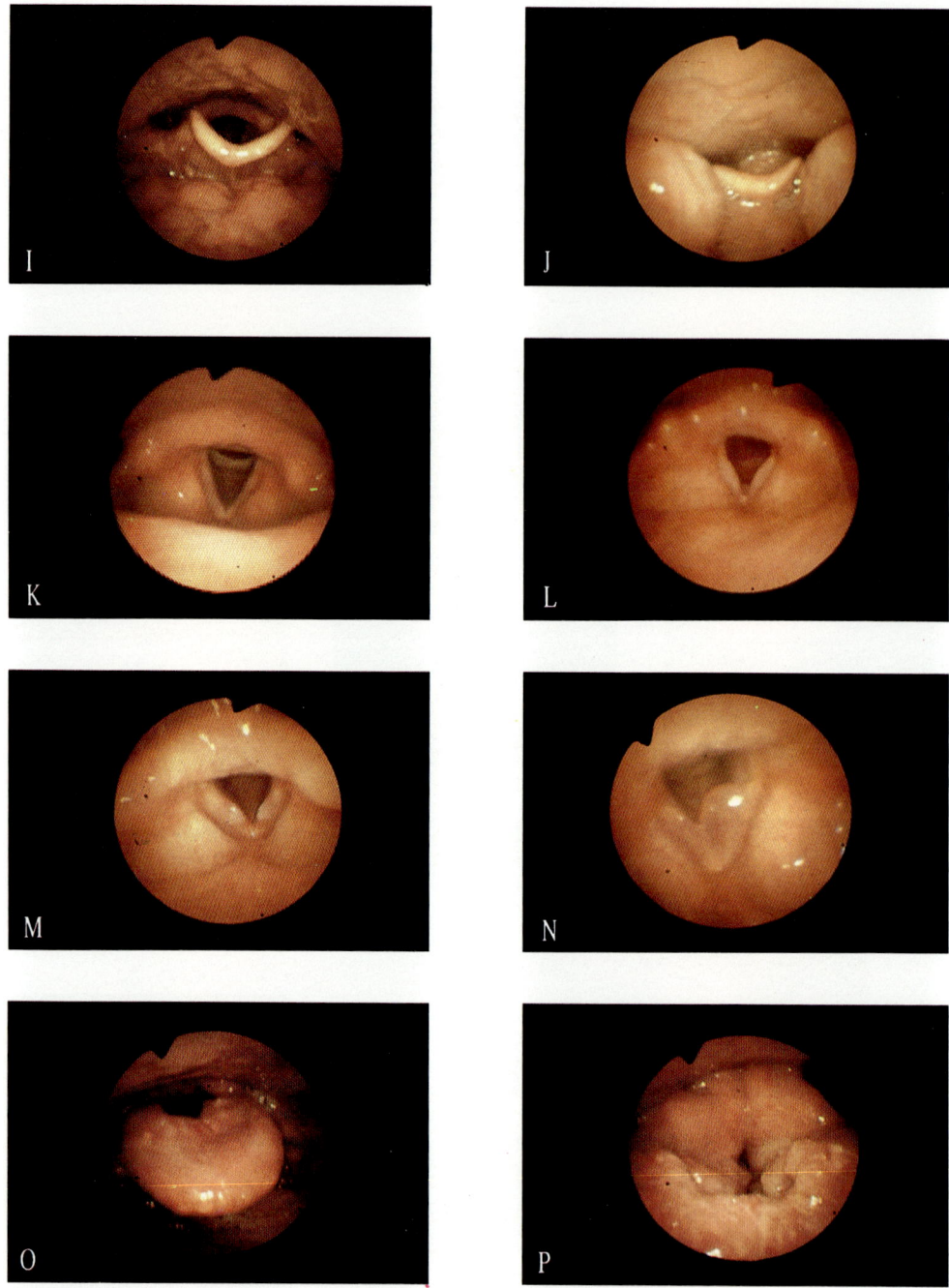

Chapter 3, Figure 7I–P

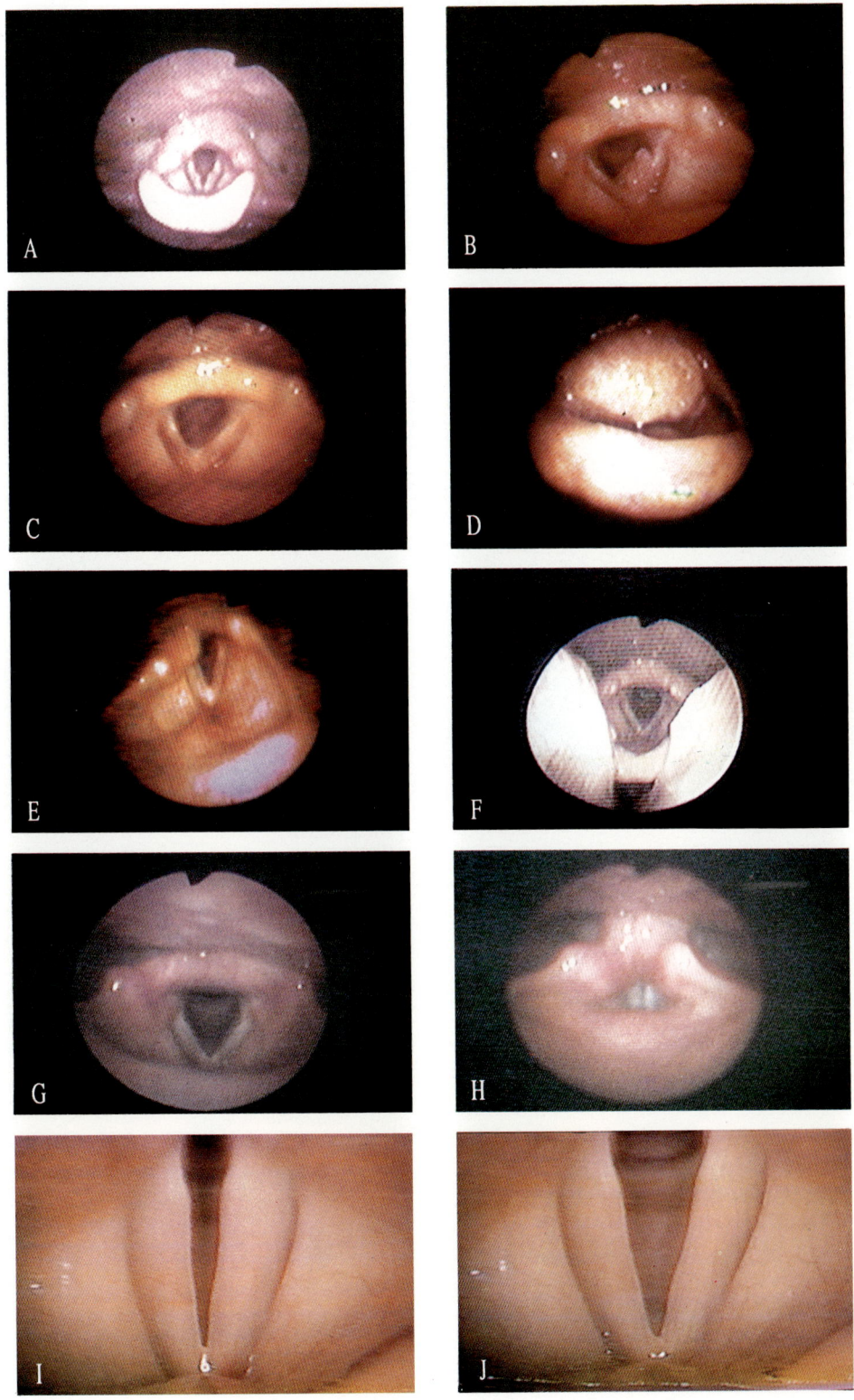

Chapter 6, Figure 6A–J

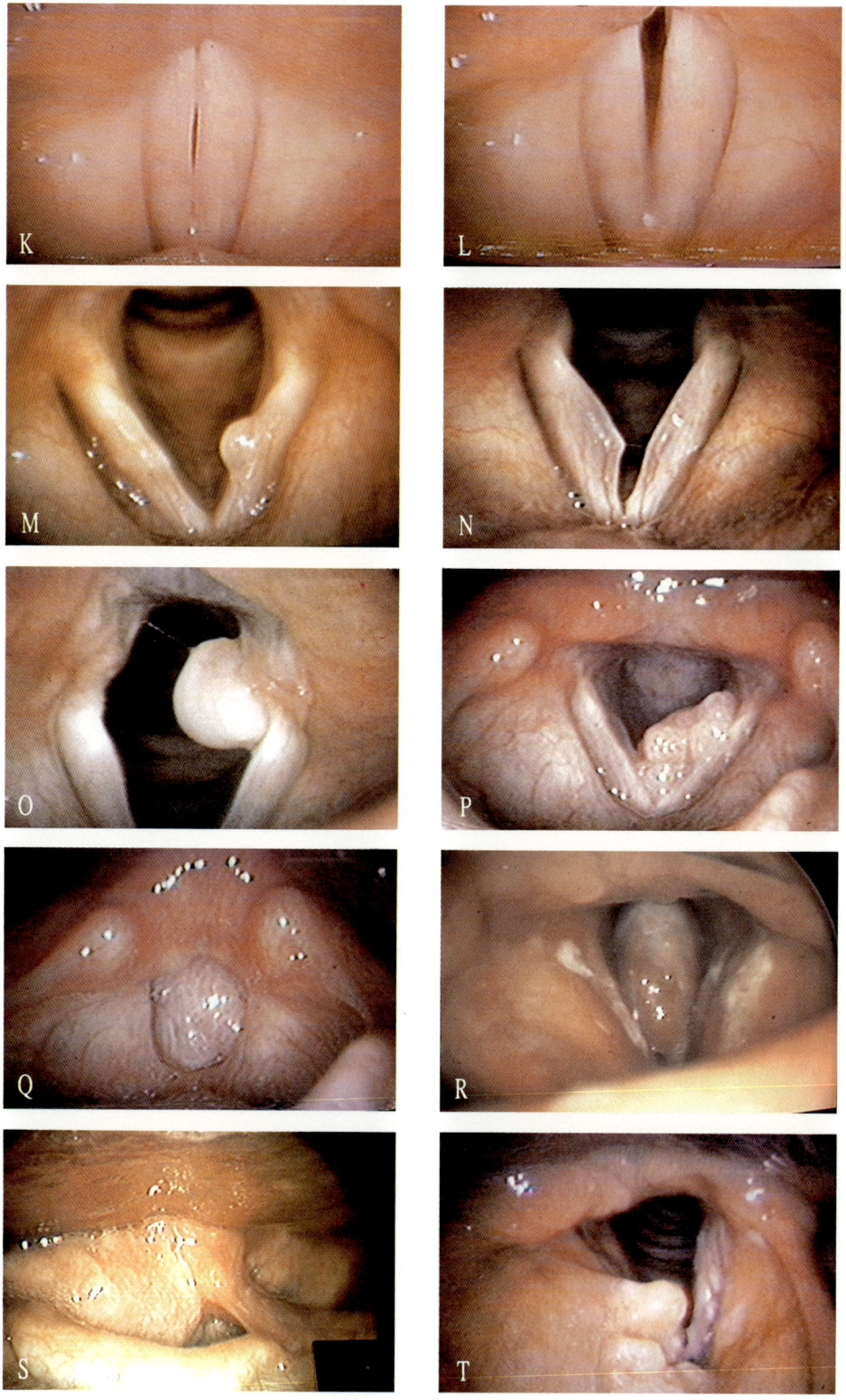

Chapter 6, Figure 6K–T

LEGENDS CHAPTER 6, FIGURES 6A–T

Fig. 6-6. Representative video images of laryngeal conditions photographed from TV monitor screen. Fiberscopic views of the larynx (1–8): (A) Laryngeal nodules. (B) Papilloma of left vocal cord. (C) Same patient 1 year after CO_2 laser surgery. Note a very small web in the anterior commissure. (D) Large carcinoma of aryepiglottic fold and arytenoid on the right side. (E) Vocal cord paralysis. (F) Larynx seen between markedly enlarged tonsils. (G) Vocal cords on deep respiration. (H) Vocal cords on phonation.
Telescopic views of the larynx (9–20): (I) Vocal cords on respiration. (J) Vocal cords on inspiration. (K) Vocal cords on phonation. (L) Vocal cords on phonation. (M) Single polyp. (N) Sessile polyps. (O) Postintubation granuloma. (P) Papilloma of a 12-year-old child. (Q) Same patient on phonation. (R) Obstructive subglottic polyp. (S) Aryepiglottic carcinoma. (T) Extensive supraglottic carcinoma.

Ambulatory Surgery and Office Procedures in Head and Neck Surgery

K.J. Lee
Thomas Vris

1
Otolaryngology—Head and Neck Physical Diagnosis

Few areas of the body provide such a complex array of structure for the skillful and knowledgeable examiner as the head and neck regions, and few examinations are as diagnostically rewarding as the systematic head and neck examination. The examination consists of two basic parts: an inspection and palpation of the external features of the head and neck region as well as an internal examination using special illumination and instrumentation.

The examiner will need a source of coaxial illumination such as a head mirror or a headlight. The coaxial principle allows the examiner's line of vision to be in the same pathway as the line of illumination. The head mirror accomplishes this by having a hole centrally placed in the mirror. This places the line of vision and the direction of the light beam on the same pathway. Certain headlights are so constructed as to allow for this coaxial illumination.

The sensitive mucosal linings of the oral and nasal cavities will frequently require topical anesthesia before an adequate examination can be carried out. The most commonly used anesthetics are:

1. 2 percent Pontocaine spray (Breon)
2. 1 percent Xylocaine spray (Astra)
3. Cetacaine (Cetylite)

It is important to wait 5–10 minutes after the application of the topical anesthetic before examining the patient. This will allow time for the local anesthetic to take effect. This is a very important step and commonly missed by the beginning students.

Mirrors are used in otolaryngology to reflect light into the larynx and the hypopharynx, as well as up into the nasopharynx beyond the soft palate. A selection of mirror sizes should be available, ranging from size Number 00 to size Number 6. A Number 4 mirror is usually very appropriate for indirect laryngoscopy examination. A size Number 1 or 2 mirror would be appropriate for nasopharyngoscopy examination.

The fiberoptic nasopharyngoscopy and laryngoscopy have become an important contribution towards the examination of the internal recesses of the head and neck region. They provide an unparalleled view of the laryngeal and nasopharyngeal structures. Adequate anesthesia is again very important before the fiberoptic nasopharyngoscope or laryngoscope is passed. The oropharynx and the nasal vestibules are carefully sprayed with topical anesthetic. Cotton pledgets soaked in a vasoconstrictive solution such as ephedrine or a topical anesthetic powder, cocaine, can be placed along the nasal mucosa to decongest the tissues. The lens of the fiberoptic nasopharyngoscope or laryngoscope should be covered with a thin film of liquid soap to prevent fogging, or the lens could be slightly warmed by dipping it in warm water prior to the insertion of the scope. A slight lubricant should be used to facilitate the passing of the scope. A detailed examination of the nasopharynx, including the eustachian tube orifices and the Rosenmüeller's fossa, can be seen. By passing the fiberoptic scope further inferiorly, a view of the hypopharynx and the larynx can be achieved.

The head and neck examination is best performed with the patient sitting forward in front of the examiner. All instrumentation and the topical anesthetics, as well as the light source, should be readily available to the seated examiner. It is always wise to sit in the position as illustrated in Figure 1-1 and not in the position as illustrated in Figure 1-2.

THE EXTERNAL HEAD AND NECK EXAMINATION

This aspect of the examination consists of inspection and palpation. Begin by noting the patient's head position. Is the head thrust forward in the sniffing position, signifying a possible upper airway obstruction—for example, due to an enlarged epiglottis, which is

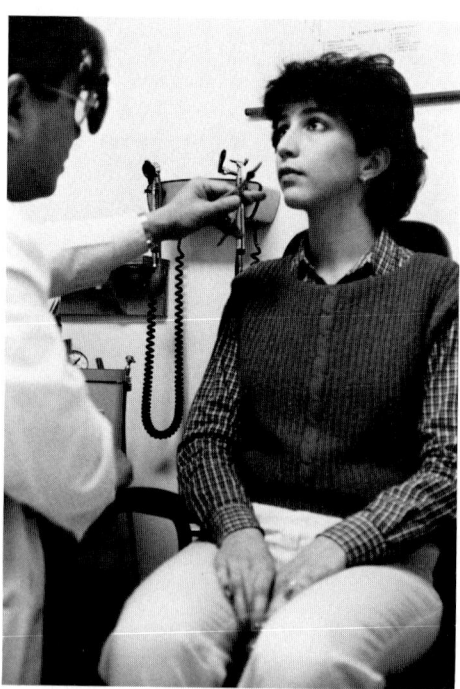

Fig. 1-1. Proper examination position of head and neck.

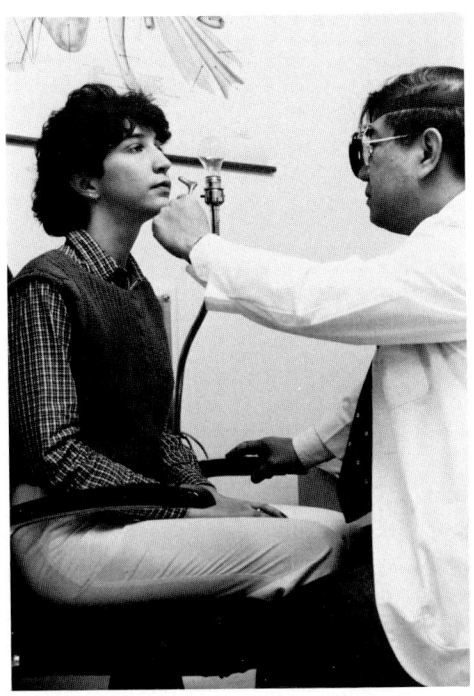

Fig. 1-2. Improper examination position of head and neck.

an anterior structure flapping posteriorly to compromise the upper airway? Please note whether or not the head is tilted to one side, possibly attributable to torticollis of the sternocleidomastoid muscle or an expanding neck mass. Before the pathology of the neck region can be appreciated by the clinician, there should be a mental picture of the anatomical structures within the neck. The hyoid bone, thyroid cartilage, cricoid cartilage, and the trachea are midline structures. The mandible superiorly, the trapezius muscle posteriorly, and the clavicle inferiorly, together with the midline structures, form the confines of a rectangle. The sternocleidomastoid muscle, which is attached to the mastoid tip superiorly and to the clavicle inferiorly, dissects this rectangular space into an anterior triangle and a posterior triangle. The anterior triangle is bordered by the mandible, the anterior margin of the sternocleidomastoid muscle, and the midline structures. The posterior triangle is bordered by the trapezius muscle, the clavicle, and the posterior margin of the sternocleidomastoid muscle. The internal jugular veins span the triangles from an inferior to superior direction. Surrounding the internal jugular veins are numerous lymph nodes. These nodes can be involved with inflammatory processes or with metastatic diseases. It would be important to describe any lymph adenopathy as low jugular nodes, mid jugular nodes, or upper jugular nodes. It would also be important to describe any neck masses in relation to the triangles mentioned above, as well as in relation to the other anatomical structures. The posterior digastric muscle and the anterior digastric muscle form a digastric sling in the upper portion of the anterior triangle. The submandibular gland is located in the anterior aspect of the digastric triangle. The digastric triangle is bordered by the posterior digastric muscle, the anterior digastric muscle, and the mandible. The carotid bifurcation or the carotid bulb is slightly below the digastric triangle. It is essential for the student to become familiar with all these structures.

An overall appraisal of the morphology and symmetry of the head and face should be made. Is there a flattening of the malar eminence suggesting an undiagnosed facial fracture, or a fullness due to neoplasia in the maxillary antrum? The normal face is roughly divided into equal thirds by horizontal lines drawn through the eyes and through the mouth. Disharmony on the middle and lower thirds of the face into relative prognathic or retrognathic configurations may reflect a malocclusion secondary to trauma or developmental malformation. Dental occlusion is generally categorized in 3 classes: Class 1 is normal; Class 2 is commonly referred to as an overbite; Class 3 occlusion is caused by relative mandibular overgrowth or prognathism, causing the mandibular teeth to be more anterior than the maxillary teeth. It is of interest to note that the mandible and certain parts of the ossicles in the middle ear are derived from the first branchial arch (mandibular arch). Hence, any malformation of the mandible may be associated with malformation of the middle ear ossicles, giving rise to a conductive hearing loss.

The skin of the head and neck region should be carefully inspected for lesions. Malignant and premalignant skin lesions are strongly correlated with sun exposure, which in most individuals is greatest to the head and neck region. Basal cell carcinoma frequently arises on the nasal dorsum, malar eminence, forehead, and eyelid, and around the auricle. The usual basal cell carcinoma is a round, elevated lesion with a rolled-up border and a central ulceration. A slight whitish discoloration may or may not be present. Squamous cell carcinoma is the next most common malignant lesion of the skin. Squamous cell carcinoma has a more flattened, scaly appearance than does the basal cell carcinoma. It is also more ulcerative. It is important to note at this junction that basal cell carcinoma is usually less aggressive than is squamous cell carcinoma. However, basal cell carcinoma that exists in the auricle within a one-centimeter radius of the external auditory canal is also very aggressive and should be treated more like a squamous cell carcinoma than a basal cell carcinoma.

Melanoma of the head and neck has a greatly improved prognosis when detected early. Hence, any pigmented nevus that has changed in recent months or has begun to ulcerate or bleed should be looked upon with great suspicion.

The examiner should also be aware of congenital benign nevi, strawberry and cavernous hemangiomata, neurofibromas, and cafe au-lait spots. It is important to note that hemangiomas in the infant do usually regress to a greater or lesser extent by the age of two. Hence, aggressive surgical treatment should not be applied to patients under the age of two unless the hemangiomas are compromising vital structures. With the advent of argon laser surgery, port wine stains, a form of hemangioma, can be very well treated. Patients with neurofibromas often develop acoustic neurinoma. Acoustic neurinoma is a form of a cerebellar-pontine angle tumor giving rise to sensorineural hearing loss, tinnitus, and vertigo.

The special features of the external head and neck that physicians normally categorize as one recognizable entity when they "learn a face" should each be inspected for structural abnormalities. Thus, the normal auricle has a natural curvature ending in an attached lobule. The size of the concha and the presence of an antihelix determine the angle at which the ear stands out from the head. The lack of an antihelical fold gives rise to a shell-shaped ear otherwise known as a lop ear. Some mothers think that the child's ear is too large and hence request an otoplasty. In most instances, it is not that the ear is too large, but, rather, that the auricle lacks an antihelical fold, giving rise to the shell-shaped appearance and thus the ear appears to be "too large." In otoplasty, the major

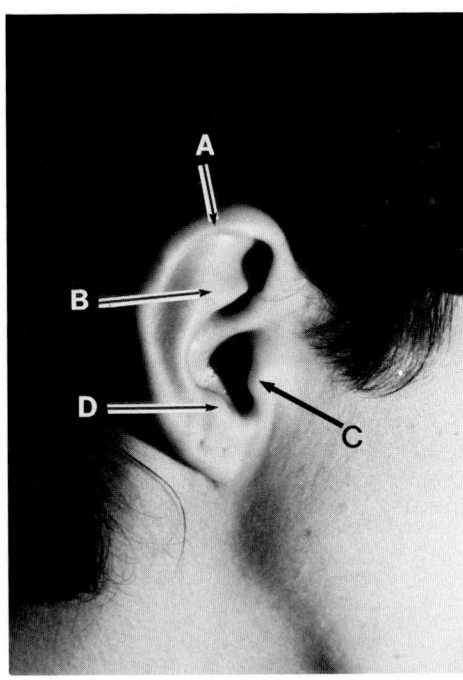

Fig. 1-3. Normal auricle (A: helix; B: antihelix; C: tragus, D: antitragus).

step is to create an antihelical fold and occasionally to remove part of the conchal cartilage to reduce the size (Fig. 1-3).

The external nose has a bony dorsum made up of the nasal bones and the nasal processes of the maxilla, which form an angle with the frontal bone at the root of the nose. Nasal gliomas or encephaloceles originating from the anterior cranial fossa may exist at this junction. The lower portion of the nose is shaped by nasal cartilages that form the tip and the alae nasi. The columella at the caudal end of the nasal septum forms the nasal labial angle with the philtrim of the upper lip. Each of these elements is of major importance in defining facial features. In the inspection of the head and neck region, the presence of periorbital edema, erythema, or chemosis should alert one to the possibility of infection in an adjacent sinus. Exophthalmos may, of course, be a sign of thyroid disease but may also reflect disease of the facial bone, such as histiocytosis or fibrous dysplasia. It is important to check for the extraocular musculature movements which are innervated by the III, IV, and VI cranial nerves. Injuries to the orbit from surrounding sinuses may cause limitation to these movements. Impairment may also be a result of facial bone fractures. Infection involving the cavernous sinus or a pituitary tumor may also give rise to limitation of the extraocular muscle movements.

Routine palpation of the head and neck should begin with the sinuses. Pressure in the medial canthal area, superior or inferior orbital rim will elicit tenderness in an infected ethmoid, frontal, or maxillary sinus, respectively. Palpation should then proceed to the preauricular and retromandibular regions. Is there a diffuse tender swelling as in parotitis, or a discrete nodule as in a parotid tumor? A deep-lobe parotid tumor may be palpated with a gloved finger lateral to the retromolar trigone intraorally. The other major salivary glands in the head and neck region are the submandibular gland and the sublingual gland. The submandibular gland can be palpated in the digastric triangle.

Each submandibular gland secretes via its duct through an orifice just lateral to the frenulum of the tongue in the anterior floor of the mouth. Frequently, an obstructing stone can be palpated and removed from the duct orifice. The Stenson's duct which drains the parotid gland is adjacent to the second upper molar on the buccal mucosa. Palpation and milking of an infected parotid gland may produce purulent discharge from the orifice of the Stenson's duct.

Of the primary salivary gland tumors, 85 percent occur in the parotid gland and two-thirds of these are benign mixed tumors. Submandibular gland tumors are malignant in about 50 percent of the cases. Tumors of the minor salivary glands which are located in the mucosal lining in the oral cavity are rare, but when they occur they are usually malignant. A parotid tumor associated with severe pain and facial weakness may imply a malignancy. Besides mixed tumors of the parotid glands (which constitute the predominant number) and the malignant tumors, Warthins' cysts are common in males between the ages of 40 and 60 and can be bilateral.

Plain film radiography can identify a calcified stone in the salivary gland regions. The use of sialograms has been advocated for many decades. Their usefulness is somewhat limited today, however. Sialography will illustrate dilated ducts implying a long-standing chronic inflammation. The sialogram may similarly outline a tumor mass. However, the decision of whether to surgically remove an infected gland or not, should not be based on sialography, but, rather, based on the clinical history of the patient. A patient with an abnormal sialography but with minimum clinical findings should not undergo surgical intervention; similarly, a patient with multiple severe episodes of infection should be treated surgically irregardless of the sialogram findings. The decision regarding whether to resect or not to resect a salivary gland tumor should be based again on clinical findings and history and not on the findings of a sialogram. In rare cases where the clinical history is borderline, sialogram perhaps may shed some light and help plan a course of treatment.

The student should be aware of the lymphatic drainage pattern in the head and neck area (Fig. 1-4). As mentioned previously, the student should be aware of the

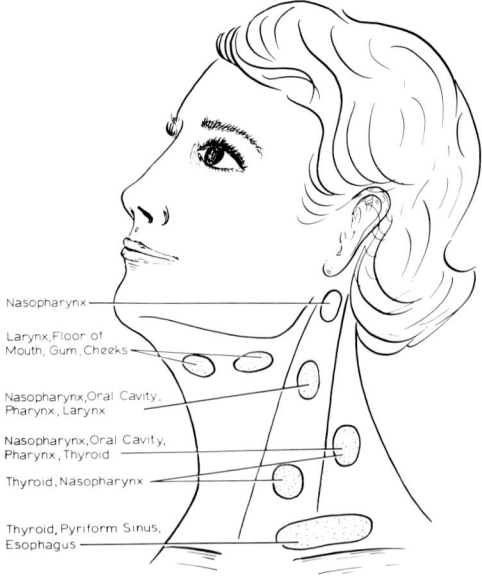

Fig. 1-4. Lymphatics of the head and neck region.

different triangles of the neck as they relate to the normal anatomical structures, particularly the internal jugular vein. When palpating neck masses, it is important to describe their size, firmness, and consistency, as well as whether they are mobile or fixed. A firm, hard mass that is fixed is more indicative of malignancy than is a more "doughy" and mobile mass, which is more suggestive of a benign lesion. A doughy mass is suggestive of a dermoid cyst. Auscultation of neck masses is also important. A mass associated with bruit may suggest a vascular tumor. Carotid body tumor is located at the bifurcation of the carotid arteries. Arteriography will illustrate a very characteristic "eggshell" appearance, which is pathognomonic of carotid body tumors. Branchial cleft cysts are congenital cystic masses usually found in the anterior triangle of the head. Such a cyst may give rise to a sinus tract into the tonsillar fossa or in the region of the pyriform sinus. A first branchial cleft sinus cyst or tract may be present as a draining sinus in the cartilaginous external auditory canal. This will give rise to recurrent external otitis of an unexplainable etiology. Hence, when treating patients with recurrent external otitis, particularly children, one should rule out the presence of a first branchial cleft sinus tract. The first branchial cleft sinus tract may have a cartilaginous core around it and may intertwine with the facial nerve. A first branchial cleft sinus cyst or tract is to be differentiated from the more common preauricular sinus tract, which occurs as a draining site just anterosuperior to the tragus. The preauricular sinus tracts are usually shallow and do not intertwine with the facial nerve.

Thyroglossal duct cysts are generally in the midline of the submental area. The distinguishing feature of these cysts is that they move with the hyoid bone on swallowing. During the fourth week of gestation, a ventral (hyoid) diverticulum of the endodermal origin can be identified between the first and second branchial arches on the floor of the pharynx. It is situated between the tuberculum impar and the copula. The tuberculum impar, together with the lingual swellings, develops into the anterior two-thirds of the tongue, while the copula is the precursor of the posterior one-third of the tongue. The ventral diverticulum develops into the thyroid gland. As the embryo develops, the thyroid diverticulum descends inferiorly and finally down to the adult position of the thyroid gland. At the sixth week of gestation, this tract or pathway of descent should be obliterated and atrophied. Should it persist through the time of birth or thereafter, a thyroglossal duct cyst is present and may become infected. This tract is intertwined with the hyoid bone and may extend to the area of the foramen cecum. A submental mass may not necessarily mean a thyroglossal duct cyst. In children, reactive lymph adenopathy is a common finding. Lipoma or dermoid cysts may be present. Rarely, the submental mass may be the only thyroid gland that is present and, hence, its excision may be detrimental to the patient's health. Prior to removal of these thyroglossal duct cysts it is therefore essential to ascertain that the patient has a normal thyroid gland in the normal position. This can be ascertained by clinical examination or with the help of a thyroid scan. Lingual thyroid may be present at the junction between the posterior one-third of the tongue and the anterior two-thirds of the tongue. This too may be the only functioning thyroid gland in that particular patient.

Cystic hygromas, large, fluid-filled lymph epithelial sacs, are common in the head and neck area in young children. These are cystic masses that transluminate easily.

The isthmus of the thyroid gland can be palpated as a distinct band of tissue lying on the trachea just below the cricoid bone. The thyroid lobes lie deep to the sternohyoid and sternothyroid muscles, and, in the absence of pathology, the thyroid lobes may be difficult to palpate. Diffuse or multinodular enlargement of the gland, as well as discrete nodules, can be palpated by pressing and spreading the strap muscles laterally with the examining fingers. It is sometimes easiest to palpate the thyroid gland by standing behind the patient.

In examining the neck, the examiner may be seated slightly to one side of the patient, facing the patient. Other examiners may prefer to palpate both sides of the neck.

THE INTERNAL EXAMINATION

The internal head and neck examination is performed to investigate the mucosally lined cavities of the head and neck through the natural orifices—the ears, nostrils, and mouth.

The Ear

The examination of the ear is most easily performed with an otoscope providing magnification and illumination. It is, however, important to first examine the auricle itself as well as the external auditory meatus prior to picking up the otoscope. If the examiner proceeds with the otoscope too soon, a lesion on the external auditory meatus or auricle may be missed. It is therefore a good habit to always examine the outer surface of the auricle carefully before using the otoscope.

The auricle is pulled slightly superioposteriorly to straighten the external auditory canal prior to introducing the otoscope. The largest possible otoscope speculum should be used. Care should be taken not to hurt the patient. The outer one-third of the external auditory canal is cartilaginous, while the medial two-thirds of this canal is osseous. The ear canal is lined with squamous epithelium and is often afflicted with external otitis, which is a form of dermatitis of the skin lining of the external auditory canal. External otitis will give an appearance of weeping eruptions and severe tenderness. The external auditory canal diameter is compromised by this disease process. If the ear canal is patent, examination of the tympanic membrane will reveal a normal tympanic membrane. In examining the external auditory canal, one should pay attention to any eruptions or lesions that may signify an adenocarcinoma, squamous cell carcinoma, or basal cell carcinoma. Keratosis obturans is a disease process in which clumps of thick, hard, whitish plaques of squamous debris originate and accumulate in the external auditory canal, almost completely obliterating the area. This is to be differentiated from cholesteatoma, which usually originates from the middle ear. Though external otitis is a very painful process for the patient, it is rarely dangerous other than in patients with diabetes mellitus. Patients with diabetes mellitus may develop a fulminating external otitis usually caused by pseudomonas aeruginosa.

Exostosis of the external auditory canal is frequently seen in patients who swim habitually in cold water. Exostosis is a firm, rounded, bony mass similar to an osteoma. If small and not occluding the external auditory canal, it need not be removed. However, when it becomes symptomatic in terms of producing either infection or a conductive hearing loss, it should be surgically removed. These whitish, bony, hard masses are not to be confused with any tumor or cholesteatoma.

The tympanic membrane is visualized next. A portion of the membrane perpendicular to the light source will reflect light back to the examiner, and this cone of light is known as the light reflex. A normal tympanic membrane will give rise to a clear light reflex, while a diseased tympanic membrane may not give this light reflex. Its significance is, however, limited. A tympanic membrane should be examined for perforations, tympanosclerotic plaques, and drainage. Students should learn to appreciate the aeration of the middle ear cavity. Normal middle ear aeration allows the tympanic membrane to be suspended with an adequate lateral-medial distance, the distance between the tympanic membrane and the promontory. Normal tympanic membrane is made of 4 layers: squamous layer laterally; 2 muscular layers; and a medial mucosal layer. A thin, retracted tympanic membrane may be made of the squamous layer alone. This thin layer may be draped over one of the ossicles, giving rise to some conductive hearing loss. Through a normal translucent tympanic membrane, one can appreciate the air space behind the tympanic membrane. It is also possible to visualize bubbles of air pockets mixed with serous effusion in patients with serous otitis media. In patients with a great deal of serous otitis media of a longstanding nature, a dark grayish or even dark bluish tympanic membrane may be visualized with some bulging effect. The bluish tympanic membrane may also reflect a high, exposed jugular bulb in the hypotympanum or a glomus tumor. In acute otitis media, an erythematous appearance with the prominence of capillaries may be visualized. A normal tympanic membrane should be mobile upon pneumomassage. This massage can be achieved with a Siegal otoscope. Patients with serous otitis media may have a less than mobile tympanic membrane.

Perforations of the tympanic membrane occurring in the anterior half are less worrisome than are perforations that exist in the posterior half of the tympanic membrane. A small, dry, anterior perforation may be fairly innocuous, giving rise to minimum infection and minimal hearing loss. A perforation in the posterior aspect may give rise to recurrent infection leading to chronic otitis media and cholesteatoma formation. When there is a perforation, it is essential that no water enter the external auditory canal, for this may lead to ear infection.

Tympanosclerosis involves a dry, hyalinized, fibrotic tissue that can be deposited on the tympanic membrane or in the middle ear. It is a reparative process after a perforation has occurred with recurrent infection. It is usually inactive and it is not to be confused with cholesteatoma, which is also a whitish clump of tissue. Cholesteatoma is usually friable, whitish, and moist, secondary to chronic or acute infection.

Penetrating injury to the tympanic membrane may give rise to a perforation without any ossicular disruption. Traumatic perforation of this sort, when kept uninfected, usually heals spontaneously. The dislocation of the malleus or incus at the time of injury will give rise to a conductive hearing loss which can be corrected subsequently. An injury to the tympanic membrane giving rise to vertiginous attacks accompanied by nausea, vomiting, ataxia, and the presence of nystagmus implies a labyrinthine fistula, most commonly due to dislocated stapes. Once a labyrinthine fistula is identified, it is important that it be repaired surgically within 24 or 48 hours in order to prevent a permanent sensorineural hearing loss. In the presence of a labyrinthine fistula, eardrops consisting of neomycin and polymyxin should not be used.

The use of a tuning fork can help to differentiate between a sensorineural hearing loss and a conductive hearing loss. Sensorineural hearing loss is one in which the end organ (the cochlea) or the neural elements are diseased. As of 1984, there is no surgical or medical cure for sensorineural hearing loss. A properly prescribed hearing aid can be helpful. Conductive hearing loss is one in which the sound is not being conducted or transmitted to the end organ. This can arise from cerumen impaction in the external auditory canal, foreign body in the external auditory canal. A perforated tympanic membrane, otitis media, chronic otitis media with or without cholesteatoma, retracted tympanic membrane with poor ventilation of the middle ear space, ossicular disruption, or otosclerosis, which is a hereditary fixation of the stapes.

The 512-hertz tuning fork is the most useful in otologic examination. It is placed firmly in a midline structure such as the forehead, the dorsum of the nose, or the anterior incisor, or on the symphysis of the mandible. In a normal individual, the sound is transmitted equally to both ears. In a patient with a conductive hearing loss in the right ear, sound is better transmitted to the right ear than in the left. In a patient with sensorineural hearing loss in the right ear, the sound is better transmitted to the left ear than to the right. This distinction is a Weber test. The Rinne test is the comparison of the loudness of the tuning fork when placed 1–2 centimeters lateral to the external auditory meatus to the loudness when placed firmly against the mastoid. The tuning fork should be placed between 1 and 2 centimeters lateral to the external auditory meatus and pressed firmly against the mastoid periosteum in the region of the antrum. A positive Rinne is one in which the patient hears the sound louder when the tuning fork is placed lateral to the external meatus than when the fork is placed on the mastoid periosteum. A positive Rinne test is a normal sign or implies a sensorineural hearing loss. When the patient hears the sound louder when the tuning fork is placed on the mastoid cortex, the Rinne test is negative, and this implies conductive hearing loss in that tested ear.

When the hearing acuity between the 2 ears varies significantly, it may be wise to mask the better-hearing ear when testing the worse ear. This can be achieved by using a Barany masking noisemaker. A Barany noisemaker should be implanted firmly in the external auditory meatus of the nontested ear while the tuning fork tests are being done on the tested ear.

When the patient has dizziness it is essential to look for spontaneous nystagmus. Nystagmus is a quick, jerky movement with a quick and a slow component. By nomenclature, the direction of the nystagmus is determined by its fast component. Hence, a nystagmus with a fast component going to the right and a slow component going back to the left is called a right-beating nystagmus. The test for nystagmus is to determine whether it is present in the straight-gaze position or in the right-lateral-gaze position or in the left-lateral-gaze direction or in more than one direction. To observe for spontaneous nystagmus, first have the patient focus on your index finger in the straight-gaze position. Presence or absence of the nystagmus is recorded, as well as the direction of the nystagmus. Subsequent to that, the index finger is brought towards the left at about a 45° angle from the midline. Do not have the patient look at an extreme lateral gaze on either side, since this will lead to what is known as a fatigue nystagmus, which is a normal finding. After having determined the presence or absence of spontaneous nystagmus in the left lateral gaze, the patient is then checked for right-lateral-gaze spontaneous nystagmus. The patient is said to have a first-degree spontaneous nystagmus when the nystagmus is present only when gazing in the direction of the fast component. A second-degree spontaneous nystagmus is present if the nystagmus is present when gazing in the direction of the fast component as well as on straight gaze. Third-degree spontaneous nystagmus is said to be present when nystagmus is present in all three directions. It is not pathognomonic, but a first-degree spontaneous nystagmus implies a periphery or labyrinthine type of a lesion. A third-degree nystagmus implies a central nervous system disorder. Second-degree nystagmus *may* imply a central nervous system disorder, but can also be due to a peripheral lesion.

Pendulum nystagmus, in which there is no fast or slow component, is usually due to a congenital benign nystagmus, as seen in patients with albinism, or in ocular nystagmus. It has little clinical significance. Patients with disassociated nystagmus or with vertical or diagonal nystagmus usually have a central nervous system disorder. Rotary nystagmus in the clockwise or counterclockwise direction is usually due to a labyrinthine disorder.

Certain patients manifest positional vertigo, that is vertigo that is present when the patient assumes a certain head or neck position. It is commonly seen when the patient rolls to one side while in bed. Positional testing is done in which the patient is brought from a sitting position on a stretcher to a recumbent position with the head hanging over the edge of the stretcher. The first test is to bring the patient down with the head hanging in the hyperextended position without turning the head to the left or the right. The next test is to bring the patient down swiftly with the head hanging in position with the right ear down. The third component of the test will be to bring the patient down swiftly with the head hanging, but with the left ear down. During all these maneuvers, the patients are asked to keep their eyes open and it is by observation of the eye movements that a diagnosis can be made. The patient with positional vertigo will usually experience violent vertigo with nausea and vomiting. The patients with positional vertigo of the benign paroxysmal type manifest what is known as a latency and a fatigue factor. There will be a latency of about 30–60 seconds between the assumption of the provocative position and the onset of the vertigo. When kept at the provocative position for more than 90 seconds, the vertiginous attack will subside. With the violent vertiginous attack, the patient will manifest a rotary nystagmus. The rotary nystagmus will again have a latency component as well as fatiguability. If the onset of the vertigo attack, as well as the rotary nystagmus, occurs right after assumption of the provocative position and is not fatiguable, a central lesion is suspected. To further study the vestibular system, electronystagmography and other rotational tests can be performed. The discussion of these sophisticated tests is beyond the scope of this text.

When a patient is suspected of having a fistula of one of the labyrinthine canals or of the vestibule, a fistula test can be performed. The fistula test is the test in which a negative and a positive pressure are applied to the external auditory canal and the middle ear space. A positive fistula test is said to occur when the presence of a negative and a positive application of pressure to the middle ear space elicits vertiginous attacks with nystagmus. A positive fistula test suggests that there is a fistula in the vestibular labyrinth. It is important to have a tight seal when performing the fistula test. It is also important to make sure that the application of positive and negative pressure is not applied too many times or it may produce a cooling effect, giving rise to a caloric stimulation (hence not a positive fistula test). When the labyrinth is exposed to cool or warm temperature, the patient may feel dizzy and may also manifest nystagmus. This is a normal caloric response and is not to be confused with a positive fistula test.

The Nose

Using a speculum and coaxial light source, the nasal vault is exposed through the nostril. Before inserting the nasal speculum, it is wise to examine the nasal vestibule and the alae. Tenderness over the nasal vestibule can be due to vestibulitis; a common offending organism is Staphylococcus aureus. Dermoid cyst is a common finding over the nasal dorsum externally with tracts leading internally spreading the nasal septum apart. After the insertion of the nasal speculum, the nasal septum is inspected for

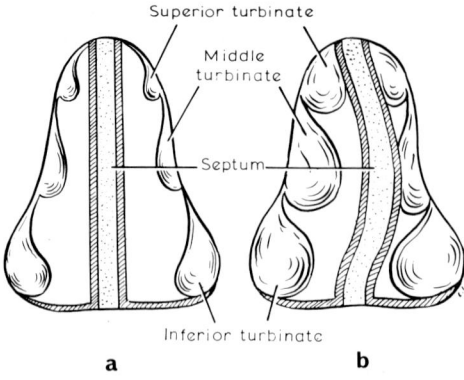

Fig. 1-5. Cross-section of the internal nose (A: normal septum; B: deviated septum and hypertrophy turbinates).

deformities, curvatures, and bony spurs. These deformities may cause nasal obstruction. Superior, middle, and inferior turbinates protrude from the lateral wall of the nose (Fig. 1-5). In a normal state of health, they are not obstructing and not edematous. In an infectious state, they may be very hyperemic. In allergy states, they may appear very "boggy," they are pale and purplish in discoloration. The nasal lacrimal duct opens anteriorly under the inferior turbinates. Nasal sinuses drain into the nasal cavity, mainly into the middle meati on both sides. Purulent discharge from the sinuses can be visualized through these meati. A nasal polyp is a roundish, greyish structure which is usually secondary to an allergic background. Most nasal polyps arise from the middle turbinates secondary to disease in the ethmoid sinuses. A choanal polyp is a large polyp in the posterior aspect of the nose or in the nasopharynx originating from the maxillary sinus. Choanal polpys usually have a stalk going into the middle meatus and through the maxillary osteum into the maxillary sinus. It is important to differentiate a polyp or a mucocele from an encephalocele, particularly in infants. A staphylococcal infection of the nasal skin of the vestibule is to be treated aggressively. The lymphatic drainage of this midface triangle is directly into the cavernous sinus. Severe staphylococcal infection of this region can lead to cavernous sinus thrombosis and hence give rise to a high mortality rate.

The Sinuses

Diseases in the sinuses can be a frequent cause of headaches. Allergic rhinosinusitis is a condition in which the mucosal lining of the sinuses are thickened or edematous, giving rise to a pressure type of a headache. The patient may have other signs and symptoms of allergy, such as sneezing, watery eyes, and congestion. These symptoms may be seasonal. One should, however, be aware that a patient may be allergic to molds and dust, which can be perennial.

Sinusitis is not to be confused with allergic rhinosinusitis. A true bacterial sinusitis gives rise to all the signs and symptoms of an infection: temperature, pain, and erythema. The most commonly afflicted are the maxillary sinuses. They will manifest maxillary pain with purulent discharge in the nasal cavity. Percussion of the maxillary region will give rise to pain in that area. Fortunately, maxillary sinusitis seldom leads to severe complications. Transillumination of the maxillary sinus may reveal an air-fluid level or opacification. Sinus x-ray is helpful in making or confirming the diagnosis.

Ethmoid sinusitis is characterized by tenderness in the medial canthal region adjacent to the nasal dorsum. Again, purulent discharge can be visualized in the nasal cavity. Severe ethmoiditis can lead to exophthalmos with limitation of extraocular eye motions, as well as periorbital edema.

Frontal sinusitis gives rise to severe frontal headache as well as tenderness when the frontal sinus is percussed. A severe case may give rise to frontal "bossing," particularly if the periosteum is thickened and there is erosion of the frontal wall of the frontal sinus. "Pott's puffy tumor" is a term used to describe a severe frontal bossing with tenderness and accumulation of edema and perhaps an abscess formation. Frontal sinusitis is flawed with severe complication because any involvement of the posterior wall of the frontal sinus can lead to brain abscess or meningitis. Again, inspection of the nasal cavity may reveal purulent discharge from the frontal sinus duct. Mucocele of the frontal sinus giving rise to headache can be easily diagnosed with x-ray.

The sphenoid sinus is a deep-seated sinus. Mucocele or infection of the sphenoid sinus may give rise to a vertex headache. Mucocele of the sphenoid sinus can be well hidden, causing patients so afflicted to suffer for a protracted period of time without proper diagnosis. When examining a patient with severe vertex headache of an unknown etiology it is good to rule out sphenoid sinus disease. This can be most easily achieved through a set of sinus x-rays, particularly the lateral sinus view and the submental-vertex view.

Dacryocystitis is an inflammation of the lacrimal sac, which is located in the inferior medial aspect of the orbit. The nasal lacrimal duct empties the lacrimal sac contents into the nasal cavity in the inferior meatus. Inflammation of the lacrimal sac gives rise to tenderness and erythema over the lacrimal sac, as well as purulent discharge in the inferior meatus.

Epistaxis

Epistaxis is a very common affliction in the field of otolaryngology. The authors feel that in an elementary differential diagnosis, the student should be made aware of how to accurately diagnose epistaxis. Epistaxis is most commonly caused by dryness of the nasal mucosa causing the abundant capillaries in the nasal mucosa to rupture. The capillaries are particularly prominent over the nasal septum. Innocuous epistaxis arising from the nasal septum can be treated with digital pressure, lubricating ointments, or, in severe cases, cauterization and anterior nasal packing. When examining the nose for epistaxis, it is important to identify the site of the bleeding. The second most common site of epistaxis is the lateral wall around the turbinates or within the turbinates. Another site of epistaxis is the superior aspect of the nasal septum in the region supplied by the ethmoid vessels. Treatment should be directed to the proper, particular site. A particularly troublesome epistaxis is what is known as a posterior epistaxis, in which the bleeding site is posterior to the line of vision when examining the anterior nares. This can be posterior to the inferior turbinate or in the choanal or even in the nasopharynx. Since this cannot be visualized anteriorly, it is almost impossible to treat with cauterization or with an anterior nasal packing. A posterior nasal packing as well as an anterior nasal packing is therefore essential. Severe epistaxis will also manifest as a bilateral bleeding, although the original site of bleeding is unilateral. It is therefore important for the examiner to accurately identify the location of the bleeding. It is important for the student or recent medical graduate to learn how to control epistaxis with an anterior nasal pack as well as with the posterior nasal pack.

The Oral Cavity

Using coaxial illumination and gloves, the oral cavity is inspected and palpated, with particular attention paid to the tongue and the floor of the mouth. Tumors of the tongue can escape visualization and, hence, palpation of the tongue is an essential component of intraoral examination. The region of the canine fossa, the upper gingiva, and the lower gingiva sulcuses should be carefully examined visually and with palpation. The orifice of Stenson's duct can be seen on the buccal mucosa adjacent to the second upper molar. The hard palate should be examined for any bony erosion. A bony growth similar to an osteoma over the hard palate is called torus palatinus, which is a very common normal finding. This is not to be confused with a soft tumor mass that may be of a minor salivary gland origin. As indicated previously, minor salivary gland tumors are usually malignant.

The soft palate should be visualized for bifid uvula or a submucous cleft. Children with a bifid, stubby uvula and a short soft palate should not undergo adenoidectomy. An adenoidectomy in such a patient can lead to severe velopharyngeal insufficiency speech. The palatine tonsils should be examined for size, cryptic formation, lodged food particles, and any other sign of chronic or acute infection. Whitish clumps on the tonsillar crypts and pharyngeal mucosa may imply acute tonsillitis or acute pharyngitis. This is to be differentiated from food deposits in the tonsillar crypts. Unilateral swelling of a tonsil with severe pain may imply peritonsillar cellulitis or peritonsillar abscess. It is important to differentiate between peritonsillar cellulitis and peritonsillar abscess. Patients with the former diagnosis have minimum or no trismus. Patients with peritonsillar abscess have severe trismus and drooling. The reason it is important to differentiate the two is because peritonsillar cellulitis should be treated with high doses of antibiotics and not with incision and drainage, while the patient with peritonsillar abscess should be drained immediately. The posterior pharyngeal wall should be observed for any bulging suggestive of retropharyngeal mass or tumors. Fortunately, most tumors of the retropharyngeal or parapharyngeal area are benign in nature and are usually of a neurogenic origin. In infectious mononucleosis with tonsillar involvement, the symmetrical tonsillar enlargement with whitish plaques and exudate is seen.

Ludwig's angina is a condition in which the anterior floor of the mouth is infected secondary to involved lymphatic spaces. Dental infection is a common etiology for Ludwig's angina. When Ludwig's angina is established, airway obstruction should be avoided either with incision and drainage or a tracheotomy.

The oral mucosa should be examined for leukoplakia, which is a whitish discoloration of the mucosal lining of a streak-like fashion. These are premalignant lesions and should be watched carefully or biopsied or removed. Lichen planus is a common affliction of the buccal mucosa; they, too, are whitish with a streak-like discoloration. These are benign lesions and perhaps are related to stress. It can be difficult to distinguish between lichen planus and leukoplakia. A biopsy may be necessary. Leukoplakia is known to be premalignant, while lichen planus is a benign process. Papilloma of the pharyngeal arches is not uncommon. These are wart-like growths on the tonsillar tissues or on the pharyngeal mucosa. They are of little significance, but can be removed at the request of the patient. Intraoral cavity melanoma is rare and can be lethal. Early detection of this discoloration will therefore be important. Squamous cell carcinoma of the tongue and oral cavity is common in elderly patients with heavy smoking and drinking histories.

The Larynx

The most challenging part of the head and neck examination is visualization of the larynx and the hypopharynx using a mirror-indirect examination. For most people, it is not necessary to preanesthetize the patient for indirect laryngoscopy with a laryngeal mirror. Occasionally, spraying the hypopharyngeal and oral pharyngeal mucosa with Pontocaine spray or Xylocaine spray may be necessary. With the patient in the upright, sitting forward position, the patient's tongue is gently grasped with a gauze and pulled anteriorly-inferiorly. A laryngeal mirror previously warmed is held up against the soft palate so that the examiner's light source is directed into the larynx through the reflection. It is important to first visualize the hypopharyngeal region, the base of the tongue, the vallecula, and the epiglottis. The lingual tonsil can be visualized at this stage. The pyriform sinuses are examined for any pooling of saliva suggesting esophageal obstruction. Any ulceration, unusual erythema, or growth on the mucosa should be identified. Subsequent to visualization of the lingual surface of the epiglottis, the laryngeal surface of the epiglottis should be examined. The aryepiglottic fold should be examined for any lesion. The arytenoid cartilages should be examined for any swelling or erythema. Besides the possibility of their being involved with any carcinomatous process, the arytenoids may be involved with rheumatoid arthritis.

The false vocal cord should be examined. Hoarseness can be secondary to the patient using the false vocal cord to phonate rather than the true vocal cord to phonate. This is usually due to laryngospasm or is of a psychological etiology. Subsequently, the vocal cord should be visualized. The vocal cords appear as 2 whitish straps with sharp edges. In health, there should be minimum erythema and minimal capillaries. They should move well with phonation and respiration. A vocal cord nodule is a callous, hyperkeratotic lesion, usually seen at the junction of the anterior and the middle third of the vocal cord. It is usually of a traumatic origin, such as secondary to smoking or voice abuse. A vocal polyp is a fluid-filled sac attached either pedunculated or sessile on the vocal cord edges. A pedunculated large polyp may not be visualized until the patient coughs or exhales strongly. Generalized hyperkeratosis of the vocal cord may be premalignant and should be watched carefully. Ulceration or exophytic lesion usually implies a carcinoma of the vocal cord. Papilloma of the vocal cord is common in children. Mobility of the vocal cord should be visualized during phonation. If a vocal cord is paralyzed, it should be noted whether it is paralyzed in the paramedian position or in the lateral position (see discussion of vagus nerve).

Cranial Nerves

The cranial nerve examination is usually included as part of a general neurological examination. It is important, however, to recognize in the head and neck examination that certain cranial nerve disorders are often a sign of disease in the head and neck region. The first cranial nerve can be tested by presenting the patient with several familiar odors for the patient to recognize and identify. The most common cause of decrease in olfaction is nasal obstruction secondary either to nasal polyps or markedly impacted deviated nasal septum. In the absence of any nasal pathology, abnormality in olfaction could imply a neurological disorder.

The third, fourth, and sixth cranial nerves should be examined carefully. The superior orbital fissure syndrome may imply an infectious process in that region or an entrapped piece of bone secondary to maxillofacial trauma. The second division of the fifth cranial nerve exits through the foramen rotundum into the pterygomaxillary space, and then traverses the roof of the maxillary antrum before finally exiting as the infraorbital nerve. If pain or numbness is thought to involve this nerve, a search should be prompted for pathology along its course. Involvement of the third branch of the fifth cranial nerve may occur in the tongue, the mandible, or in the infratemporal fossa.

The seventh cranial nerve shares the internal auditory canal with the eighth cranial nerve. It also travels through the temporal bone in the middle ear and mastoid, exiting from the stylomastoid foramen and dividing into its facial branches amidst the parotid gland. A careful examination of the seventh cranial nerve is of vital importance. It is also important to separate a peripheral facial paralysis from a central facial paralysis. Peripheral facial paralysis involves the whole face, while a central facial paralysis will involve the lower two-thirds of the face but not involve the frontalis muscle. In examining the patient who suffers facial paralysis, it is first important to determine whether it is a partial paralysis or a total paralysis. It is equally important to ascertain an etiology for the facial paralysis. An acoustic neurinoma or a facial nerve neurinoma should be excluded. Subsequent to that, any middle ear disease, such as cholesteatoma, mastoiditis, or acute otitis media should be diagnosed or ruled out. Lesions in the external auditory canal or the parotid region should again be identified or ruled out. Facial nerve neurinoma usually gives rise to facial twitching followed by facial weakness and paralysis; it can be firmly diagnosed with polytomography of the facial nerve and a computed axial tomography (CAT) scan. Acoustic neurinoma usually gives rise to a sensorineural hearing loss, loss of discrimination, and dizziness, followed by facial paralysis. This again can be identified with sophisticated audiological evaluation, and by a CAT scan with air cisternogram. When a facial paralysis is diagnosed without any known etiology, then the diagnosis of Bell's palsy is pronouced. It should be emphasized that a diagnosis of Bell's palsy should not be made until all known etiologies are ruled out. Bell's palsy implies a facial paralysis of an unknown etiology.

The next step in working up the patient with facial paralysis is to do what is known as topography mapping. The greater superficial petrosal nerve is a branch of the facial nerve at the vicinity of the geniculate ganglion in the middle fossa. Hence, a patient's facial nerve paralysis and decreased tearing imply that the lesion is central to the geniculate ganglion region. The finding that a patient with facial paralysis maintains normal tearing implies that the lesion is distal to the geniculate ganglion. The stapedius reflex test can be performed by the audiologist to ascertain whether the lesion is proximal or distal to the stapedius nerve, which is a branch of the facial nerve in the vicinity of the stapes. The chorda tympani is the branch of the facial nerve just proximal to the stylomastoid foramen. Here again, the testing of the taste sensation would help to topographically identify the site of lesion. The more serious student in this field should refer to the bibliography to study more regarding the Schirmer's test, the different electrical stimulation tests, and the salivary flow tests.

It is important to mention in this basic text that the patient with facial nerve paralysis showing signs of degeneration should have the facial nerve decompressed before it is degenerated, in order to achieve an improved prognosis. Similarly, a patient with a traumatic facial nerve injury secondary to contusion or edema of the nerve can be followed with electrical stimulation. Should the electrical stimulation suggest imminent nerve degeneration, then a facial nerve decompression is again warranted. If the tests do not imply imminent degeneration, however, careful watching may suffice. A patient with an immediate onset of facial nerve paralysis following trauma or surgery should have the nerve explored and resutured to get a better functional result. It is possible to do nerve grafting or a hypoglossal-facial nerve anastomosis for those patients with permanent facial nerve paralysis.

Recurrent laryngeal nerve paralysis can be identified through the indirect laryngoscopy. Patients with thyroid tumors or thyroid surgery may manifest hoarseness secondary to recurrent laryngeal nerve paralysis. Patients who have no head and neck diseases but who manifest hoarseness secondary to a left vocal cord paralysis should receive a pulmonary consult and tomograms of the left upper lobe to rule out a left upper lobe or mediastinal lesion or a hypertrophied left ventricle.

Cranial nerves nine, ten, and eleven may be involved with a jugular foramen tumor such as glomus jugulare. The hypoglossal canal which is adjacent to the jugular foramen may be eroded, giving rise to hypoglossal nerve involvement. A glomus jugulare tumor usually presents at its early phase with a pulsatile bruit in the ear as well as with a bluish hue or tinge when the tympanic membrane is inspected. As the disease progresses, cranial nerves nine, ten, eleven, and twelve may be involved.

BIBLIOGRAPHY

Lee L, Lee KJ: A study of facial proportions and sketching of facial contours. Ear Nose Throat J 58:12-30, 1979

Lee KJ: Differential Diagnosis in Otolaryngology. New York City: Arco Publishing Company, 1978

Lee KJ: Essential Otolaryngology-Head and Neck Surgery (3rd ed.). New York City: Medical Examination Publishing Company, 1983

Lee KJ: Comprehensive Surgical Atlases and Text in Otolaryngology-Head and Neck Surgery (5 vols.). New York City: Grune & Stratton, 1983

Paparella M, Shumrick D: Textbook of Otolaryngology (3 vols.). Philadelphia: W.B. Saunders Company, 1980

Stewart D. Fordham
Robert P. Rowe

2

Office Photography

The adage that one picture is worth a thousand words sums up the great value of photography to facial surgery. Properly exposed pictures complement the written chart and actually enhance the physician's ability to treat facial problems on an outpatient basis. This fact was initially appreciated in the first recorded picture of an orbital blow-out fracture on December 18, 1888. In fact, at the first international Congress of Plastic Surgery in Stockholm, Galles stated: "I have been asked to speak about the important advances in plastic surgery. I think the most important advance is photography."

At first, medical literature relied most on drawings and illustrations to record facial problems. This form of recording was somewhat limited, however, because of variability in reproduction and the time factors involved. At the same time, photography began to advance at a rapid pace. Lens resolution was greatly improved and film reproduction characteristics rapidly progressed. Single-lens reflex camera (SLR) bodies have now been designed that integrate the latest technology into a system that allows somewhat amateur photographers to take professional-type pictures. Consequently, medical photography has reached a high level of sophistication in the office setting; it can be considered to have almost the same significance as x-rays in dealing with facial disorders. They have both become a necessity in treating patients in multiple-stage operations—not only in planning procedures, but also in evaluating results. In performing outpatient procedures, it is therefore useful to have appropriate photographs prominently displayed for reference and comparison purposes. This chapter will discuss the full utilization of office photography. The aim is to review various aspects of photography, so that the reader will increase in confidence and ability, and therefore enhance skills in this modality, another tool in the surgical armamentarium.

What are the reasons for the frequent routine use of photography in the office? Of course, it is first used for comparison purposes. How could a better method be developed to remind the patient of the presurgical state and to enable the physician to judge the results of certain techniques? This enhances the ongoing learning experience as well as allowing the physician to determine if results meet expectations. That is why exact comparisons are so helpful. In addition, pictures are a definite and sought-after form of documentation for medico-legal purposes, so extra copies should be stored in both the chart and in private files. Teaching, in most instances, likewise depends on these pictures. By consulting and referring to such photographs, the physician has the unique opportunity to thoroughly analyze disorders or possible complications so that a redirection or revision of a treatment plan may be promptly instituted.

What is the advantage of having the physician take the photographs? First, it provides a relaxed period for interaction with the patient. Casual conversation about what the patient thinks of his facial appearance in general and his particular facial problem in particular can be elicited and so elucidate the patient's concern with a particular area. Then too, the surgeon can closely study a specific region and, in so doing, take additional pictures or vary the technique in order to bring these areas into prominent relief. Since the involved doctor is most likely to benefit from the overall use of photography, it may be best for the doctor to be responsible for its production. At least by beginning this way, if a photography assistant is later required because of time constraints, the physician will be somewhat familiar with this area and will be better able to evaluate the assistant's skills, and to communicate with the technician, and will also be in a good position to solve any problems or difficulties. Control over the parameters that affect the picture can greatly influence its quality and eventual usefulness.

DEVELOPING PHOTOGRAPHIC SKILLS

Costs are always a factor. One can purchase an uncomplicated Kodak camera with coning attachments, which is both simple and inexpensive, or one can even use a Polaroid special portrait camera that requires minimal care or expertise. Alternatively, a high-priced Hasselblad camera with high-detail resolution can be considered. What shall be enumerated here however, is a basic but quality approach to outpatient photography that will allow the surgeon to produce excellent pictures in any situation with limited effort. This will eventually prove to be worth any initial expenses involved, in that it will produce material that can be used and filed for a long period of time; will start the surgeon with good habits that can be built upon; and will provide a core of equipment that can later be expanded, depending on requirements. If one is going to go through the bother of taking photographs, why not make it worth the effort? Almost as useful as good medical instruments for surgery, excellent cameras improve office practice in general, last longer than less expensive cameras, and would be able to meet your future needs.

Elucidating the subject of medical photography can be organized around the pneumonic CAMERAS.

C—color film
A—adjustments
M—magnification
E—equipment
R—reproduction
A—accessories
S—standards

C—COLOR FILM

For the 35 mm camera, there is a wide variety of color film available. Proper selection depends on these factors: light—whether natural or artificial; subject—static or moving; and prints versus slides. This last choice is a matter of preference, depending in part on how one prefers to display the image. Generally, the slides (reversal film) are most economical and also have a vibrance and brightness range that cannot be equalled by an image on paper. Slide film, however, requires more careful exposure than does print film since slight variations in exposure can be compensated when prints are produced from negative film. Slides are a better medium for lecturing and can easily be magnified on a projector. Prints are more easily stored in a patient's chart and can even be converted into slides.

Whatever film is selected, the degree of sensitivity to light must be considered. This speed is expressed in ISO numbers ranging from 25 for slower, less sensitive film, to 1000 for very sensitive, high-speed or fast film. A doubling in the light sensitivity of the film is represented by a doubling of the ISO number, which is the same as the older system of ASA numbers (a second number after the ISO digits comes from the European DIN system). The slower a film (lower ISO), the more light is needed for exposure, and the more grain-free the resulting image will be, thus providing maximum clarity and detail. Only slide film can be "pushed" to double its sensitivity, and processed accordingly, but this process does result in some loss of image quality.

Films carry an expiration date. High temperature and humidity accelerate the aging process. Storing film at reduced temperature does slow down this process, but one must remember to return film to room temperature at least two hours before opening the seal to prevent condensation.

Remember to load and unload the film only in subdued light and keep it in a light-tight container between use. Care should be taken not to touch the film itself. In general, use of name-brand film such as Kodak or Fuji will prevent potential variation in film curves or characteristics. There is no distinct advantage in using black and white film (which can also be produced by using internegatives or color slides), except to create mood or emphasize the effect of shadows. Daylight film is most commonly used in preference to tungsten. Any film should not be sent through x-ray inspection machines at airports. Instead, keep the film in lead-lined pouches. Also, shoot and develop the entire roll as soon as possible. (Don't always wait for the last few frames to be completed.)

A—ADJUSTMENTS

Factors that can readily be changed are: filters, background, lighting and subject. The patient should be placed in a relaxed position on a comfortable and easily movable, adjustable chair with a back. No makeup, distracting clothes, or accessories should interfere. The hair must be cleared from the face.

Lighting is crucial and can be incidental from the background or reflected by flash. Strict lighting rules produce the most constant results and can change the entire picture. The lighting can alter the appearance of a subject through changes in intensity and direction. For a studio, three properly positioned, synchronized slave strobe lights can be placed at 45° to either side of the patient, with another overhead. The front- and sidelighting techniques give the subject depth and volume, while at the same time ensuring that every detail is visible. Shadows are eliminated by using neutral-colored umbrellas to reflect the flash as the light is spread over a wide area and strikes the subject from many different angles. This produces a soft and even texture and yet remains somewhat directional, producing subtle shadows that also give a three-dimensional form (Fig. 2-1).

For the background, a neutral light green or blue is optimal, with white a second choice. This can be provided by seamless paper purchased in camera stores or by a large window shade that can be pulled down as needed.

For photographing lesions in the mouth or for close-ups of skin abnormalities, a ring flash is useful. This spreads the light onto the center of a small surface.

M—MAGNIFICATION

In order to make use of a focal length lens angle long enough to yield no distortion, as well as to permit the photographing of the entire face, a designated area should be set aside in the office.

To render the face in proper perspective, a 100 mm portrait lens is recommended. This can fill the frame with a light image without noticeable distortion. This lens allows the photographer to stand back from the subject and still get a close-up view. This provides a type of psychological advantage, since the patient will not tend to feel as camera-conscious and will be more natural and comfortable. Since it does have a somewhat limited depth of field, however, the focusing must be accurate. (To take comparable photos with the usual 50 mm lens, the camera would be so close that the scale would be distorted.)

Even if a small area on the face or oral cavity is to be photographed, a larger overall

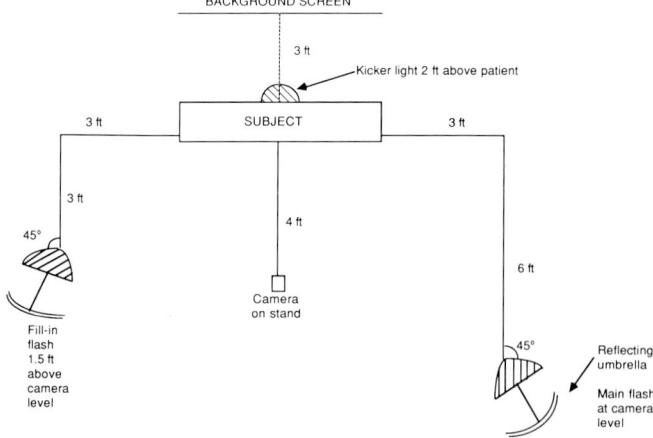

Fig. 2-1. Portrait studio: the flashes are connected to each other by direct wiring or are activated by photoelectric slave units positioned on the more distant flash. A top light (kicker) is activated upon shutter release and creates a three-dimensional effect while eliminating background shadows. A simple alternative plan combines a camera-mounted flash with a strong overhead light and/or synchronized kicker unit.

picture is usually desirable for overall perspective. Limited areas can then be magnified with the macro component of the lens or special close-up magnifier diopter lenses that can be added in multiple increments, depending on the amount of magnification desired. With the latter, however, there tends to be minimal distortion about the periphery.

E—EQUIPMENT

The 35 mm SLR camera has a through-the-lens viewing system that permits the subject to be framed with great accuracy. Also, near-to-far sharpness can be seen and controlled while focusing. This through-the-lens type viewing arrangement allows assessment of the immediate effect of changing a lens or using a particular filter. In this system, viewing and focusing is performed through the exact same lens that casts the image on the film. Reflex comes from the word "reflection" and indicates that the image seen in the viewfinder is bounced off a mirror in the optical path between the lens and the eye (Fig. 2-2).

This camera contains circuitry for metering the light and adjusting the aperture and/or speed settings for proper exposure (exposure = illumination × time). Although these can be operated manually, programmed cameras with fully automatic exposures are the authors' preference. If cost is a consideration, however, then a shutter priority system should be considered. Any well-known brand can fulfill these requirements.

Expensive cameras should be treated as are similar-type laboratory instruments. An annual preventive maintenance program is suggested. The camera should be protected from dust and dirt. Clean the inside only with a soft brush or air syringe. Remember to change batteries at least once a year. Become thoroughly familiar with your camera and read the instruction manual carefully before operating. Ordinarily, keep the camera room at a moderate temperature and humidity; when not in use for a few weeks, however, this equipment should be stored in a plastic bag and/or case.

R—REPRODUCTION

For accuracy and validity, comparison views standardized with respect to positions, lighting, and exposure should be strictly adhered to for pre- and postoperative shots. As

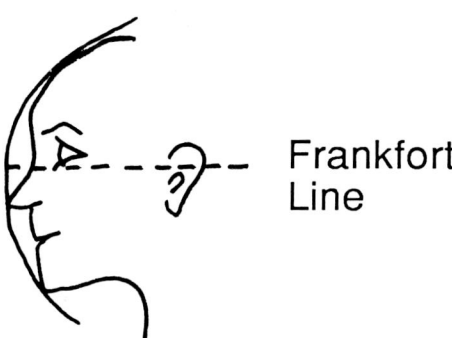

Fig. 2-2. Frankfort line: this line is used for all frontal and lateral views. The vertical axis is maintained on the frontal view by aligning it with the midsagittal plane. True laterals are checked by superimposing the eyebrows or by sighting across the two corners of an open mouth. For facial pictures: take each at the same distance for comparisons; go from the top of the head to the bottom of the neck; reveal the exact nose-ear relationship by tucking hair behind the ear; for the oblique view, align the lateral border of the face with the tip of the nose; and for the nasal basal view, place the nasal tip in the interbrow area.

is known, there is a tendency to take the initial picture under lighting and exposure conditions that show the deformity at its worst, while subsequent photos are taken under more favorable conditions.

The medical photograph is a visual record and so must be able to represent either a point in time alone or to represent part of an ongoing, comparable recording over a more prolonged period. Consistent quality, position, and reliability must therefore be ensured, just as in any scientific pursuit.

The studio method helps ensure proper and constant lighting and positioning. If possible, it is best to use a headrest for the patient to prevent potential movement. The face should be placed in a position in accordance with the horizontal Frankfort line (a line drawn from the tragus to the medial canthus and parallel to the floor—Fig. 2-2) and the midsagittal planes of the face. Use of fixed points behind the camera assist the patient in holding a fixed position. For maximum consistency, a cone can be fashioned for the face or area of interest, to eliminate extraneous details. All other variable factors such as film type, developing laboratory, etc. should be held as constant as possible. Developed pictures should be placed in a plastic folder and stored in a dark, cool place to prevent possible fading. (This gradually occurs over 10–15 years for Ektachrome and 25–35 years for Kodachrome slides.)

Finally, standardized projections and positions must be maintained. Consider the routines listed in Table 2-1, with an explanation of the various primary views below.

1. *Full face view*—The patient should have the eyes open and should look directly into the camera. Remove personal accessories. Unless specifically desired, the patient should be at rest and not smiling.
2. *Lateral profile view*—Avoid hyperextension or hyperflexion of the neck. Always include some part of the ear for better orientation.
3. *Oblique view*—Align the tip of the nose with the edge of the far cheek.
4. *Base view*—The neck should be in extreme hyperextension. Attempt to align the tip of the nose with the transeyebrow line.
5. *Intraoral view*—Plastic cheek retractors are recommended. Do not pull too hard on the retractors, so that lip distortion is minimized.
6. *Operating room view*—Positioning is limited so include familiar anatomic landmarks to enhance viewer orientation. Eliminate bloody towels, extra instruments, and gloved fingers. A metric ruler or scalpel handle included in the frame with the lesion or specimen helps to identify size relationships.

A—ACCESSORIES

Various accessories may prove useful. Lens caps for both the front and rear of all lenses are really a necessity to prevent dust distortion. This is likewise true for an equipment case with foam padding or rubber inserts for storing and/or transporting the camera system. A motor winder is also helpful to advance the film at 2–3 frames/second and might prevent inadvertent movement and at the same time allow rapid-sequence exposure. Also required is a sturdy tripod at least three to five times heavier than the camera and allowing for multiple adjustment and angulations. A 2-foot long cloth-covered cable release should contribute to flexibility as well as limit any motion on releasing the shutter. A databack which records the date and/or initials on the film is quite beneficial in recordkeeping and for comparisons. An ultraviolet, skylight filter is

Table 2-1
Suggested (or Common) Standardized Projections and Positions in Facial Plastic Surgery

Rhinoplasty
   vertical full face
   right and left laterals
   right and left 45° obliques
   basal view of nasal pyramid
   optimal
     front face with neck hyperextended
     close-up front face
     laterals with smiling

Blepharoplasty
   vertical full face
   eyes open and horizontal
   eyes looking up
   eyes closed
   right and left laterals
   close-ups: front face and both obliques

Rhytidectomy
   full face and neck
   right and left laterals
   right and left 45° obliques
   full face: smiling, eyes closed tightly, pursed lips
   optional: neck hyperextended or teeth clenched to demonstrate bands

Otoplasty
   vertical full face
   right and left laterals
   vertical back of head (use headband)
   antihelix
   close-up: both ears 45° anterior and posterior

Scar of Skin Lesion
   full face
   scar—include facial landmark with magnification
   both laterals
   optional: close-up and basal

Scalp (including transplant)
   vertical full face
   right and left lateral
   forehead
   top of head—hair combed normally and away from defect
   back of head

routinely used to cover and protect the lens. If fluorescent light is utilized, as in either mirror office procedures or in photographing x-rays, then an FLD filter will prevent discoloration and result in a more natural light. An orange-colored filter (or other similar variations) can produce differently colored teaching slides by means of photographing the object in question on Kodak SO-279 film and then mounting the negative for projection. Slides composed of white letters on a blue background can also be made with Diazo film. If objects are stationary, then a copy stand is an excellent means of duplication. In addition, a special device can be purchased to place on top of the lens to conveniently copy slides. In fact, an attachment has been devised that can be placed on the camera body itself and attached to the microscope observer tube in conjunction with high-speed film. Finally, the basic camera can be placed in a sterile plastic bag, one that is used for underwater photography, so that multiple pictures can readily be taken by the surgeon during a sterile outpatient procedure. The above are the most common and useful accessories, but numerous others are available. In this regard, perusal of a large photographic catalog may be helpful, depending on the camera configuration and on one's special needs.

S—STANDARDS

It is imperative to have a simple but comprehensive photographic consent form. This should be dated, signed by the patient or guardian, if the patient is a minor, and witnessed. It can read as follows: "The undersigned hereby authorizes the attending physician to photograph or permit other designated persons to photograph [patient's name] and agrees that the negatives and/or prints prepared from such photographs may be published, displayed, or otherwise used as deemed necessary either before or after the date of this authorization, in any manner they may consider proper."

Always consider the patient. This is especially important for those with embarrassing abnormalities. The patient should be adequately informed of the purpose of these pictures and the intent of their use.

Rarely, a civil legal action may be brought by the patient for failure to use reasonable skill or care that results in damage. Thus, it behooves the photographer to take special care to check that the apparatus is in good working order and not likely to damage the patient in any way, i.e., a patient suffering from epilepsy may have an attack precipitated by repeated flashes. In addition, it must be recognized that certain patients may become lightheaded or faint during this procedure. The physician-photographer has a responsibility to see that the patient is not represented in any undignified fashion. Remember that the patient is not an actor but may be ill, anxious, or even self-conscious about the entire process.

A filing system should be devised from which the photographs are readily extractable and in which serial studies can be placed adjacent to each other for fast comparison. A fireproof, locked cabinet is ideal. If possible, duplicates should be stored in a separate area.

It is prudent to insure the camera system, for exact replacement value, on a separate insurance policy and wise to record the serial numbers of each component.

Concerning the purchase of the system, it is wise to buy high-quality equipment from a reliable dealer. Discounts can be obtained by mail-ordering from dealers in New York City who regularly advertise in magazines like *Modern Photography*. Decide on the brand name of the system desired. If cost is a factor, it is most important to have the best lens possible. Camera bodies can be upgraded or manual models can be used along with other, lower grade accessories until a better configuration is feasible.

Furthermore, courses in or reading about new developments in photography may be beneficial in improving techniques. Societies devoted to biomedical photography provide another means for developing expertise and for associating with others who have the same difficulties or interests.

BASIC STEPS IN MEDICAL PHOTOGRAPHY

A discussion of the initial steps in taking pictures follows. Some of this may be a review, but the ideas are worth reemphasizing.

First, purchase a quality 35 mm SLR camera with a grid-type viewing system that is particularly useful for coned camera alignment and proper patient positioning. Affix a motor-driven mechanism to conveniently speed film transport. Place a databank onto the posterior camera and set the correct dates.

Attach a quality, high-resolution 100 mm macrolens to enable the subject to appear natural and nondistorted by parallax error. This will allow an extended focusing distance that is especially useful during surgery. Place a skylight clear filter on top of the lens to prevent contamination.

Lighting for portraiture is optimally applied in a studio using special flash attachments from several different sources. This is best set up with the assistance of a camera store. Usually, single-source frontal lighting is simple and adequate but involves some loss of detail. This should fit in a "shoe" holder on top of the camera so that it can be synchronized with the exposure, which is automatically set at 1/60 sec. Alternatively, if fluorescent lights illuminate, then an FLD special filter can be placed on the lens instead of the flash.

Slide film is usually preferred for medical records because of cost, storage size, and possible later presentation or teaching. For the portrait, Kodachrome 64 should be loaded carefully into the camera, with care taken to ensure that it easily fits into the carriage to the opposite spool. This type of film has excellent color reproduction, fine grain, superior sharpness, and long durability, and can easily be transferred to prints. For all other purposes, Ektachrome 400 should suffice. This allows the camera to be handheld in low lighting conditions; however, it may tend to fade in about 10–15 years and so additional copies may have to be made.

A plain, uncluttered background is preferred. If a specimen is the object, place it on a blue towel with a paper ruler adjacent (to prevent the glare of metal or plastic). If pictures are taken during surgery, take a moment to clean up the surrounding area. For facial photos, a medium blue pastel color does not reflect or absorb too much light and is complementary to skin tones. Another option is to flood the subject with bright lights so that the exposure is decreased. This tends to black out the surrounding area.

Check the camera settings: be sure the proper film number is dialed, the camera and lens are on automatic, the light meter is turned on, and the film is fully wound. In an operation, the equipment can be handled with a second set of larger gloves or with a sterile plastic aperture drape. A stand can be utilized when appropriate. In any case, it is best for the physician to take the pictures to ensure that the area of interest is included and in focus as well as for consistency, which is the keystone of successful pictures.

CONCLUSION

Patient photography in the office is valuable for a variety of reasons. It may be a starting point to document the course of a disease or accident, or may be used to document or support a diagnosis. The photographic illustration of the presurgical condition and/or the history of a condition definitely is more beneficial than is any detailed description. All this seems to underline the importance of photography for medico-legal

Table 2-2
Fundamental Concepts of Office Photography

1. 35 mm single-lens reflex camera with a high-quality 100 mm portrait lens. The patient can be directly viewed at a comfortable working distance without distortion.
2. Kodachrome 64 film for facial portraits and Ektachrome 400 with an FLD filter for specimen and operative pictures under fluorescent lights.
3. Multiple electronically coordinated flashes for portraits. Camera-connected flash for all others, with a ring flash for cavity or oral photographs.
4. Careful patient positioning with a neutral, nonglare background. Strive for consistency and avoid misrepresentation. Use the Frankfort plane horizontal and multiple projections.
5. Critical evaluation of technique. Keep accurate records and correlate with surgical worksheets.

records, for instruction, and for analysis. The limits of the application of photography in the office milieu are reached when exact values and statements are pictorially refined and defined.

The greatest utilization of outpatient photography will be for facial problems. Some offices may need, however, to explore and record other areas with respect to surgery of the head and neck, and so endoscopic and/or microscopic photographic devices will be required. The physician should at least supervise all photographic procedures. In cases of specialized photography, it is imperative for the physician to be directly involved because of the physician's knowledge of endoscopic procedures and related anatomy, and because of the need to recognize certain features of interest.

As a physician's practice expands, more equipment and more than one camera system may be necessary. A certain area of the office should be set aside as a studio for taking standardized pictures with a controlled lighting flash system and 100 mm lens. The hand-held camera with an FLD filter can be used in conjunction with fluorescent lights, including x-ray photography. To maintain consistent standards in medical photography, remember the ideas elucidated in Table 2-2.

Continued developments in camera equipment and office photography are to be expected. In fact, the basic camera system may be soon replaced and/or modified with video recording devices, perhaps in conjunction with computers. This should further expand the scope and usefulness of medical photography in the office.

BIBLIOGRAPHY

Barreras RD, Kraus EM: Iowa Guide to Basic Photographic Techniques for the Otolaryngologist. Iowa City: Department of Otolaryngology and Maxillofacial Surgery, 1982

Converse JM: Reconstructive Plastic Surgery. Philadelphia: W. B. Saunders Company, 1977

Davidson TM: Photography in facial plastic and reconstructive surgery. Photogr Assoc 47:59–67, 1979

Dickason WL, Hanna DC: Pitfalls of comparative photography in plastic and reconstructive surgery. Plast Reconstr Surg 58:166–175, 1976

Eastman Kodak Company (Ed.): How to Take Good Pictures. New York City: Ballantine Books, 1982
Eastman Kodak Company (Ed.): The Joy of Photographing People. Boston: Addison-Wesley Publishing Company, 1983
Hansell P (Ed.): A Guide to Medical Photography. Baltimore: University Park Press, 1979
Hansell P, Ollerenshaw R (Eds.): Longmore's Medical Photography (8th ed.). London: Focal Press, 1969
Karlan MS: Photographic documentation techniques. Ear Nose Throat J 58:21-29, 1979
Krugman ME: Photoanalysis of the rhinoplasty patient. Ear Nose Throat J 60:56-59, 1981
Morello DC, Converse JM, Allen D: Making uniform photographic records in plastic surgery. Plast Reconstr Surg 59(3):366-372, 1977
Simpson C: Cannon SLR Cameras. Tucson: HP Books, 1983
Simpson C: Understanding Photography. Tucson: HP Books, 1974
Thomas JR, Tardy MD, Przekop H: Uniform photographic documentation in facial plastic surgery. Symposium on the aging face. Otolaryngol Clin North Am: 13(2):367-381, 1980

Eiji Yanagisawa
Koichi Yamashita

3
Fiberoptic Nasopharyngolaryngoscopy

Fiberoptic (fiberscopic) nasopharyngolaryngoscopy is a very useful office procedure. It is of great value in studying the function and pathology of the nasal cavity, the nasopharynx, and the larynx. It is essential for proper laryngeal examination of children and adults with hypersensitive gag reflex.

Since the introduction of flexible fiberoptic laryngoscopy by Sawashima and Hirose in 1968,[1] the flexible fiberscope has been used for evaluation of various conditions of the larynx, including evaluation of voice therapy, postlaryngectomy speech and rehabilitation, stuttering, spastic dysphonia, pre-intubation evaluation of the obstructive upper airway, and difficult endotracheal intubation.[2-17] It has also been used for evaluation of various conditions of the nasal cavity and the nasopharynx, including endonasal surgery, pre- and postoperative evaluation for tympanoplasty and sleep apnea, and endoscopic YAG-Nd laser surgery.[16-17]

Fiberoptic nasopharyngolaryngoscopy is a quick, simple way to examine the upper respiratory tract with only minimal discomfort to the patient.

EQUIPMENT

Commonly used flexible fiberscopes are the Olympus ENF-P flexible rhinolaryngofiberscope, and the Machida ENT-4L or 3L flexible nasopharyngolaryngoscope (Fig. 3-1). Other flexible fiberscopes, such as the Olympus ENF-L (4.8 mm in diameter), and the Olympus ENF-LD (4.8 mm in diameter and provided with an instrument channel), are also available (Table 3-1).

The Olympus ENF-P fiberscope is a slim scope, 3.7 mm in diameter. It gives a wide angulation range, specifically 130° up and 90° down, providing easy and comfortable maneuverability (Fig. 3-2). Simple thumb movement control of tip bending in the ENF-P is an obvious advantage over designs with the knob on one side of the control head that call for two-handed control (Fig. 3-3A&B). This is particularly true when this scope is used with a still or video camera. The Machida ENT-4L fiberscope has an outer diameter

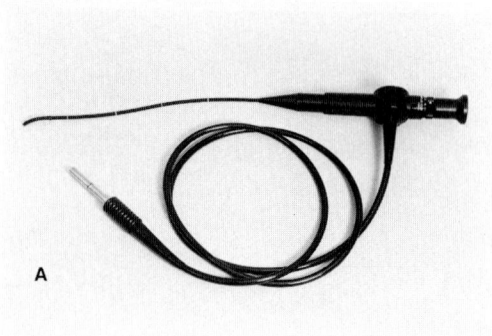

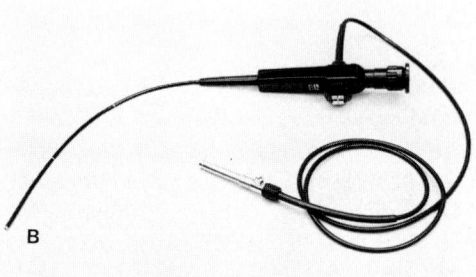

Fig. 3-1. (A) Olympus ENF-P flexible nasopharyngolaryngoscope. (B) Machida ENT-4L flexible nasopharyngolaryngoscope.

of 4 mm and tip angulation of 130° up and 90° down (Fig. 3-2). The Machida ENT-3L fiberscope has an outer diameter of 3.3 mm, with deflection angulation of 100° up and 100° down. The Wolf and Karl Storz Companies have introduced new fiberscopes at the time of this writing. The Wolf flexible Naso-pharyngo Laryngoscope (Model 5940.50) has a 3.5 mm rounded distal end tip with an extra-wide field of view of 105°, useful for visualizing the nasopharyngeal area. It has an angulation capability of 140° up and 90° down (Table 1). Teaching attachments for the second viewer are available for both Olympus and Machida fiberscopes. The Olympus ENF-P fiberscope is the choice of the authors.

Table 3-1
Specifications of Flexible Fiberoptic Nasopharyngolaryngoscopes

	Olympus ENF-P	Olympus ENF-L	Machida 4L	Machida 3L	Olympus LB	Wolf
Diameter of insertion tube	3.7 mm	4.4 mm	4 mm	3.3 mm	4.8 mm	3.5 mm
Field of vision	75°	75°	70°	60°	70°	105°
Bending angle						
up	130°	130°	130°	100°	160°	140°
down	90°	90°	90°	100°	90°	90°

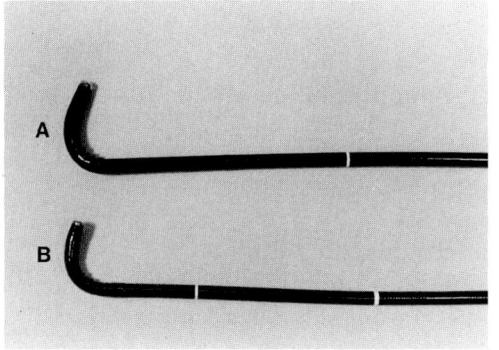

Fig. 3-2. Tip angulation range. Both Machida ENT-4L (A) and Olympus ENF-P (B) provide a wide angulation range of 130° up and 90° down. Note, however, that the Olympus ENF-P has the shorter bending section. This tight bending radius is of great advantage in the convoluted nasal cavity, where significant structures are at all angles.

For routine examination, each instrument company has its own recommended light source: Olympus ILK-3 light source (Olympus), Machida LH-150 (Machida), Karl Storz 481-C miniature light source (this requires different adaptors for different scopes), and Pilling Illuminator 2X (Fig. 3-4). When more than 2 endoscopes are used, the Pilling Illuminator 2X is highly recommended because it has built-in adaptors for the light cable plugs for most other endoscopes available today. For still and video photography, it may be necessary to use more powerful light sources, such as Karl Storz xenon light source 487C, Olympus CLE-F10, or Olympus CLV-F10.

PREPARATION

The examiner must thoroughly explain the endoscopic procedure to the patient prior to the examination. This will help to eliminate some of the fears the patient may have. For unusually anxious patients, it may become necessary to give sedatives prior to the examination.

The patient should be warned about the effect of topical anesthesia, the feeling of numbness, difficulty in swallowing, and feeling of choking. It is important to assure the patient that these sensations are expected and temporary. The patient should be advised not to eat or drink for approximately 30 minutes following the procedure, until the effects of the topical anesthetic have subsided.

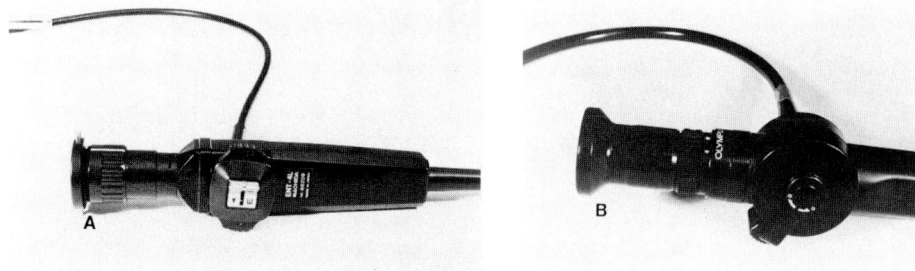

Fig. 3-3. Control units of the fiberscopes. (A) Control unit of the Machida ENT-4L fiberscope with a knob on one side of the control head. (B) Thumb control knob of the Olympus ENF-P is situated at the bottom of the unit. Simple thumb movements control tip bending—an obvious advantage over two-handed control designs that have a knob on one side of the control head.

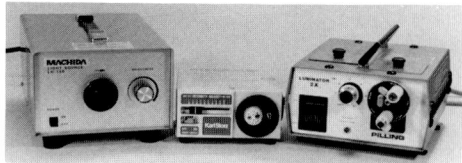

Fig. 3-4. Standard light sources (from left to right): Machida LH-150 light source, Karl Storz 481-C miniature light source, and Pilling Luminator 2X. Olympus ILK-3 light source is not shown.

Past medical history, such as previous reaction to local anesthesia, bleeding tendency, and recent heart ailment, should be carefully considered.

Although the complications from this procedure are extremely rare, emergency upper airway equipment and emergency medication should be near at hand. It is also important to have an assistant present during the examination in case of unexpected complications. One of the authors experienced 2 cases of laryngospasm in over 1000 consecutive fiberscopic examinations.

Prior to the procedure, the examiner should check the fiberscope for any damage or malfunction. Make sure that the instrument is clean, particularly the lens tip. The scope should be focused for the examiner's eye by adjusting the diopter ring.

TECHNIQUE

The patient and examiner sit facing each other (Fig. 3-5A&B). The nose is first examined and sprayed with 3 percent ephedrine in order to allow the examiner to admit the fiberscope without traumatizing the hypertrophied turbinates and for optimal visualization. The side of the nose without septal spur and with widest air passage is chosen. The nose is lightly anesthetized with 2 percent Pontocaine (Breon) (tetracaine hydrochloride) or 4 percent Xylocaine (Astra) spray. The lens of the fiberscope may be dipped in warm water prior to the insertion of the scope to prevent fogging. The distal end of the fiberscope is then lightly lubricated with K-Y Jelly to facilitate the easy passage of the

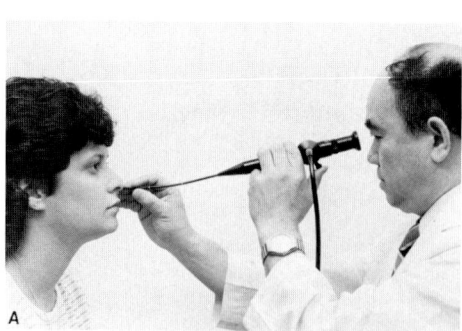
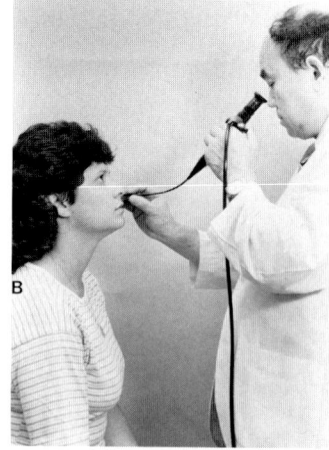

Fig. 3-5. Technique of fiberscopic nasopharyngolaryngoscopy. (A) Both patient and examiner sit facing each other. The examiner inserts the fiberscope into the nose with one hand, while adjusting the tip angulation with a thumb control knob of the Olympus ENF-P fiberscope with the other hand. (B) The fiberscope is inserted with the examiner in a standing position.

scope. The examiner can perform the procedure either in a sitting or a standing position, depending upon the examiner's preference (Fig. 3-5).

The scope is inserted into the nose and advanced toward the nasopharynx along the floor of the nose (Figs. 3-6 and 3-7). When there is a large inferior septal spur, it is advisable to pass through the middle meatus above the spur (Fig. 3-6). As soon as the scope reaches the choana, the fiberscope is turned slightly laterally to examine the orifice of the eustachian tube (Fig. 3-6). In many instances, the torus tubaris and the eustachian tube orifice come into view without any tip angulation. Then, the tip is angled to visualize the eustachian tube orifice on the opposite side. The eustachian tube orifice is examined at rest and upon swallowing (Fig. 3-6). When the patient swallows, the soft palate is elevated by the levator muscle and the posterior lip of the tubal torus is pulled back and upward and the opening of the tubal orifice is clearly observed (Fig. 3-6). The fossa Rosenmüller, the eustachian tube orifice, and the torus tubaris are well visualized.

After the examination of the nose and the eustachian tube orifice, the tip of the scope is straightened at the choana. Then, the flat posterior nasopharyngeal wall comes into view (Fig. 3-6). In the case of children, the adenoidal tissues become clearly visible.

The tip of the fiberscope is then bent downward and advanced slightly. At this time, the patient is instructed to breath through the nose. This allows the soft palate to fall away from the posterior nasopharyngeal wall. With the palate in the relaxed state, the posterior aspect of the soft palate and the uvula can be examined (Fig. 3-6). The patient is then asked to swallow or say "eee." The process of the closure of the nasopharynx by elevation of the soft palate and elevation of the torus tubaris and the lateral pharyngeal walls can be clearly visualized (Fig. 3-6). In the patient with velopharyngeal incompetence, such as cleft palate, the nasopharynx cannot be closed. This examination is also very useful for the evaluation of the patient with sleep apnea and/or snoring. With the patient imitating snoring, the vibration of the uvula can be readily visualized.

When the scope is passed slightly downward, the panoramic view of the base of the tongue, the epiglottis, the hypopharynx, and the larynx is clearly seen (Fig. 3-6).

The scope is advanced to the level of the epiglottis. The epiglottis, even though anatomically anomalous, does not usually interfere with the visualization of the larynx. However, slight irritation of the epiglottis (if not properly anesthetized), may provoke gagging or coughing. The base of the tongue, the vallecula, the pyriform sinus, and the posterior pharyngeal wall are carefully examined for a possible tumor.

Clouding of the lens of the fiberscope may be caused by mucus in the hypopharynx. This can be easily removed by having the patient swallow, which will help to wipe out the small distal lens of the fiberscope. Another way to clear the clouding of the lens is to move the tip of the fiberscope back and forth in such a way that the lens tip wipes against the posterior wall of the hypopharynx or the base of the tongue.

The larynx is then examined thoroughly on both phonation and respiration (Fig. 3-6). Once the larynx is in view, it is possible to observe the larynx for an extended length of time while the patient is asked to swallow, cough, and phonate. The laryngeal surface of the epiglottis and the anterior commissure can also be visualized without difficulty.

The fiberscope can be advanced further and the close-up view of the vocal cords becomes possible. Although the fiberscope can be easily passed through the glottis, it is not advisable to do so in the office situation because of the possibility of laryngospasm. When such a close-up examination is advisable, it is necessary to give adequate topical anesthesia to prevent laryngospasm.

Upon completion of the laryngeal examination, the fiberscope is removed gently.

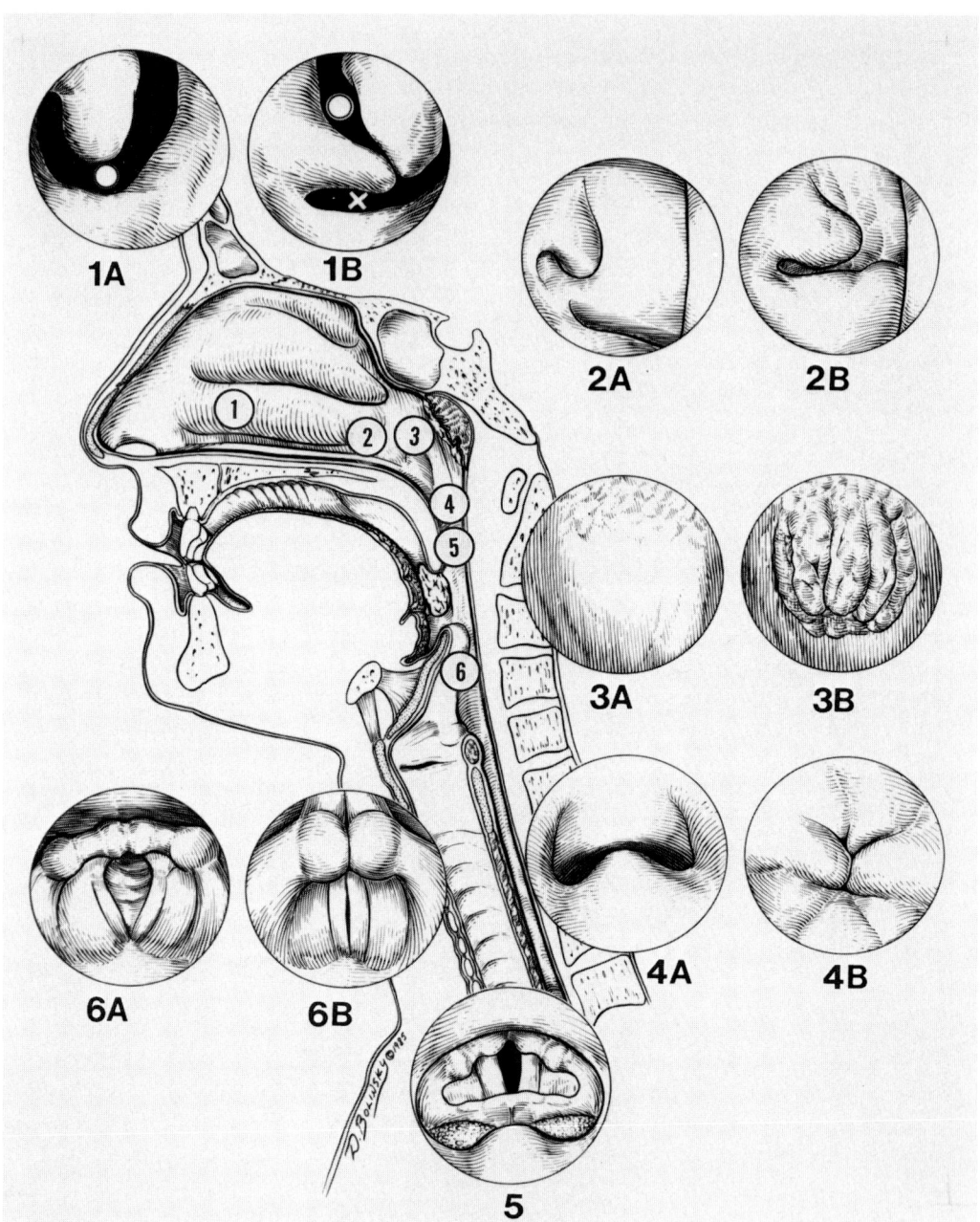

Fig. 3-6. Anatomical structures seen during fiberscopic nasopharyngolaryngoscopy.

(1) The tip of the scope in the anterior portion of the nasal cavity. (A) The fiberscope is passed along the floor of the nasal cavity below the inferior turbinate. (B) When there is a large inferior septal spur, the scope is passed above the spur or through the middle meatus.

(2) Eustachian tube orifice. (A) The torus tubaris and eustachian tube orifice at rest. (B) The torus tubaris and tubal opening during swallowing. Note the change of position of the torus as the soft palate is elevated.

(3) The posterior wall of the nasopharynx. (A) Flat posterior nasopharyngeal wall in an adult. (B) Adenoidal tissues in a child.

Endoscopy of the Eustachian Tube

Systematic endoscopic examination of the eustachian tube and its lumen by the flexible fiberscope was described by Yamashita.[17] He demonstrated various pathological conditions of the tubal orifice and the tubal lumen.

The observation of the tubal orifice can be performed using a conventional fiberscope, such as the Olympus ENF-P or ENF-L. For examination of the lumen beyond the tubal orifice, a fiberscope with a channel, such as the Olympus ENF-LD, is necessary. Air is insufflated through the channel to open the tube, permitting insertion of the fiberscope. The air tank is attached to the scope by an adaptor. Air is insufflated by occluding the aperture of the adaptor with the finger. The pressure of the air can be controlled by the degree of occlusion by the finger. The tip of the fiberscope has to be placed precisely in the tubal orifice.

Air is insufflated to widen the tubal orifice as the tip of the fiberscope is inserted into the eustachian tube orifice and the internal wall is observed. The sound of the air is constantly monitored by an auscultation tube placed against the ear canal of the side being examined. This method is called pneumatic endoscopy of the eustachian tube.[17]

In this way, the hidden pathology of the eustachian tube orifice and lumen can be detected (Fig. 3-7).

CLINICAL APPLICATIONS

The anatomical structures seen and to be examined during the entire course of fiberscopic nasopharyngolaryngoscopy are (from above downward) the nasal septum, the nasal turbinates, the ostia of paranasal sinuses, the nasopharynx, the torus tubaris, the Rosenmüller fossa, the posterior surface of the soft palate and the uvula, the pharyngeal and lingual tonsils, the base of the tongue, the valleculae, the epiglottis, the hypopharynx, and the larynx.

Any disease process involving these anatomical structures can be evaluated by the flexible nasopharyngolaryngoscope. These include infection, trauma, congenital anomalies, granulomatous diseases, and benign and malignant tumors.

Fiberscopic nasopharyngolaryngoscopy is particularly useful for the evaluation of the function of the eustachian tube, the soft palate (velopharyngeal incompetence), and the larynx. Laryngeal function such as phonation, respiration, glottal effort, coughing, and swallowing can be effectively examined. It is also useful for identification of bleeding of an unknown site in the upper airway; preoperative evaluation of patients with sleep apnea and snoring; identification of specific sinuses in case of active sinusitis—by observing pus coming out of the ostium or actually visualizing the pus within the sinus;

---

(4) The view of the nasopharynx from above. (A) At rest. Note the posterior surface of the soft palate and uvula and patent nasopharynx. (B) During swallowing. Note complete closure of the nasopharynx by elevation of the soft palate, medial and upward elevation of the torus tubaris, and the lateral pharyngeal walls.

(5) Panoramic view of the base of the tongue, the hypopharynx, and the larynx with the tip of the scope at the level of the uvula.

(6) The view of the larynx with the tip of the scope at the level of the epiglottis. (A) The larynx in aspiration. (B) The larynx in phonation.

diagnosis of pathological conditions in and around the tubal orifice and the tubal lumen; hypertrophy of adenoids in relation to the eustachian tube orifice; biopsy of the nasopharynx—by passing the biopsy forceps via the ipsilateral or contralateral nasal cavity; diagnosis of unilateral or bilateral choanal atresia; and diagnosis of foreign bodies in the upper respiratory tract.

More recently, the flexible fiberscope has been used for therapeutic purposes such as endonasal sinus surgery, pneumatic endoscopy of the eustachian tube, and YAG-Nd laser treatment of the eustachian tube orifice and of the nasopharynx.[16,17]

CARE OF THE FIBERSCOPE

It is always necessary to clean the fiberscope immediately after its use, because mucus and blood dry quickly and then cleaning becomes very difficult.

The insertion tube of the fiberscope should be carefully wiped down with surgical soap (pHisoHex—Winthrop) first and then it should be washed off under lukewarm running water and dried with 70 percent alcohol. The control unit should be wiped off with a gauze pad moistened with 70 percent alcohol. The fiberscope should not be washed or cleaned with extremely cold (below 40°F) or extremely hot (above 130°F) water. Extreme temperature variations can cause the optical lens to separate from the image bundle. Do not use too much force when wiping down the insertion tube during cleaning, because over a period of time the insertion tube covering may stretch, causing wrinkles at the distal bending section.

Avoid unreasonable lateral pressure on the instrument, especially on the insertion tube, because such pressure can cause breakage within the flexible insertion tube. This can happen when a heavy object such as the light source is placed on the insertion tube or when the carrying case is closed with the insertion tube partially hanging out of the case.

Do not force the angulator beyond its limitation, because this can cause distortion and possible breakage of internal wires.

Do not bend the insertion tube sharply, because this will destroy the image bundle light guide system and the control mechanism within the insertion tube.

When disinfection of the entire instrument is desired, the fiberscope may be immersed in Cidex (activated dialdehyde) or Sporicidin (alkaline glutaraldehyde) for 10 minutes. the fiberscope should be carefully rinsed in water to remove any residual solution, particularly in the eyepiece area. For the Machida scope, the white cap of the light guide plug must remain on the Luer-Lok at all times to prevent fluid invasion. This is not necessary when the instrument is gas sterilized. Avoid immersion of the scope for longer than 10 minutes, because prolonged immersion may loosen the hermetically sealed components, allowing fluid invasion.

Remember that sterilization of the fiberscope by autoclaving will totally destroy the fiberscope. It is suggested that only ethylene oxide gas be used for sterilization. For a detailed method of sterilization, the examiner should follow the recommendations by the respective instrument company.

ADVANTAGES AND DISADVANTAGES

The distinct advantages of flexible fiberscopic nasopharyngolaryngoscopy are that (1) single insertion of the tube will permit examination of the entire upper respiratory tract in less than a few minutes; (2) the patient's discomfort is minimal; (3) the procedure is simple and easy as compared to the rigid telescopic examination; (4) it has increased accessibility because of its flexibility; (5) it has a lower instance of trauma to the soft tissues and of accidental injuries; (6) it may save general anesthesia in the hospital or surgicenter, particularly for children and adults with hypersensitive gag reflex; therefore, it will be *cost-effective* and will decrease anesthetic complications; (7) simplified documentation by photography and videography is possible; (8) preoperative sedation is not necessary; (9) very little anesthesia is necessary; and (10) it is a time-saving procedure and better accepted by patients than is rigid telescopic examination. Any other distinct advantage is the ability to document the function of the eustachian tube, the soft palate, and the larynx.

There are very few disadvantages of fiberscopic nasopharyngolaryngoscopy except perhaps for its cost. The scope costs approximately $3,000 at the time of this writing. The other disadvantage is that the image obtained through the fiberscope is much smaller than is that obtained by the rigid telescope and the resolution of the image is much less clear. Accordingly, the photographic and videographic images are inferior to those obtained by the rigid telescope.

DOCUMENTATION

Fiberscopic nasopharyngolaryngoscopy can be documented by still, movie, and video cameras. Satisfactory methods of still and video photography have been described by Selkin and others.[18-22]

Fiberscopic still photography can be achieved in the following manner: The Olympus OM-2 35 mm single-lens reflex camera with autowinder, clear glass focusing screen 1-9, and 2X teleconverter is attached to the Olympus ENF-P flexible fiberscope, using the Olympus SMR endoscopic coupler. The Karl Storz xenon cold light fountain (487C) is used as a light source. Kodak Ektachrome 400 ASA Daylight film is used. The ASA indicator of the camera is set to 400 and the camera is set on automatic mode. The fiberoptic cable of the fiberscope is connected to the xenon light source. As the fiberscope is advanced to the epiglottis, the laryngeal image is centered in the viewfinder of the camera and the photographs are taken both on respiration and phonation. The exposure is bracketed using the exposure compensation dial situated on the top of the camera. The picture is taken at -1 and -2 because the size of the image on the 35 mm screen by a fiberscope has a tendency to overexpose the laryngeal image. The xenon light source is set at the highest filming mode during the photography. In this way, relatively satisfactory pictures can be obtained (Fig. 3-7).

Videographic documentation during fiberoptic nasopharyngolaryngoscopy will be described in the chapter on videolaryngoscopy.

CONCLUSION

Fiberoptic (fiberscopic) nasopharyngolaryngoscopy is a valuable office procedure for the examination of the nasal cavity, the nasopharynx, the hypopharynx, and the larynx. It allows visualization of the entire course of the upper respiratory tract in a few minutes.

The procedure is fast, nontraumatic, and comfortable. The results are often rewarding.

This procedure may eliminate, in some cases, the need for direct laryngoscopy under general anesthesia. The child, even under 3 years of age, can be safely examined in the office.

Fiberoptic nasopharyngolaryngoscopy is essential for the proper examination of the larynx of young children and adults with hypersensitive gag reflex.

Photographic and videographic images taken through the fiberscope are inferior to those obtained by the rigid telescope.

REFERENCES

1. Sawashima M, Hirose H: New laryngoscopic technique by use of fiber optics. J Acoust Soc Am 1968; 43:168-9
2. Davidson TM, Bone RC, Nahum AM: Flexible fiberoptic laryngobronchoscopy. Laryngoscope 1974; 84:1876-82
3. Brewer DW, McCall G: Visible laryngeal changes during voice therapy: fiber-optic study. Ann Otol Rhinol Laryngol 1974; 83:423-7
4. Brewer DW, Gould LV, Casper J: Fiber-optic video study of the post-laryngectomized voice. Laryngoscope 1975; 85:666-70
5. Williams GT, Farquharson IM, Anthony J: Fiberoptic laryngoscopy in the assessment of laryngeal disorders. J Laryngol Otol 1975; 89:299-316
6. Silberman HD, Wilf H, Tucker JA: Flexible fiberoptic nasopharyngolaryngoscope. Ann Otol Rhinol Laryngol 1976; 85:640-645
7. Conture EG, McCall GN, Brewer DW: Laryngeal behavior during stuttering. J Speech Hear Res 1977; 20:661-8
8. Parnes SM, Lavorato AS, Myers EN: Study of spastic dysphonia using videofiberoptic laryngoscopy. Ann Otol Rhinol Laryngol 1978; 87:322-6
9. Tobin HA: Office fiberoptic laryngeal photography. Otolaryngol Head Neck Surg 1980; 88:172-3
10. Witton TH: An introduction to the fiberoptic laryngoscope. Can Anaesth Soc J 1981; 28:475-8
11. Chapey R, Salzberg A: The speech clinician's use of fiberoptics in indirect laryngoscopy. J Commun Disord 1981; 14:87-90
12. Sessions DG: Recent advances in surgery of the larynx and trachea. Head Neck Surg 1982; 5:42-52
13. Welch AR: The practical and economic value of flexible system laryngoscopy. J Laryngol Otol 1982; 96:1125-9
14. Silberman HD: The use of the flexible fiberoptic nasopharyngolaryngoscope in the pediatric upper airway. Otolaryngol Clin North Am 1978; 11:365-71
15. Maniglia AJ: Vocal rehabilitation after total laryngectomy: a flexible fiberoptic endoscopic technique for tracheoesophageal fistula. Laryngoscope 1982; 92:1437-9
16. Inouye T: Fiberoptic examination of the larynx and esophagus. Trans Amer Broncho-Esophagol Assoc 1984; pp. 123-127
17. Yamashita K: Endonasal flexible fiberoptic endoscopy. Rhinology 1983 (Sept.); 21:233-237
18. Selkin SG: The otolaryngologist and flexible fiberoptics: photographic considerations. J Otolaryngol 1983; 12:223-227
19. Selkin SG: "How I do it:—Head and Neck and Plastic Surgery." A targeted problem and its solution. Flexible fiberoptics for laryngeal photography. Laryngoscope 1983; 93:657-658
20. Selkin SG: Polaroid instant endo camera EC-3. Otolaryngol Head Neck Surg 1983; 91:331-333
21. Yanagisawa E: Videolaryngoscopy using a low cost home video system color camera. J Biolog Photogr 1984; 52:9-14
22. Yanagisawa E, Owens TW, Strothers G, et al: Videolaryngoscopy—a comparison of fiberscopic and telescopic documentation. Ann Otol Rhinol Laryngol 1983; 91:354-358

Jacob Loke
S.Y. So

4

Fiberoptic Bronchoscopy

The invention of the fiberoptic bronchoscopy by Ikeda[1] allows the physician flexible and easy access to the tracheobronchial tree under local anesthesia and enables the bronchoscopist to visualize directly the anatomy of the upper airways (pharynx, larynx, and trachea) and the lower airways.[2] Abnormal mucosal patterns or endobronchial lesions can be brushed or biopsied to obtain cytological or tissue specimens. Peripheral or lung parenchymal lesions in which there are no visible endobronchial abnormalities can be evaluated by performing brushings or transbronchial biopsy with the use of fluoroscopic guidance.[3,4] Bronchial washings[5] of an abnormal lung segment are valuable in patients suspected of having a malignant process or in those immunosuppressed patients[6] in whom fungal, protozoan, or mycobacterial disease is being considered in the differential diagnosis. Using the wide-channel bronchoscope, suction of tenacious mucus secretions in the tracheobronchial tree that cause lobar collapse or atelectasis can be done.[7] In patients with foreign body in the proximal or lower airways, removal of the foreign body is achieved with different grasping forceps.[8] Prior to the fiberoptic bronchoscope, the rigid bronchoscope refined and modified by C. Jackson[9] was used in the endoscopic examination of the tracheobronchial tree. Since the development of the flexible bronchofiberscope, however, the latter has replaced the rigid bronchoscope as in the instrument of choice in bronchoscopic examination. There are certain clinical conditions, such as in the management of massive hemoptysis, biopsy of vascular tumors, and removal of foreign bodies in the pediatric age group, in which the rigid bronchoscope is still preferred.[3,10]

Fiberoptic bronchoscopy can be performed in the office or hospital setting. Irrespective of the locations, adequate resuscitative facilities, including emergency medications for resuscitation, electrocardiograph (ECG) monitor, defibrillator, suction apparatus, and oxygen, should be available. However, when transbronchial biopsy or forceps biopsy procedures are contemplated, the admission of the patient to the hospital is strongly recommended, especially the high-risk patient with cardiopulmonary disease; although these procedures have been shown to be safe when performed on an outpatient basis in 1428 patients.[11] There are different types of fiberoptic bronchoscopes[2,3,12] that are produced. The latest fiberoptic bronchoscope (Olympus BF Type 10, Type P10, and Type 1T10, or Pentax FB-15H) allows the bronchoscope to be totally immersible in strong disinfectants, and has a bigger image size and superior angulation or bending radius for biopsy forceps in the upper lobes compared to the previous model of bronchoscope. For visualization of the distal and peripheral bronchi, the BFP10 (distal end outer diameter of 4.8 mm) is preferred over the BF1T10 with an outer diameter of 5.9 mm. However, the inner diameter channel of the BFP10 is smaller, 2.0 mm, compared to 2.6 mm of the BF1T10. The BF10 has a distal end outer diameter of 5.3 mm and inner diameter channel of 2.0 mm. An inner diameter of 2.6 mm is superior for suctioning to the 2.0 mm orifice and bigger biopsy and grasping forceps can be inserted through the larger channel. For the study of the distal small airways of the lung, Tanaka et al.[13] have devised a fiberscope (BF1.8T) with an apical diameter of 1.8 mm, although with no lumen or channel system. This small bronchofiberscope is designed to be passed through the 2.6 mm channel of the Olympus BF1T10. An extra bulb for the light source for the fiberoptic bronchoscopic system should be available.

The bronchoscopist should have a thorough knowledge of the different parts of the fiberoptic bronchoscope in order to avoid malfunction of the suction channel and costly repair of the instrument through neglect in cleaning or handling, i.e., abuse of the instrument by forceful manipulation or bending it, since the fiberoptic bundles can be broken. The distal objective lens should be cleaned or wiped with alcohol, and the bronchoscopic system, including the suction capability, should be tested before the procedure is performed on a patient. An adequate knowledge of the anatomy of the tracheobronchial tree[2] is a prerequisite for a bronchoscopist, who should also be able to identify an abnormal muscosal pattern or endobronchial pathology. Without knowing the "road map" of the segmental or subsegmental orifice to a particular lung segment,[14] especially in peripheral lung lesions, multiple attempts (which are time-consuming) may be needed to localize the lesion with the bronchial brush, and at times a false negative biopsy result may be achieved. The practice of the procedure using an "old" bronchoscope in a lifelike lung mannequin model[15] would provide the physician or surgeon the opportunity to become familiar with the anatomy of the tracheobronchial tree and the technique of the procedure.

What are the indications for fiberoptic bronchoscopy? The most common indication is the need to diagnose carcinoma of the lung in patients who present with cough,[16] hemoptysis,[17,18,19] and an abnormal chest roentgenographic finding suggestive of bronchial carcinoma. The latter includes a central (hilar) lesion, a lung infiltrate with lobar or segmental collapse, delayed resolution of a pneumonia, or recurrent pneumonitis in the same lung area. In 600 patients who had fiberoptic bronchoscopy, Zavala[4] found bronchogenic carcinoma was the most commonly encountered disease, accounting for 55 percent of the total cases. Other indications include staging the patient with bronchogenic carcinoma to determine the extent of the disease,[5,20,21] patients with abnormal sputum cytology,[5] peripheral lung lesion,[5,22] diffuse lung disease,[23-26] bacterial,[4,27] fungal,[6,28] and protozoan infection[6,29,30] in nonimmunosuppressed and immunocompromised patients,[30,31] suspected cases of pulmonary tuberculosis in which sputum smears for acid fast bacilli are negative,[32-34] upper or central airway obstruction,[35-37] acute inhalation injury,[38] difficult endotracheal intubation, foreign bodies[3,8] retention of secretions and atelectasis,[7,39,40] bronchography,[14] and lung abscess.[41]

A clinical examination and laboratory evaluation of the patient is essential before the patient is subjected to a fiberoptic bronchoscope. Routine arterial blood gases are performed in patients with chronic obstructive airway disease or in those patients with dyspnea. In patients who gave a history of bronchial asthma, bronchodilator therapy should be administered to avoid laryngospasm and bronchospasm.[42] Oxygen therapy is given by nasal prongs to patients with cardiopulmonary disorder to prevent arterial hypoxemia[43,44] and cardiac arrhythmia.[45,46] For high-risk patients with cardiac or respiratory disease, electrocardiographic monitoring is performed in addition to inserting an intravenous peripheral access line. Coagulation studies (prothrombin time, partial thromboplastin time) and platelet count are routinely done, especially in patients with liver disease or in immunosuppressed patients who are on chemotherapy. In patients with low platelets who are immunosuppressed or uremic,[23,47] forceps biopsy is not recommended because of the high incidence of severe bleeding. Platelet transfusions (5 packs) before and during the procedure are indicated in those patients with low platelet count (less than 50,000/cm); and bronchial washings are then performed without a forceps biopsy or transbronchial biopsy. Gentle bronchial brushings may be performed after the instillation of the topical adrenaline 1:20,000 solution onto the involved site. Other contraindications to forceps biopsy procedures are pulmonary hypertension and severe bleeding diatheses. Fiberoptic bronchoscopy should not be performed in those patients who are not medically stable, or in those patients who are not cooperative with the procedure despite adequate sedation.

    The fiberoptic procedure and its complications[16,48] are explained to the patient. The patient is placed on nothing by mouth for 4–6 hours before the procedure. Premedication consists of Demerol (Winthrop), 25–100 mg, and Atropine (Winthrop), 0.4–1.0 mg given by the intramuscular route, 30–60 minutes before the fiberoptic bronchoscopy. Additional medication for sedation, such as diazepam or morphine can be given by the intravenous route. Low dose of the above medications should be given to avoid hypotension, too much sedation, and respiratory depression. Local anesthetics[49] in the form of 4 percent lidocaine or 10 percent lidocaine solution (Xylocaine—Astra) are sprayed onto the oral pharynx. If one is performing the procedure through the transnasal approach,[50] 2 percent lidocaine spray and jelly is applied to the most patent nostril. The author (JL) prefers the transoral approach[51] in addition to inserting the bronchoscope through an endotracheal tube with a mouthguard in place. Additional 2 percent lidocaine solution is instilled onto the vocal cord area before the distal tip of the bronchoscope is passed through the vocal cords into the trachea. The endotracheal tube (with or without a cuff) is rotated in a downward manner through the bronchoscope to be positioned about 3–4 cm above the carina. Prior to the endotracheal intubation through the bronchoscope, the mobility of the vocal cords should be observed to detect any vocal cord paralysis or dysfunction. One–2 percent lidocaine solution is instilled into the right and left main stem bronchi. The amount to be instilled for topical anesthesia will depend on the amount of coughing that is present. The total dose of topical lidocaine solution that can be given is 200–400 mg[49,52] in order to avoid toxicity of the drug such as signs of tremulousness, dizziness, and talkativeness. The placing of an endotracheal tube (preferably 8.5 mm) will allow the bronchoscope to be withdrawn freely in cases of "red out" or tenacious secretions or blood clots obstructing the view of the objective lens; then the channel of the bronchoscope is cleaned or flushed or another bronchoscope can be reinserted rapidly into the airway.[14] Inspection of the uninvolved side of the lung should be done before proceeding to the involved one. It is recommended that 1 percent lidocaine solution with adrenaline solution (1:20,000) be instilled onto friable erythematous mucosa area before bronchial brushings or forceps biopsy procedure is performed.

For visible endobronchial lesions in 106 patients from the Memorial Sloan-Kettering Cancer Center, the diagnostic yields for a malignant lesion from bronchial brushings and forceps biopsies were 92 percent and 93 percent, respectively.[53] Washings have a relative diagnostic yield of 79 percent, compared to 68 percent for sputum cytology. The performance of two or more of the above procedures resulted in a diagnostic yield for carcinoma in visible endoscopic tumors of 98 percent. In 484 Chinese patients with bronchial carcinoma, the yield from washings was 76 percent; from brushing, 74 percent; and from biopsy, 82 percent (total yield: 94 percent) in cases of visible endoscopic tumors.[54] Fluoroscopy is not needed during the procedure for central or visible endobronchial lesions.

For peripheral lung lesions or lung infiltrate in which no endobronchial lesion is seen, location of the lesion should be done initially with the bronchial brush (with the covered sheath) under fluoroscopic guidance. The patient lies on a rotating bed which can be moved before a C-arm fluoroscope, thus providing a biplane location of the peripheral lung lesion. The location of the forceps biopsy is checked fluoroscopically and the involved area is biopsied. The forceps biopsy is withdrawn through the channel of the bronchoscope and if there is significant bleeding, the bronchoscope can be wedged[23] into the segmental orifice and suction and adrenaline solution are applied. In certain situations, the bronchoscope can be removed and another bronchoscope inserted rapidly[14] for suctioning and control of bleeding. The injection of 1:20,000 adrenaline solution into the selected segmental orifice is performed before the forceps biopsy is applied to the area. If there is significant bleeding after bronchial brushings, forceps biopsy may be deferred. For bleeding during the procedure, the rotating bed is turned such that the bleeding side of the lung is in the decubitus position. Generally, 3 bronchial brushings and 3 bronchial biopsy procedures are done in addition to bronchial washings. The bronchoscopic specimens are sent mainly for cytological and tissue examination[54,55] in patients suspected of having lung malignancy. One may send the bronchial washings for tuberculosis culture or fungal studies depending on the clinical suspicion of the case. Bacteriologic cultures are not done.[56] It should be noted that lidocaine has antibacterial properties,[57] so that lidocaine solution to the airways should not be used sparingly if bacteriological cultures are contemplated from the bronchial aspirate. Expiratory chest roentgenogram is routinely done in patients who have peripheral transbronchial lung biopsy to check for the presence of pneumothorax. In immunosuppressed patients in whom bleeding tendency is present, bronchoalveolar lavage[6] of a particular lung segment can be performed with 50–150 ml of normal saline to evaluate for the presence of protozoan, mycobacterial, cytomegalovirus, and certain types of fungal infection. The usual amount, instilling 300 ml of saline as lavaged fluid in a relatively healthy patient, may not be tolerated by a patient with pulmonary disease and arterial hypoxemia, and may precipitate respiratory failure. After the procedure, in patients with chronic obstructive airway disease, naloxone 0.4 mg is given intravenously to prevent respiratory depression with the use of narcotic sedation. The patient is not allowed to eat or drink for 2–3 hours and oxygen therapy is continued for a few hours, especially in patients who have bronchoalveolar lavage. For peripheral lung lesion of less than 1 cm and even less than 2 cm in diameter, percutaneous needle biopsy under fluoroscopy[58] or CT (computed tomographic) guidance may provide an acceptable yield for cytological diagnosis if special bronchography and curette biopsy procedures are not available.[14]

In the staging of bronchogenic carcinoma, Wang et al.[21,59] developed a flexible aspiration needle that can be inserted through the bronchoscope to penetrate the carinal or main bronchi in order to assess the presence or absence of tumor involvement in the mediastinum. This technique is also useful when there is extrinsic compression of the bronchi with no visible endobronchial lesion. There was no serious complication of bleeding with the transbronchial needle aspiration. The above procedure should be performed by a bronchoscopist who has been trained in this technique.

Recently, two forms of therapeutic intervention with laser technology have been used with the fiberoptic bronchoscope in the treatment of bronchogenic carcinoma. One is the use of hematoporphyrin derivative phototherapy in the treatment of lung cancer[60,61] and may be used as an alternative to surgical resection in selected patients. The other major development is the use of the neodymium-YAG laser[35-37,62,63] in the therapy of patients with malignant and benign lesions obstructing the central airways: larynx, trachea, and major bronchi. In patients with recurrent bronchogenic carcinoma with major airway obstruction that causes severe dyspnea and hypoxemia, and in cases in which the patient has received the maximum dose of radiation therapy, the use of laser photoresection of the obstructive lesion would open the airways and be a form of palliative therapy. In some patients with lung cancer, laser therapy of endobronchial lesion can be performed as the initial therapy. In benign laryngeal and tracheal disorders, lung function studies have shown an improvement after the laser therapy.[63] Major complications of laser therapy are hemorrhage, tracheoesophageal fistula or perforation, and pulmonary infection. Dumon et al.[35] used the YAG laser with the rigid bronchoscope rather than the flexible fiberoptic bronchoscope in the majority of their cases, with most of their patients receiving general anesthesia. Kvale and his group[63] utilized the flexible fiberoptic bronchoscope with the YAG laser and emphasized the need for skillful technique and anesthetic management and post-treatment intensive care therapy in high-risk patients with central airway obstruction.

There are complications associated with fiberoptic bronchoscopy without the use of the laser therapy and these include fever, pneumonitis, hemorrhage, laryngospasm, bronchospasm, hypoxemia, respiratory failure, pneumothorax, cardiac arrhythmias, and death. The fever is usually self-limited[3,64] and requires no antibiotic therapy, although a fatal case of pneumonitis and septicemia[65] has been reported after fiberoptic bronchoscopy. Careful screening of patients and good clinical judgment in the fiberoptic bronchoscopy procedure should avoid the major complications that are associated with fiberoptic bronchoscopy.

REFERENCES

1. Ikeda S: Flexible bronchofiberscope. J Jap Bronchoesophago Soc 19:54-63, 1968
2. Ikeda S: Atlas of Flexible Bronchofiberscopy. Tokyo: Igaku Shoin Ltd., 1974
3. Sackner MA: Bronchofiberoscopy. Am Rev Respir Dis 111:62-88, 1975
4. Zavala DC: Diagnostic fiberoptic bronchoscopy: Techniques and results of biopsy in 600 patients. Chest 68:12-19, 1975
5. Loke J, Matthay RA, Ikeda S: Techniques for diagnosing lung cancer: A critical review. Clin Chest Med 3(2):321-329, 1982
6. Stover DE, Zaman MB, Hajdu SI, et al: Bronchoalveolar lavage in the diagnosis of diffuse pulmonary infiltrates in the immunosuppressed host. Ann Intern Med 101:1-7, 1984
7. Barrett CR Jr: Flexible fiberoptic bronchoscopy in the critically ill patient. Methodology and indications. Chest 73(S), no. 5:746-749, 1978

8. Cunanan OS: The flexible fiberoptic bronchoscope in foreign body removal. Experience in 300 cases. Chest 73(S), no. 5:725–726, 1978
9. Jackson C: Tracheal-bronchoscopy, Esophagosocopy and Gastroscopy. St. Louis MO: Laryngoscope Company, 1907
10. Mitchell DM, Collins JV: Fiberoptic bronchoscopy (no. 2). In Flenley DC (Ed.): Recent Advances in Respiratory Medicine. Edinburgh, London: Churchill Livingstone, pp. 91–104, 1980
11. Ackart RS, Foreman DR, Klayton RJ, et al: Fiberoptic bronchoscopy in outpatient facilities, 1982. Arch Intern Med 143:30–31, 1983
12. Loke J, Matthay RA: Endoscopy A. Bronchoscopy. In Glenn, Baue, Geha, et al. (Eds.)(Phoracic and Cardiovascular Surgery). Norwalk, CT: Appleton-Century-Crofts, pp.43–48, 1983
13. Tanaka M, Satoh M, Kawanami O, et al: A new bronchofiberscope for the study of diseases of very peripheral airways. Chest 85:590–594, 1984
14. Ono R, Loke J, Ikeda S: Bronchofiberoscopy with curette biopsy and bronchography in the evaluation of peripheral lung lesions. Chest 79:162–166, 1981
15. King EG, Sproule BJ, Yamamoto I: A teaching model for bronchoscopy. Chest 70:72–73, 1976
16. Fulkerson WJ: Fiberoptic bronchoscopy. N Engl J Med 311:511–515, 1984
17. Smiddy JF, Elliott RC: The evaluation of hemoptysis with fiberoptic bronchoscopy. Chest 64:158–162, 1973
18. Weaver LJ, Solliday N, Cugell DW: Selection of patients with hemoptysis for fiberoptic bronchoscopy. Chest 76:7–10, 1979
19. Gong H Jr, Salvatierra C: Clinical efficacy of early and delayed fiberoptic bronchoscopy in patients with hemoptysis. Am Rev Respir Dis 124:221–225, 1981
20. Robbins HM, Morrison DA, Sweet ME, et al: Biopsy of the main carina. Staging lung cancer with the fiberoptic bronchoscope. Chest 75:484–486, 1979
21. Wang KP, Terry PB: Transbronchial needle aspiration in the diagnosis and staging of bronchogenic carcinoma. Am Rev Respir Dis 127:344–347, 1983
22. Radke JR, Conway WA, Eyler WR, et al: Diagnostic accuracy in peripheral lung lesions. Factors predicting success with flexible fiberoptic bronchoscopy. Chest 76:176–179, 1979
23. Zavala DC: Transbronchial biopsy in diffuse lung disease. Chest 73(S), no. 5:727–733, 1978
24. Andersen HA: Transbronchoscopic lung biopsy for diffuse pulmonary diseases. Results in 939 patients. Chest 73(S), no.5:734–736, 1978
25. Reynolds HY, Fulmer JD, Kazmierowski JA, et al: Analysis of cellular and protein content of bronchoalveolar lavage fluid from patients with idiopathic pulmonary fibrosis and chronic hypersensitivity pneumonitis. J Clin Invest 59:165–175, 1977
26. Crystal RG, Bitterman PB, Rennard SI, et al: Interstitial lung diseases of unknown cause, disorders characterized by chronic inflammation of the lower respiratory tract (second of two parts). N Engl J Med 310:235–244, 1984
27. Wimberly NW, Bass JB Jr, Boyd BW, et al: Use of a bronchoscopic protected catheter brush for the diagnosis of pulmonary infection. Chest 81:556–562, 1982
28. George RB, Jenkinson SG, Light RW: Fiberoptic bronchoscopy in the diagnosis of pulmonary fungal and nocardial infections. Chest 73:33–36, 1978
29. Coleman DL, Dodek PM, Luce JM, et al: Diagnostic utility of fiberoptic bronchoscopy in patients with Pneumocystis carinii pneumonia and the acquired immune deficiency syndrome. Am Rev Respir Dis 128:795–799, 1983
30. Stover DE, White DA, Romano PA, et al: Diagnosis of pulmonary disease in acquired immune deficiency syndrome (AIDS), role of bronchoscopy and bronchoalveolar lavage. Am Rev Respir Dis 130:659–662, 1984
31. Matthay RA, Greene WH: Pulmonary infections in the immunocompromised patient. Med Clin N Am 64:529–551, 1980

32. Danek SJ, Bower JS: Diagnosis of pulmonary tuberculosis by flexible fiberoptic bronchoscopy. Am Rev Respir Dis 119:677–679, 1979
33. Wallace JM, Deutsch AL, Harrell JH, et al: Bronchoscopy and transbronchial biopsy in evaluation of patients with suspected active tuberculosis. Am J Med 70:1189–1194, 1981
34. So SY, Lam WK, Yu DYC: Rapid diagnosis is of suspected pulmonary tuberculosis by fiberoptic bronchoscopy. Tubercle 63:195–200, 1982
35. Dumon JF, Shapshay S, Bourcereau J, et al: Principles for safety in application of neodymium-YAG laser in bronchology. Chest 86:163–168, 1984
36. McDougall JC, Cortese DA: Neodymium-YAG laser therapy of malignant airway obstruction: A preliminary report. Mayo Clin Proc 58:35–39, 1983
37. Joyner LR Jr, Maran AG, Sarama R, et al: Neodymium-YAG laser treatment of intrabronchial lesions. A new mapping technique via the flexible fiberoptic bronchoscope. Chest 87:418–427, 1985
38. Moylan JA, Adib K, Birnbaum M: Fiberoptic bronchoscopy following thermal injury. Surg Gynecol Obstet 140:541–543, 1975
39. Marini JJ, Pierson DJ, Hudson LD: Acute lobar atelectasis: A prospective comparison of fiberoptic bronchoscopy and respiratory therapy. Am Rev Respir Dis 119:971–978, 1979
40. Mahajan VK, Catron PW, Huber GL: The value of fiberoptic bronchoscopy in the management of pulmonary collapse. Chest 73:817–820, 1978
41. Sosenko A, Glassroth J: Fiberoptic bronchoscopy in the evaluation of lung abscesses. Chest 87:489–494, 1985
42. Sahn SA, Scoggin C: Fiberoptic bronchoscopy in bronchial asthma: A word of caution. Chest 69:39–42, 1976
43. Albertini RE, Harrell JH, Kurihara N, et al: Arterial hypoxemia induced by fiberoptic bronchoscopy. JAMA 230:1666–1667, 1974
44. Matsushima Y, Jones RL, King EG, et al: Alterations in pulmonary mechanics and gas exchange during routine fiberoptic bronchoscopy. Chest 86:184–188, 1984
45. Shrader DL, Lakshminarayan S: The effect of fiberoptic bronchoscopy on cardiac rhythm. Chest 73:821–824, 1978
46. Katz AS, Michelson EL, Stawicki J, et al: Cardiac arrhythmias: Frequency during fiberoptic bronchoscopy and correlation with hypoxemia. Arch Intern Med 141:603–606, 1981
47. Zavala DC: Pulmonary hemorrhage in fiberoptic transbronchial biopsy. Chest 70:584–588, 1976
48. Pereira W Jr, Kovnat DM, Snider GL: A prospective cooperative study of complications following flexible fiberoptic bronchoscopy. Chest 73:813–816, 1978
49. Fry WA: Techniques of topical anesthesia for bronchoscopy. Chest 73(S), no. 5:694–696, 1978
50. Harrell JH II: Transnasal approach for fiberoptic bronchoscopy. Chest 73(S), no. 5:704–706, 1978
51. Sanderson DR, McDougall JC: Transoral bronchofiberoscopy. Chest 73(S), no. 5:701–703, 1978
52. Perry LB: Topical anesthesia for bronchoscopy. Chest 73(S), no. 5:691–693, 1978
53. Martini N, McCormick PM: Assessment of endoscopically visible bronchial carcinomas. Chest 73(S), no. 5:718–720, 1978
54. Lam WK, So SY, Hsu C, et al: Fibreoptic bronchoscopy in the diagnosis of bronchial cancer: Comparison of washings, brushings and biopsies in central and peripheral tumours. Clin Oncol 9:35–42, 1983
55. Kvale PA: Collection and preparation of bronchoscopic specimens. Chest 73(S), no. 5:707–712, 1978
56. Bartlett JG, Alexander J, Mayhew J, et al: Should fiberoptic bronchoscopy aspirates be cultured? Am Rev Respir Dis 114:73–78, 1976

57. Wimberley N, Willey S, Sullivan N, et al: Antibacterial properties of lidocaine. Chest 76:37–40, 1979
58. Westcott JL: Direct percutaneous needle aspiration of localized pulmonary lesions: Results in 422 patients. Radiology 137:31–35, 1980
59. Wang KP, Brower R, Haponik EF, et al: Flexible transbronchial needle aspiration for staging of bronchogenic carcinoma. Chest 84:571–576, 1983
60. Cortese DA, Kinsey JH: Hematoporphyrin derivative phototherapy in the treatment of bronchogenic carcinoma. Chest 86:8–13, 1984
61. Hayata Y, Kato H, Konak C, et al: Hematoporphyrin derivative and laser photoradiation in the treatment of lung cancer. Chest 81:269–277, 1982
62. Toty L, Personne CL, Colchen A, et al: Bronchoscopic management of tracheal lesions using the neodymium yttrium aluminium garnet laser. Thorax 36:175–178, 1981
63. Kvale PA, Eichenhorn MS, Radke JR, et al: YAG laser photoresection of lesions obstructing the central airways. Chest 87:283–288, 1985
64. Pereira W, Kovnat DM, Khan MA, et al: Fever and pneumonia after flexible fiberoptic bronchoscopy. Am Rev Respir Dis 112:59–64, 1975
65. Beyt BE, King DK, Glew RH: Fatal pneumonitis and septicemia after fiberoptic bronchoscopy. Chest 72:105–107, 1977

Myron H. Brand
Frank J. Troncale

5

Fiberoptic Esophagoscopy

The introduction of flexible fiberoptic endoscopy in the early 1960s revolutionized the physician's ability not only to discover disorders of the esophagus, but also to intervene in a therapeutic way. Over the past two decades, flexible fiberoptic technology has expanded rapidly, enabling endoscopists to perform esophagoscopy rapidly, safely, and with minimal patient discomfort. Diagnostic acumen has been improved and this has been coupled with an evolution of practice patterns. Formerly, the endoscope had a wide diameter (13.4 mm) which could only be used with moderate to heavy patient sedation in a hospital environment. Today, coupling the new thinner fiberendoscope (8.2 mm) with knowledge and experience gained over the past 25 years, the fiberoptic esophagoscope (FE) has moved into an outpatient office setting.

Modern esophagoscopy has become such an integral part of the evaluation of patients with suspected disorders within the esophagus that many physicians have now made it their initial diagnostic study. The major benefits of this examination derive from the endoscopist's ability to directly visualize the esophageal mucosa, coupled with the capabilities of making permanent photographic records, of obtaining biopsy material, and of intervening therapeutically. Fiberoptic esophagoscope examinations have become so integrated into the modern evaluation of esophageal disease that as of 1982 approximately one million examinations had been performed.[1]

ADVANTAGES OF FIBEROPTIC ESOPHAGOSCOPY
(Table 5-1)

The rapid acceptance of the FE into modern medical practice stems from its advantages over the rigid esophagoscope and barium studies. Rigid endoscopy requires heavy sedation (to overcome patient discomfort) and an in-hospital setting. Fiberoptic esophagoscopy, on the other hand, may be performed with a minimum of analgesia, is well-accepted by patients, and is ideally suited for the outpatient office setting. Rigid esophagoscopy has not, however, become extinct entirely, since it can be recommended still for removing sharp foreign bodies from the proximal one-third of the esophagus.[2] It also has utility for esophageal sclerotherapy in treatment of bleeding esophageal varices, but even this has largely been replaced with the flexible instrument.[3]

The barium swallow examination, although safe, allows only limited evaluation of the esophageal mucosa. Not even the introduction of the newer double contrast techniques has led to the ability to identify superficial or small mucosal lesions. Esophagitis, esophageal ulcers, esophageal varices, and Mallory-Weiss tears are commonly missed with barium techniques.

Numerous recent studies, including those by Dooley,[4] Cameron,[5] Tedesco,[6] and Martin,[7] have documented the diagnostic superiority of flexible endoscopic examinations in the diagnosis of mucosal gastrointestinal (GI) lesions. There are, however, conditions in which barium studies should be performed prior to endoscopy: esophageal motility disorders, cricopharyngeal dysfunction, esophageal diverticula, and esophageal stricture. In these circumstances, the x-ray findings will aid the endoscopist in performing a safer, more accurate study.

GUIDELINES FOR ESTABLISHMENT OF GASTROINTESTINAL ENDOSCOPY AREAS

The performance of safe and accurate outpatient office esophagoscopy is dependent upon meeting five major guidelines. These guidelines, suggested by the American Society for Gastrointestinal Endoscopy (ASGE), include:

1. A properly trained endoscopist
2. Properly trained ancillary personnel
3. Modern equipment
4. An adequately furnished endoscopy area
5. An informed and cooperative patient

The Endoscopist

Modern endoscopic equipment is complex and delicate and requires not only training in the technical performance of the examination, but also an appreciation of the indications, limitations, and risks of the examination. The endoscopist must be able to

Table 5-1
Advantages of Office
Fiberoptic Esophagoscopy

Cost-effective
Rapid, accurate diagnosis
Safety
Convenient for patient and physician
Well accepted by patient

perform the exam with a minimum of patient discomfort and correctly interpret the endoscopic findings. Guidelines for training in endoscopy have been suggested by the ASGE.*

Ancillary Personnel

The gastrointestinal endoscopy assistant plays a vital role in the safe completion of an outpatient fiberoptic esophagoscopy. It is the function of the assistant (prior to the examination) to insure that all equipment and instrumentation is functional and properly disinfected.

A suggested regimen for the proper disinfection of the FE includes both mechanical and chemical cleaning. Other responsibilities include discussing the procedure with the patients and reassuring them. A brief medical history is taken with specific reference to drug allergies, glaucoma, or a history of cardiac or pulmonary problems. If there is a history of cardiac valvular disease, appropriate antibiotic prophylaxis is required.[8,9]

Before, during, and after the procedure, the endoscopy assistant's responsibility is to monitor the patient's vital signs. If, during the examination, biopsies or brush cytology are necessary, these endoscopic accessories will be manipulated in conjunction with the physician. The assistant will be responsible for proper labeling and handling of all specimens obtained. Post-procedure special instructions should be given to the patient, which usually include abstaining from all food or beverages for about 2 hours until the posterior pharyngeal anesthetic dissipates. The patient will also be warned about operating any machinery or automobiles for 24 hours if any sedation or tranquilizers were given at the time of the procedure.

Functional Modern Equipment

A complete endoscopic system is comprised of the FE, a high-intensity cold light source, two continuous suction apparatuses, and endoscopic accessories which include biopsy forceps, cytology brushes, and an endoscopic camera (Figures 5-1A and 1B).

Modern endoscopists have a variety of instruments from which to choose, but all operate on the same basic principles. The insertion shafts are pencil-thin, usually about 1 meter in length, and composed of two sets of glass fiber bundles and a flexible tip controlled by wire cables. The diameter of the insertion shafts varies in modern endoscopes from 8 to 12 mm (Table 5-2). The two sets of glass optical bundles allow light to travel on one set of bundles from the light source to the esophagus, with the other set allowing the illuminated image to travel back to the examiner. The wire cables allow the endoscopist to control tip bending. (The newer endoscopes bend as far as 240°.) The FE are forward viewing, with a field of vision of about 100°. Within the FE shaft there are usually two specialized channels, one for air/water insufflation and the other for biopsy/suction.

Several manufacturers make light sources that are small and inexpensive. Halogen bulbs producing 150 watts provide adequate illumination for routine office use, although bigger units are needed if teaching or photographic attachments are used.

---

*A copy of these guidelines may be obtained by writing the ASGE at 13 Elm Street, Manchester MA, 01944.

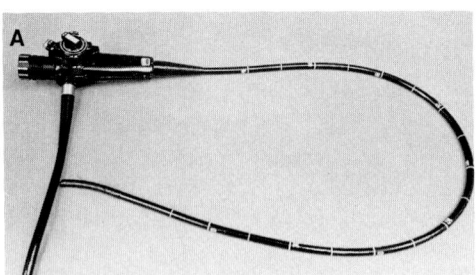
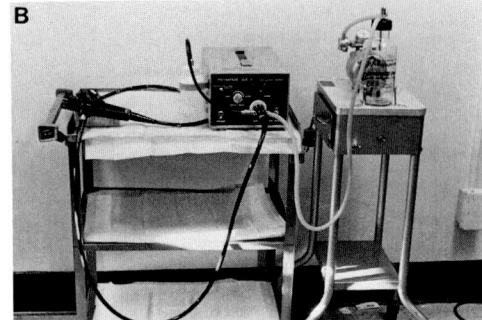

Fig. 5-1. A. Flexible, thin-caliber office esophagoscope. 5-1B. Office equipment, including endoscopic portable cart, esophagoscope, cold light source, and suction apparatus.

Two portable suction pumps are necessary! One will attach to the FE (to remove excess secretions), and the other will attach to a dental-type mouth suction (to remove pooled saliva from the mouth).

Biopsy forceps and a cytology brush are indispensable accessories, and there should be present an endoscopic camera, either 35 mm or Polaroid, for photographic documentation of the findings.

In addition to modern, well maintained equipment, the endoscopist must have an adequately furnished endoscopy suite, including the procedure room and a recovery area. The procedure room should include an adjustable examination table, cabinets for storage of instruments, drug storage (narcotic), portable suction apparatus, and a sink for cleaning the instruments. Cardiopulmonary resuscitation equipment must be available and functioning properly. Both the physician and endoscopist assistant must have Red Cross certification in cardiopulmonary resuscitation. A recovery room should be present in close proximity to the endoscopy procedure room.

Table 5-2
Selected Endoscopes for Office Practice

	Channel Size	Diameter	Field of View	Bending up/down	Angle R/L
ACMI					
AG R	2.5 mm	9.8 mm	90°	180°/120°	120°/120°
AG RF	2.5 mm	9.8 mm	90°	180°/180°	180°/180°
Pentax					
FG-23H	2.2 mm	7.9 mm	104°	180°/180°	100°/100°
FG 34J	3.5 mm	11.5 mm	105°	180°/180°	100°/100°
Olympus					
GIF XP10	2.0 mm	7.9 mm	100°	210°/90°	100°/100°
GIF XQ10	2.8 mm	9.8 mm	100°	210°/90°	100°/100°
Fujinon					
UGI FP2	2.7 mm	9.5 mm	105°	210°/90°	90°/90°
UGI F2	2.8 mm	11.0 mm	105°	210°/90°	90°/90°
Welch-Allen					
81105	2.8 mm	11.8 mm	90°	180°/120°	120°/120°

Informed and Cooperative Patient

Prior to the endoscopic procedure, the patient should be clearly told the reasons for the esophagoscopy and the possible risks, and written consent obtained. It should be stressed that the more time spent explaining the procedure and reassuring the patient, the more cooperative the patient will be. An uncooperative patient should not undergo office esophagoscopy.

INDICATIONS FOR OFFICE FIBEROPTIC ESOPHAGOSCOPY (Table 5-3)

The indications for office diagnostic esophagoscopy are broad.[10] In general, if there is a suspicion of an esophageal mucosal defect, i.e., esophagitis, ulcer, mass, or varix, the physician should proceed directly to endoscopy. Those patients who give a history of severe heartburn or odynophagia should be endoscoped prior to barium swallow. If the patient complains of solid or liquid dysphagia, or both, then a barium swallow should be the initial diagnostic study of choice, with endoscopy to follow. An esophagoscopy will also be performed if there is a suspicion of esophageal mucosal pathology (even if the barium swallow is normal) or to clarify an abnormality seen on barium swallow examination. Hematemesis is an indication for endoscopy, but, depending upon the amount of bleeding and the clinical circumstances, it may be wisest to perform this study in a hospital setting.

THE EXAMINATION

Once the decision to perform endoscopy is made, the physician will need to decide whether the study should be done as an office procedure or in a hospital environment. Those factors which will enter into the decision include the patient's age and the underlying medical condition. In general, those patients below age 15 or above age 70 are best studied in a hospital setting, as are those with cardiopulmonary problems, i.e., emphysema, arteriosclerotic heart disease, or cardiac arrythmias. A patient who is uncooperative should not be endoscoped at all (Table 5-4).

Preparation for endoscopic examination will begin at the initial office consultation. The physician should explain the indications and risks of the procedure and answer all questions. Time should be spent reassuring the patient that this is a simple and safe diagnostic study.

Table 5-3
Indications for Office Esophagoscopy

Odynophagia
Dysphagia
Abnormal barium swallow
Chronic severe reflux complaints
Chest pain of unclear origin (cardiac evaluation negative)
Suspected foreign body in distal esophagus

Table 5-4
Contraindications to Office Endoscopy

Uncooperative patient
Cardiopulmonary disease (recent M.I. unstable
 cardiac rhythm, significant COPD)
Significant hematemesis
Bleeding disorder
Suspected foreign body lodged in cervical
 esophagus
Suspected Zenker's diverticulum

At the initial consultation, the physician will need to determine if special precautions are necessary, e.g., if there is a history of drug allergies, glaucoma, or cardiopulmonary problems, or a need for antibiotic prophylaxis. It is suggested that physicians have an esophagoscopy booklet available to the patient, which explains the procedure, including preparation, risks, and postesophagoscopy instructions. (Such a booklet is available from the ASGE.) At the conclusion of the patient's initial office consultation, the patient will be asked to return at a scheduled date and time for the planned endoscopic examination. The patient should arrive after an 8-hour fast and bring a friend or relative who can drive the patient home. The need for a companion is emphasized, since the patient will likely receive intravenous sedatives and will not be allowed to drive an automobile for 24 hours post-procedure.

When a patient arrives, the prescribed period of fasting will be verified. The vital signs are checked and conditions requiring special precautions previously noted are identified, i.e., glaucoma, cardiopulmonary problems, and need for antibiotic prophylaxis. The endoscopy assistant reviews the procedure with the patient once again. A written consent is obtained by the physician if not previously taken in the initial office interview. The patient is asked to remove dentures and bridgework, and the posterior pharynx is then anesthetized with a topical anesthetic. Those recommended include Pontocaine (Breon), Cetacaine spray (Cetylite), Tessalon pearls (Du Pont), or Dyclone gargle (Astra). These medications reduce gagging while the scope is being introduced into the posterior pharynx. Next, an intravenous line is placed either with a heparin lock or a microdrip infusion. These lines insure access to the circulation for premedication and for medication reversal, if necessary.

The premedications given are dependent upon the patient's age, anxiety level, and cardiopulmonary status. In general, younger patients require more sedation than do elderly patients. Elderly patients and those who have had a previous endoscopic examination often will only require topical pharyngeal anesthesia.

The amount of intravenous premedication should be individualized. It is suggested that atropine, 0.6 mg I.V., be given to those patients without tachycardia, glaucoma, or an enlarged prostate. This medication will decrease salivation, help prevent reflex bradycardia, and decrease gastric motility. Usually a combination of Demerol (Winthrop) and Valium (Roche) will be given separately by the intravenous route. Since there are synergistic effects between the two drugs, it is recommended that only 25 mg of Demerol be given initially before any intravenous Valium. Once the effect of the Demerol is assessed, Valium can then be added in 1–2 mg increments. A suitable endpoint, pharyngeal anesthesia, can be determined by inserting the gloved finger gently into the posterior pharynx. If the gag reflux has been abolished, the patient needs no further medication, and is ready to swallow the instrument.

A few words about Valium are in order. It is an ideal medication for flexible esophagoscopy because it has a rapid onset of action and a wide therapeutic range.[11] Its amnesic properties are particularly welcome, especially since many patients need repeated examinations. The major drawback of intravenous Valium is a 10 percent risk of chemical thrombophlebitis of the infusion site. Thus, prior to giving the drug, the patient should be warned of this side effect as it may be particularly troublesome. To minimize this side effect, Valium should only be given in a large vein in the arm. In addition to the pharyngeal relaxation mentioned above, other desirable side effects are patient relaxation, decrease of anxiety, and sedation. Oversedating can be avoided by pausing 30–60 seconds between increments. In the event of excessive medication effects, Demerol can be reversed by intravenous naloxone (4 mg ampules). I.V. physostigmine is said to reverse the central nervous system effects of Valium, but the authors have no personal experience with its use.

With the patient positioned securely on the left side, the endoscopy assistant flexes the patient's neck. The FE is then passed gently into the posterior pharynx with the index finger of the physician's left hand, as the tongue is kept depressed and the endoscope tip guided toward the midline, as posteriorly as possible.

With the endoscope tip in the correct position, the patient is then asked to swallow and the scope is gently advanced through the cricopharyngeus muscle. The FE should never be passed against resistance. During the advancement of the instrument, if the patient gags or has respiratory difficulty, the scope should be rapidly removed. After reassurance, and a few minutes rest (and possibly more sedation), the endoscopist should again attempt passage of the instrument.

Once the esophagus has been entered, the lumen should be gently insufflated so all mucosal surfaces can be clearly seen. The FE should not be advanced blindly, i.e., without a clear view of the lumen, since this could lead to perforation. In order to prevent aspiration into the trachea, the endoscopist should be on the alert for pooled secretions within the lumen and remove them quickly through the suction channel. If gastric juice is noted to be freely refluxing into the esophagus, the head of the patient's bed should quickly be elevated so that gravity will aid in preventing aspiration.

The esophageal mucosa usually begins at about 20 cm from the incisors and is normally grayish-pink colored. Within the proximal esophagus, one can usually appreciate aortic pulsations on the left lateral wall.

The gastroesophageal junction is normally present at 40 cm from the incisors and is marked by an irregular, sawtoothed, squamocolumnar junction (Z line) (Fig. 5-2).

It will be difficult for the endoscopist to appreciate motility disturbances or extrinsic compression on the esophagus (unless extreme). Normally, the esophageal lumen will have a tendency to collapse without frequent insufflations of air. Contraction rings, unless they have caused the lumen to narrow enough to prevent passage of the instrument, will appear and disappear with peristalsis.

BENIGN ESOPHAGEAL CONDITIONS (Table 5-5)

The common benign conditions include hiatal hernias, esophageal rings, esophagitis, Barrett's epithelium, esophageal strictures, and esophageal varices. The malignant

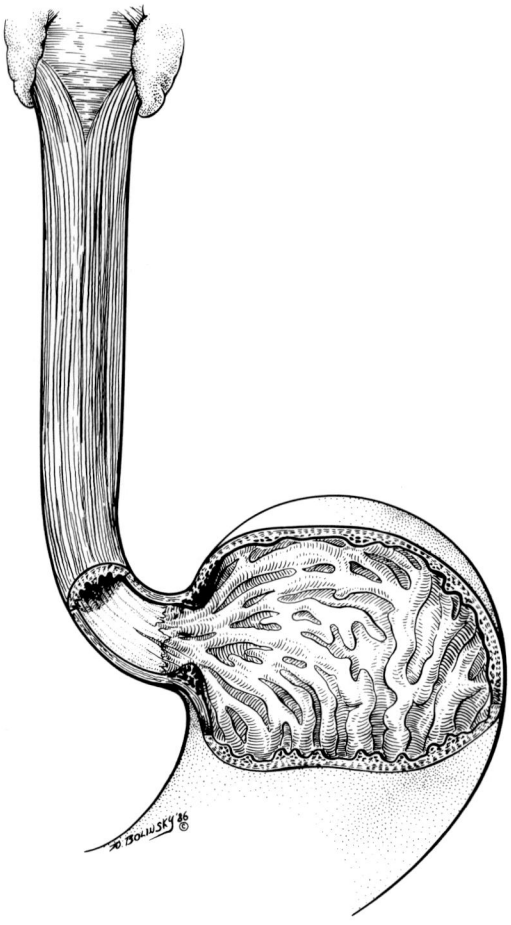

Fig. 5-2. The gastroesophageal juncton is normally present at 40 cm. from the incisors and is marked by an irregular, saw toothed, squamo columnar junction. (Z-line)

conditions include primary neoplasms originating within the esophagus or extending up from the gastric fundus.

When a hiatal hernia is present, the gastroesophageal junction will be located proximal to the usual 40 cm distance from the mouth, signifying that the upper stomach is above the level of the diaphragm. The diaphragmatic hiatus is usually recognized as a circular indentation of the distal end of the herniated stomach. By having the patient sniff, the narrowing caused by the diaphragmatic pinchcock on the herniated stomach can be confirmed. The presence of a hiatal hernia alone on a barium examination is not

Table 5-5
Common Benign Conditions of the Esophagus

Hiatal hernia with lower esophageal ring
Gastroesophageal reflux with esophagitis
Barrett's esophagitis (premalignant)
Mallory-Weiss tear
Esophageal varices

an indication for esophagoscopy, since it is of little clinical significance unless it is associated with gastroesophageal reflux.[12] On the other hand, if esophagitis is suspected from the history, the esophagoscopy is the most accurate means of making the diagnosis. Commonly, esophagitis is due to the reflux of acid peptic juice, with rarer causes being viral, caustic, monilial, or drug-induced (so-called "pill" esophagitis) in origin. Esophagitis, regardless of etiology, is characterized by mucosal erythema, friability, exudate, and ulcerations. These findings may be limited to one wall or present concentrically. When esophagitis is found, it should be confirmed histologically by a pinch biopsy and brush cytology. This is because occasionally primary esophageal malignancy can be confused with esophagitis, and because both herpes and monilia are best diagnosed by histology.

Barrett's epithelium is thought to be a consequence of chronic reflux esophagitis.[13,14] This type of metaplastic columnar epithelium is one of the responses of the esophagus to chronic peptic injury. Endoscopically, this epithelium is characterized as salmon-colored (gastric) epithelium extending up from the esophagus from the GE junction; or it can appear as islands of reddened mucosa surrounded by inflamed squamous mucosa.[15] The significance of Barrett's epithelium is that it represents a premalignant change signaling the need for close endoscopic follow-up of the patient.[16]

This epithelium is often found in the presence of deep esophageal ulcers or esophageal strictures.

Benign esophageal strictures are the end result of chronic peptic injury or, more rarely, radiation damage.[17] They may prevent the endoscopist from entering the stomach, depending on the luminal diameter. They are characterized by a narrowed lumen bordered by erythematous, friable, ulcerated esophageal mucosa. All esophageal strictures should be biopsied and brushed for cytology on initial discovery to rule out malignancy. The esophageal brush cytology of a stricture may be more accurate for diagnosing malignancy than is a biopsy, because one can often insert the tip of the brush (carefully) through the stricture. One note of caution is that if there is a significant amount of peptic inflammation present it may be difficult for the cytopathologist to differentiate regenerative (benign) from malignant cytologic changes. To obtain more representative esophageal biopsies from an esophageal stricture, it is often necessary to dilate the esophageal stricture and then repeat the endoscopy to obtain tissue from its more distal aspects.

Finally, esophageal varices are recognized as submucosal blue-gray vascular projections entering the esophagus at the level of the gastroesophageal junction. They signify the presence of portal hypertension and should initiate an evaluation of the liver and portal circulation. Because these varices have thin walls, they should never be biopsied for fear of initiating severe hemorrhage.

MALIGNANT ESOPHAGEAL CONDITIONS (Table 5-6)

Primary esophageal or gastric malignancy with esophageal involvement usually presents with odynophagia (pain on swallowing) or dysphagia. These complaints should always trigger esophageal evaluation to include esophagoscopy and barium swallow. These malignancies may involve one wall only, or they may concentrically constrict the esophageal lumen. They may appear as flattened and plaque-like, or as exophytic and bulky. As previously mentioned, on occasion, areas of esophagitis or stricture may be confused with malignancy. It should be emphasized that multiple biopsies (six or more) should be taken from various areas of the lesion to avoid sampling errors.[18]

Table 5-6
Common Malignant Conditions
of the Esophagus

1° Esophageal malignancy (squamous)
2° involvement of distal esophagus from fundal gastric adenocarcinoma
1° adenocarcinoma of esophagus arising in area of Barrett's epithelium

---

THERAPEUTIC OPTIONS

In addition to diagnosis, flexible fiberoptic esophagoscopy gives the endoscopist several therapeutic options.[19] In an office setting, the most common ones would include removal of foreign bodies and dilatation of benign strictures. Sclerosis of esophageal varices, laser phototherapy, and bipolar electrocoagulation can also be done on outpatients, but are best performed in a hospital setting in view of the risks associated with these patients.

Acute food impactions (usually poultry or beef) within the distal esophagus are a common clinical problem, and they are always associated with an underlying organic cause such as a lower esophageal ring or a stricture (benign or malignant). These foreign bodies can usually be removed by the FE with the aid of an endoscopic wire (polypectomy) snare. If the underlying pathology is not known to the endoscopist, then the foreign body should not be blindly pushed into the stomach. Attempts to do so may not be successful, and if a malignancy is present with an eccentric lumen, esophageal perforation could result. Once the obstruction is relieved, the underlying cause for the obstruction can be noted and appropriate treatment started. In the case of a ring[20] or stricture,[21] bougienage is the initial treatment of choice.

Sharp foreign bodies (such as pins) impacted within the distal esophagus require special care, since they frequently penetrate the mucosa. In general, they are safe to remove even if they have penetrated; however, great care must be taken to keep a tight grip on them lest they fall into the tracheobronchial tree during removal of the instrument through the cricopharyngeal sphincter. Their removal is greatly simplified by the use of an "overtube."[22] This is a hollow plastic tube with an inner diameter slightly larger than the esophagoscope. The technique involves having the patient swallow the overtube first so that the distal end is in the mid to upper esophagus (not deeper, since the gastroesophageal junction can be easily damaged by blind passage of the overtube's leading edge). The FE is then passed through the overtube and the foreign body grasped tightly. It is slowly brought back to the tip of the FE and both the FE and the foreign body (attached to the forceps) are pulled into the protective sheath of the overtube. The overtube with the FE and the foreign body are then removed in one motion while the operator keeps firmly grasping pressure on the foreign body. This maneuver prevents laceration of the mucosa by the foreign body, since it is safely encased in the overtube.

As has been past practice, sharp foreign bodies impacted within the cervical esophagus should be removed with the rigid esophagoscope under general anesthesia.

The FE also allows the clinician to dilate tight esophageal strictures with the use of a guidewire. These wires are introduced under direct vision through the esophagoscope into the stricture and, with fluoroscopic help, their position in the stomach can be

Table 5-7
Risks of Office Endoscopy

Oversedation
Drug reaction
Aspiration pneumonia
Cardiac or pulmonary depression
*Esophageal perforation
*Esophageal bleeding
*Infection

*rare

verified. The wires are long enough so that the scope can be removed, leaving the wire in place. Over these wires, stiff plastic dilators may be passed, their size gradually increasing in a serial fashion.[23] An older acceptable technique is to pass metal olives over the wires, also best performed under fluoroscopic guidance to avoid perforation.

COMPLICATIONS

The complication rate of esophagoscopy is small but real (Table 5-7). The major complications include oversedation or allergic reactions from medications, cardiopulmonary complications, esophageal perforations, bleeding, and infection.[24-26]

The most frequent complication from fiberoptic esophagoscopy is related to medications used during the procedure. The risk of a drug-induced (Valium) chemical phlebitis at the I.V. site is about 10 percent. In addition, Valium and Demerol may precipitate severe cardiopulmonary depression (0.06 percent).[25] Recent studies have shown that there is a 2–5 percent reduction in arterial oxygen desaturation during esophagoscopy.[27] The resultant hypoxia is potentially dangerous, since it may precipitate cardiac arrythmias, particularly in patients with pre-existing heart disease.

Aspiration pneumonia is also a risk, especially in patients with free gastroesophageal reflux, esophageal obstruction, or oversedation. Patients must always be told to contact their physicians should they develop a cough or fever postendoscopy.

Esophageal perforation (0.03 percent) occurs rarely, usually in the setting of cervical osteophytes or esophageal strictures.[25] It should be emphasized again that the endoscope should never be passed either into the esophagus or through a stricture if resistance is encountered. If a barium swallow is available prior to the examination, this study should be reviewed, since often it will help the endoscopist spot potential problems in advance.

Esophageal bleeding (0.03 percent) usually arises after a target biopsy.[25] This complication is rare and the risks are minimized if appropriate coagulation studies are drawn prior to the procedure (and esophageal varices are avoided).

Infection is also quite rare after endoscopy (0.08 percent). The risk of bacteremia from esophagoscopy is between 5 and 8 percent and is usually that of mouth flora.[28] Some have recommended that only patients with cardiac prosthetic valves, joint prosthesis, and recently placed arterial grafts be given prophylactic antibiotics, however, the authors feel that all patients with significant valvular disease be treated so as not to risk even a small chance of bacterial endocarditis (Table 5-8).

Table 5-8
Prophylaxis for Esophagoscopy

I. Congenital heart disease, rheumatic heart disease, acquired valvular heart disease, IHSS, mitral valve prolapse with mitral insufficiency.
   A. Adults—aqueous crystalline penicillin G (1 million units I.M.) mixed with procaine penicillin G (600,000 units I.M.) 30 minutes–1 hour prior to the procedure, then penicillin V 500 mg P.O. Q6H × 8 doses.
or
   B. Penicillin V 2 grams orally 30 minutes prior to procedure, then 500 mg Q6H × 8 doses.[a]

II. Cardiac prosthetic valves, joint mechanical prosthesis, aortic grafts
   A. Adults—aqueous crystalline penicillin G (2 million units I.V.) or ampicillin 1 g I.V. plus gentamycin (1.5 mg/kg, not to exceed 80 mg) I.V. 30 minutes prior to examination. Both antibiotics to be repeated Q8H × 2 after the procedure.[b]

[a] If penicillin-allergic, use erythromycin 1 g P.O. 1 hour prior to procedure, then 500 mg P.O. Q6H × 8 doses.
[b] If penicillin-allergic, use vancomycin I.V. 500 mg Q8H for 2 doses post-procedure.

SUMMARY

The ability to diagnose and treat esophageal diseases has improved markedly over the past 20 years. The introduction of the small-caliber flexible upper endoscope now offers the ability to shift most diagnostic and therapeutic endoscopy exams from the hospital to the office setting.

Over the next few years, as endoscopes become even thinner, procedures such as laser phototherapy and sclerosis of esophageal varices will become common office practice.

REFERENCES

1. Vennes JA, Silverstein FE: Upper gastrointestinal fiberoptic endoscopy. In Schleisenger MH, Fordtran JS (Eds.): Gastrointestinal Disease (3rd ed.). Philadelphia: W.B. Saunders Company, pp. 1599–1617, 1983
2. Jackson C, Jackson CL: Diseases of the Air and Food Passages of Foreign Body Origin. Philadelphia: W.B. Saunders Company, 1937
3. Sivak M Jr: Sclerotherapy for esophageal varices. In Silvis MS (Ed.): Therapeutic Gastrointestinal Endoscopy (1st ed.). New York City and Japan: Igaks-Shoin, pp. 31–66, 1985
4. Dooley C, Larson A, Stace N, et al: Double contrast barium meal and upper gastrointestinal endoscopy. Ann Intern Med 101:538–545, 1984
5. Cameron AJ, Ott BJ: The value of gastroscopy in clinical diagnosis. Mayo Clin Proc 52:806–808, 1977
6. Tedesco F, Griffin J, Crisp W, et al: "Skinny" upper gastrointestinal endoscopy—The initial

diagnostic tool: A prospective comparison of upper gastrointestinal endoscopy and radiology. J Clin Gastroenterol 2:27–30, 1980
7. Martin TR, Vannes JA, Silvis SE: A comparison of upper gastrointestinal endoscopy and radiology. J Clin Gastroenterol 2:21–25, 1980
8. Antimicrobial prophylaxis for surgery. The Medical Letter 21(18):Sept. 7, 1979
9. Goldman L: Cardiac risks and complications of non-cardiac surgery. Ann Intern Med 98:504–513, 1983
10. Colcher H: Current concepts: Gastrointestinal endoscopy. N Engl J Med 293:1129–1131, 1975
11. Mayer I: Endoscopic premedications. Endoscopy Review, March-April:38–51, 1985
12. Richter JE, Castell DO: Gastrointestinal reflux. Ann Intern Med 97:93–103, 1982
13. Mangle JC: Barrett's esophagus: An old entity rediscovered. J Clin Gastroenterol 3:347–356, 1981
14. Bonnick CA, Eastwood GL: Barrett's esophagus. Surv Dig Dis 1:229–242, 1983
15. Burbige EJ, Radigan JJ: Characteristics of the columnar-cell lined (Barrett's) esophagus. Gastrointest Endosc 25(4):133–136, 1979
16. Naef AP, Savary M, Ozzello L: Columnar lines lower esophagus: An acquired lesion with malignant predisposition. J Thorac Cardiovasc Surg 70(5):826–835, 1975
17. Pope C E II: Gastroesophageal reflux disease. In Schleisenger MH, Fordtran JS (Eds.): Gastrointestinal Disease (3rd ed.). Philadelphia: W.B. Saunders Company, pp. 449–476, 1983
18. Bruni HC, Nelson RS: Carcinoma of the esophagus and cardia. J Thorac Cardiovasc Surg 70:367, 1975
19. Silvis S (Ed): Therapeutic Gastrointestinal Endoscopy (1st ed.). New York City and Japan: Egaku-Shoin, 1985
20. Spiro HM: Primarily structural disorders. In: Clinical Gastroenterology (3rd ed.). New York City: McMillan, pp. 88–128, 1983
21. Buchin PJ, Spiro HM: Therapy of esophageal stricture: A review of 84 patients. J Clin Gastroenterol 3:121–128, 1981
22. Spurling TJ, Zaloga GP, Richter JE: Fiberendoscopic removal of a gastric foreign body with overtube technique. Gastrointest Endosc 29:226–227, 1983
23. Dumon JF, Meric B, Dupin B, et al: A New Endoscopic Method of Esophageal Dilation: Savary Bougies. Wilson Cook Med. Inc., pp. 1–7, 1985
24. Shahmir M, Shuman B: Complications of fiberoptic endoscopy. Gastrointest Endosc 26:86–89, 1980
25. Health and Public Policy Committee, American College of Physicians. Ann Intern Med 102:266–269, 1985
26. David R, Graham D: Endoscopic complications. Gastrointest Endosc 25(4):146–149, 1979
27. Lieberman E, Wverker C, Katon R: Cardiopulmonary risk of esophagogastroduodenoscopy. Gastroenterol:468–472, 1985
28. Norfleet R, Mitchell P, Mulholland D: Does bacteremia follow upper gastrointestinal endoscopy? Am J Gastroenterol 76:420–422, 1981

Eiji Yanagisawa

6
Videolaryngoscopy

Videolaryngoscopy—a videographic documentation of the laryngeal examination with simultaneous voice recording using a color video camera—is a most useful office procedure for the clinical practice of laryngology. Videolaryngoscopy can be accomplished using either a flexible fiberscope or a rigid telescope. It allows excellent visualization and documentation of the physiological function and pathological conditions of the larynx. It is of significant value for better understanding of the laryngeal disorders.

Since the introduction of flexible fiberoptic laryngoscopy by Sawashima and Hirose in 1968,[1] the flexible fiberscope has been widely used for evaluation of various conditions of the larynx, including evaluation of speech therapy, postlaryngectomy speech, difficult endotracheal intubation, and pre- and postoperative evaluation for obstructive upper airway, even for endoscopic YAG-Nd laser surgery.[2-17]

One of the most significant advances in endoscopic documentation was the development of the telescope with the new rod lens system by Hopkins.[18] The air-containing spaces between the conventional series of lenses have been replaced with glass rods, with polished ends separated by small "air lenses." The optics of this new system are such that light transmission and magnification are significantly increased, thereby providing a brighter and more easily perceived image and an improved resolution of depth. The attractive feature of this telescopic system is the ease with which the video camera can be coupled with the telescope. Telescopic videolaryngoscopy has been widely used for examination and documentation of laryngeal diseases.[18-32] A simple method of videolaryngoscopy, using a right-angled telescope and a low-cost home video color camera, was introduced by Yanagisawa et al. in 1981.[24]

Fiberscopic and telescopic videolaryngoscopy can be performed in one setting or independently. In this chapter, a comparison of fiberscopic and telescopic videolaryngoscopy will be made.

AMBULATORY SURGERY AND ISBN 0-8089-1803-6 Copyright © 1986 by Grune & Stratton, Inc.
OFFICE PROCEDURES IN HEAD AND NECK SURGERY All rights of reproduction in any form reserved.

EQUIPMENT

Laryngoscopes

Flexible Fiberscopes

Commonly used flexible fiberscopes are the Olympus ENF-P flexible rhinolaryngofiberscope (nasopharyngolaryngoscope-Fig. 6-1), and the Machida ENT-4L or 3L flexible nasopharyngolaryngoscope. Other flexible fiberscopes, such as the Olympus ENF-L, with wider diameter of 4.8 mm and the Olympus ENF-LD, with a 4.8 mm diameter and an instrument channel, are also available. For the specifications of these flexible fiberscopes, the readers are referred to Table 3-1 in Chapter 3 on fiberoptic nasopharyngolaryngoscopy. At the time of this writing, Richard Wolf and Karl Storz Instrument Companies have introduced new fiberscopes.

The Olympus ENF-P fiberscope is the author's choice. The diameter of the insertion tube of this fiberscope is 3.7 mm. It gives the wide angulation range, specifically 130° up and 90° down, providing easy and comfortable maneuverability. Simple thumb movement control of tip bending in the ENF-P appears to be an obvious advanage over designs with a knob on one side of the control head that calls for two-handed control. This is particularly true when the scope is used with the video camera.

Rigid Right-angled Telescopes

Right-angled telescopes most commonly used today are (1) the Berci-Ward indirect laryngopharyngoscope with Hopkins telescope (Karl Storz 8702D); (2) the telelaryngopharyngoscope with Hopkins telescope (Karl Storz 8704D) or the Karl Storz telelaryngopharyngoscope especially designed for photography, cinematography, and television (H8704FJ); (3) the Stuckrad magnifying laryngoepipharyngoscope (Richard Wolf); and (4) the Nagashima SFT-1 laryngoscope (Fig. 6-1). The author primarily uses the Nagashima SFT-1 laryngoscope for office telescopic videolaryngoscopy.

The Nagashima laryngoscope is a single, integrated laryngoscope composed of a telescope and a light transmission system (Fig. 6-1). It measures 24.5 cm in length and 9 mm in outer diameter. The angle of the prism at the tip of the telescope is 70°, providing a right-angled view of the larynx. The rectangular outlets on each side of the lens offer

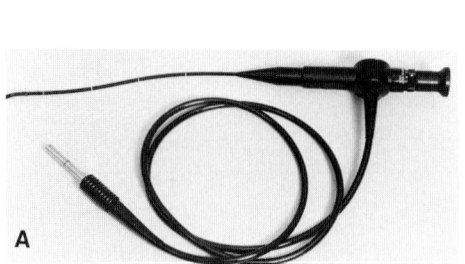
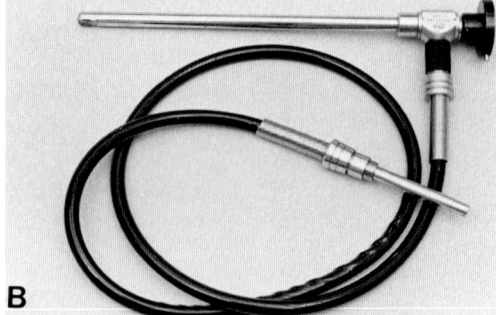

Fig. 6-1. Laryngoscopes. (A) Olympus ENF-P flexible fiberscope. (B) Nagashima SFT-1 rigid telescope.

Videolaryngoscopy

Table 6-1
Comparisons of Fiberscopic and Telescopic Videolaryngoscopy

	Fiberscopic Videolaryngoscopy	Telescopic Videolaryngoscopy
Image resolution	fair–good	excellent
Patients' acceptance	excellent	very good
Normal speech	excellent	impossible
Phonation (vocal cord vibration)	very good	excellent minute detail
Respiration	excellent	excellent
Effort closure (coughing)	very good	very good—excellent
Swallowing	very good	impossible to swallow with tongue pulled
Singing	excellent, particularly for singers and professionals	poor, "distorted" voice
Pathology		
clarity	very good	excellent
upper border of tumor	excellent	excellent
lower border of tumor	very good	poor

well-balanced illumination of the viewing field. Each measures approximately 2 × 4 mm. The front lens diameter measures 4 × 3 mm.

Video Cameras

There are many fine-quality miniature color video cameras specifically designed for medical use (Circon, Zeiss-Circon, Olympus OTV-E, Sony DXC-1850, Hitachi, etc.). More recently, "three-tube" cameras, such as the Ikegami ITC-350M and the Hitachi DK5050, have been introduced. The cost of these cameras ranges from $10,000 to $30,000. While they are ultracompact and convenient, the cost of these cameras is often prohibitive to most otolaryngologists. The author has advocated the use of reasonably priced home video system cameras for videolaryngoscopy and has obtained excellent results.[24,31,32] It is important to emphasize that not all home video cameras can be used for videolaryngoscopy. A camera equipped with a detachable lens, a C-mount coupler, and an adjustable or detachable hand grip should be chosen for this technique. At the time of this writing, the author is using the PK-973 Newvicon color video camera (Fig. 6-2). This camera is equipped with a built-in microcomputer character generator to display the title, the date, and the name of the patient, and was found to be quite satisfactory for both fiberscopic and telescopic videolaryngoscopy.

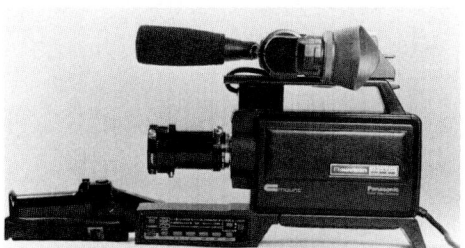

Fig. 6-2. Panasonic home video color camera. The zoom lens of the camera is removed and replaced with a video camera adapter, to which a fiberscope or a telescope is attached. In this photograph, the Nagashima video adapter is attached to the camera.

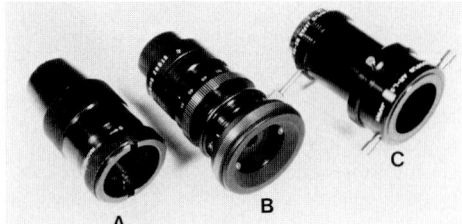

Fig. 6-3. Video adapters. (A) Nagashima video adapter (f-60 mm). (B) Karl Storz zoom lens adapter (35–70 mm). (C) Olympus video adapters: AR-L2 plus MC-08.

The author also tried the new JVC GX-N8U color home video camera. This camera has an automatic focusing device, but the lens is not detachable. With the use of an adapter, however, either a fiberscope or a rigid telescope can be attached to the front of the lens. Surprisingly good video images have been obtained.

Video Adapters

The Olympus video adapter AR-L2 with MC-08 adapter or Karl Storz 35–70 mm zoom lens video adapter was used for the Olympus ENF-P fiberscope (Fig. 3-C & B). The Nagashima video adapter (f-60 mm) was used for the Nagashima telescope (Fig. 3-A).

Light Source

The xenon cold light fountain (Karl Storz 487C—Fig. 6-4A), which produces approximately 6000 K, is recommended for both fiberscopic and telescopic video documentation. However, the Panasonic PK-973 home video camera is so light-sensitive that standard light sources, such as the Olympus ILK-3, Machida LH-150, Karl Storz 481-C, or Pilling Luminator 2X (Fig. 6-4B), may suffice for telescopic videolaryngoscopy. For fiberscopic documentation, however, the more powerful light sources, such as the Karl Storz xenon light source 487C, Karl Storz metal haloid arc (484C), Olympus CLE-F10, or Olympus CLV-F10, are still necessary to produce consistently high-quality video images.

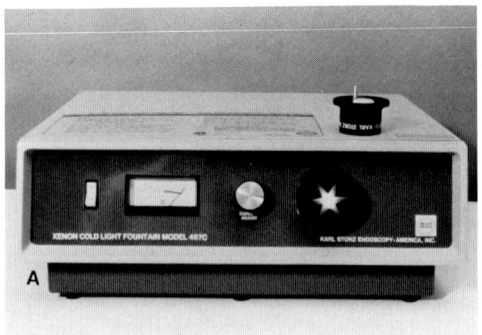 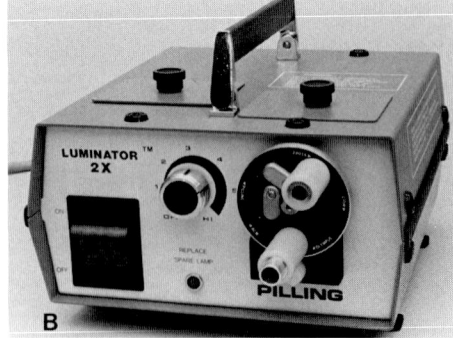

Fig. 6-4. Light sources. (A) Xenon cold light fountain 487C (Karl Storz). (B) Pilling Luminator 2X.

Video Recorder and Monitor

Technically, any three-quarter-inch or one-half-inch video recorder can be used. The author uses the Sony three-quarter-inch VO-5600 U-matic videocassette recorder. This is a front-loading tape transport system that allows high-speed search at 5 times normal playback speed in forward and reverse directions. One of the distinct advantages of this particular recorder is that while searching the previously videotaped material, the video images are cleary visible on the TV monitor. This is a very useful, time-saving advantage for videolaryngoscopy.

Voice can be simply recorded by plugging the audio output connector of the camera cable to a videocassette recorder. For high-fidelity voice recording, however, the author recommends the use of a separate external microphone that can be directly connected to the cassette recorder.

TECHNIQUE

Fiberscopic Videolaryngoscopy (Transnasal)

The Olympus ENF-P fiberscope is connected to the video camera via the Olympus AR-L2 with MC-08 adapter or Karl Storz 35–70 mm zoom lens adapter.

The patient sits facing the examiner. The examiner may perform the procedure either in a sitting or standing position (Fig. 6-5A). The nose is first examined and sprayed with 3 percent ephedrine to admit the fiberscope without traumatizing hypertrophied turbinates. The side of the nose without septal spur and with widest air passage is chosen. The nose is lightly anesthetized with 2 percent tetracaine hydrochloride or 4 percent Xylocaine spray (Astra). The tip of the flexible fiberscope is lightly lubricated and inserted into the nose gently (Fig. 6-5A). While observing the monitor or the viewfinder of the camera, the fiberscope is gradually advanced until it reaches the posterior wall of the nasopharynx. Then, the tip is bent downward and the fiberscope is gradually advanced until it reaches the posterior wall of the nasopharynx. The tip is then bent further downward and the fiberscope advanced. The epiglottis is soon visible.

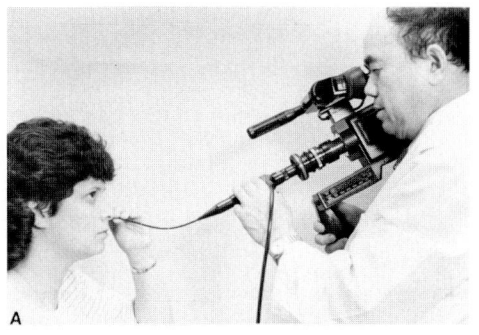
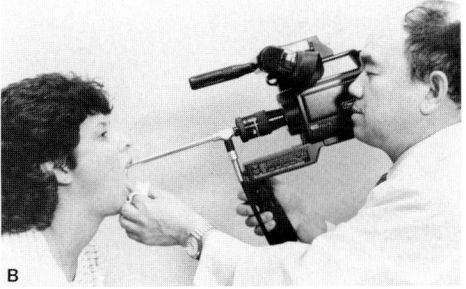

Fig. 6-5. (A) Technique of fiberscopic videolaryngoscopy. Examiner holds the fiberscope and adjusts position of the tip of the fiberscope with one hand while holding the camera in the other hand. (B) Technique of telescopic videolaryngoscopy. The larynx is viewed and centered on the screen of the TV monitor.

The scope is passed to the level of the epiglottis, the larynx is centered on the screen, and the patient is ready for videotaping.

Every effort should be made to stabilize the camera and the laryngoscope in order to prevent image movement during videotaping. In some cases, the camera has been mounted on a tripod and the patient has passed the fiberscope into the nose with one hand while adjusting the control knob of the fiberscope with the other hand.

Telescopic Videolaryngoscopy (Transoral)

The patient and the examiner sit facing each other (Fig. 6-5B). The soft palate and the posterior half of the tongue are topically anesthetized with a 2 percent tetracaine hydrochloride (Pontocaine—Breon) solution or a 4 percent Xylocaine solution.

The Nagashima telescope is connected to the video camera via the video adapter and its fiberoptic cable is attached to the xenon illuminator. The tip of the telescope is dipped in warm water and dried, in order to prevent fogging of the lens during the examination. The video camera and the illuminator are turned on. The examiner holds the video camera in one hand and inserts the telescope into the mouth, while holding the patient's tongue with the other hand (Fig. 6-5B). When the desired image appears on the monitor screen, video recording is begun. The laryngeal image is centered on the screen using the television monitor or the viewfinder of the camera. The light intensity is adjusted according to the video image desired.

For both fiberscopic and telescopic videolaryngoscopy, the larynx is routinely videotaped on respiration and phonation.

RESULTS

Fiberscopic videolaryngoscopy produces quite adequate images of anatomical structures and pathological conditions of the nasal cavity, the nasopharynx, and the larynx (Fig. 6-6); the images produced by a fiberscope are generally smaller and less clear. The function of the eustachian tube, the soft palate, and the larynx can be well demonstrated (Fig. 6-6).

Telescopic videolaryngoscopy provides larger images of higher resolution than and of a quality superior to those produced by fiberscopic videolaryngoscopy (Fig. 6-6). Certain functions of the larynx can be well demonstrated. Comparison of fiberscopic and telescopic videolaryngoscopic findings are shown in Table 6-1.

COMMENTS

Both fiberscopic and telescopic videolaryngoscopy have advantages and disadvantages (Table 6-1).

One of the most significant advantages of fiberscopic videolaryngoscopy is the ease of the examination. Fiberscopic videolaryngoscopy is the procedure of choice for children or hypersensitive adult patients whose larynx cannot be examined either by a mirror or a telescope. The use of the fiberscope may prevent unnecessary direct laryngoscopy under general anesthesia for these patients.

Fiberscopic videolaryngoscopy is of great value for voice analysis of functional and organic disorders and for evaluation of the physiological functions of the larynx. Respiration, phonation, glottal effort closure (coughing, lifting, Valsalva procedure, defecation), normal speech, whistling, and swallowing can be studied effectively with the fiberscope. It is very useful for the voice therapist or speech pathologist in the evaluation and documentation of pathology and in counseling for such functional disorders as spastic dysphonia, psychogenic dysphonia, and stuttering. Fiberscopic videolaryngoscopy is very useful for singers who wish to study and improve their own methods of singing. It also allows observation and documentation of disorders of the upper airway structures, such as the nasal cavity, the nasopharynx, and the posterior surface of the soft palate, as well as the larynx.

Telescopic videolaryngoscopy provides much clearer, sharper, brighter, and larger images of the larynx than does fiberscopic videolaryngoscopy. For documentation of anatomical and structural changes of the larynx, telescopic videolaryngoscopy is far superior in the author's experience. The most significant advantage of telescopic videolaryngoscopy is the clear video image of high resolution which can be very satisfactorily photographed. With the use of a new video printer (Mitsubishi P60U video printer), the laryngeal image on the TV screen can be instantaneously copied and a hard copy can be given to the patient or sent to a referring physician or a radiotherapist.[33] Although telescopic videolaryngoscopy is not ideal for the evaluation of speech and singing, the vibration of the vocal folds on phonation is much more clearly visualized on the screen than by fiberscopic videolaryngoscopy. Stroboscopic laryngoscopy can be more effectively carried out by using the telescope than by using the fiberscope. Very early lesions of laryngeal tumors, which may escape the physician's attention by fiberscopic examination, can be detected by telescopic examination.

Some of the disadvantages of fiberscopic videolaryngoscopy are that: (1) it provides smaller, less clear, more distorted pictures of the larynx, (2) it requires a more powerful light source (xenon) for videotaping because of the small diameter of the insertion tube, and (3) it may not demonstrate minor mucosal changes and early lesions of the vocal cords clearly.

Some of the disadvantages of telescopic videolaryngoscopy are that: (1) children and some adults with hyperactive gag reflexes may not tolerate the procedure; (2) fogging of the telescopic lens is more common; and (3) normal speech and singing voice are distorted and impossible to document.

INDICATIONS

Indications for fiberscopic and/or telescopic videolaryngoscopy include:

1. Evaluation and documentation of physiological functions of the larynx. For this purpose, fiberscopic documentation is definitely most valuable, although glottal effort, such as coughing, can be very effectively studied by telescopic examination.
2. Evaluation and documentation of organic disorders of the larynx, such as infection, tumor, congenital anomalies, trauma, etc. For the precise evaluation of structural changes of the larynx, telescopic examination is the choice, except for those young children and adults with hypersensitive gag reflexes.
3. Evaluation and documentation of functional disorders of the larynx, such as spastic dysphonia, psychogenic dysphonia, and stuttering. Fiberscopic examination is the choice.

4. Evaluation of voice therapy and teaching of singers (fiberscopic).
5. Difficult endotracheal intubation (fiberscopic).
6. Live viewing with simultaneous recording at head and neck tumor conferences or other teaching exercises for medical students, interns, and residents (fiberscopic or telescopic or both).
7. Documentation for permanent record, publication, teaching, research, and medicolegal purposes (fiberscopic or telescopic or both).
8. Preoperative and postoperative comparison of various laryngeal disorders (fiberscopic or telescopic or both).
9. Comparison of laryngeal tumor, before and after radiotherapy (fiberscopic or telescopic or both).

CONCLUSION

Videolaryngoscopy is a very valuable office procedure for evaluation and documentation of the function and pathology of the larynx to help better understand disorders of the larynx.

Video laryngoscopy permits voice and video recording. This is particularly valuable for preoperative and postoperative voice analysis and documentation of progressive improvement or regression of laryngeal disorders. It is of great value for patient counseling, planning treatment, teaching, research, and permanent records.

Both fiberscopic and telescopic videolaryngoscopy have advantages and disadvantages. For teaching institutions and serious laryngologists, the combined use of a fiberscope and a telescope is recommended. If the clinician must choose one in clinical practice, then the fiberscope should be the choice because fiberscopic videolaryngoscopy, in spite of some limitations, can document both the function and the pathology of the larynx at the same time, in most cases.

REFERENCES

1. Sawashima M, Hirose H: New laryngoscopic technique by use of fiber optics. J Acoust Soc Am 43:168-169, 1968
2. Davidson TM, Bone RC, Nahum AM: Flexible fiberoptic laryngobronchoscopy. Laryngoscope 84:1876-1882, 1974
3. Brewer DW, McCall G: Visible laryngeal changes during voice therapy: Fiber-optic study. Ann Otol Rhinol Laryngol 83:423-427, 1974
4. Brewer DW, Gould LV, Casper J: Fiber-optic video study of the post-laryngectomized voice. Laryngoscope 85:666-670, 1975
5. Williams GT, Farquharson IM, Anthony J: Fiberoptic laryngoscopy in the assessment of laryngeal disorders. J Laryngol Otol 89:299-316, 1975
6. Silberman HD, Wilf H, Tucker JA: Flexible fiberoptic nasopharyngolaryngoscope. Ann Otol Rhinol Laryngol 85:640-645, 1976
7. Conture EG, McCall GN, Brewer DW: Laryngeal behavior during stuttering. J Speech Hear Res 20:661-668, 1977
8. Parnes SM, Lavorato AS, Myers EN: Study of spastic dysphonia using videofiberoptic laryngoscopy. Ann Otol Rhinol Laryngol 87:322-326, 1978
9. Tobin HA: Office fiberoptic laryngeal photography. Otolaryngol Head Neck Surg 88:172-173, 1980

10. Witton TH: An introduction to the fiberoptic laryngoscope. Can Anaesth Soc J 28:475–478, 1981
11. Chapey R, Salzberg A: The speech clinician's use of fiberoptics in indirect laryngoscopy. J Commun Disord 14:87–90, 1981
12. Sessions DG: Recent advances in surgery of the larynx and trachea. Head Neck Surg 5:42–52, 1982
13. Welch AR: The practical and economic value of flexible system laryngoscopy. J Laryngol Otol 96:1125–1129, 1982
14. Silberman HD: The use of the flexible fiberoptic nasopharyngolaryngoscope in the pediatric upper airway. Otolaryngol Clin North Am 11:365–371, 1978
15. Maniglia AJ: Vocal rehabilitation after total laryngectomy: A flexible fiberoptic endoscopic technique for tracheoesophageal fistula. Laryngoscope 92:1437–1439, 1982
16. Inouye T: Fiberoptic examination of the larynx and esophagus. Trans Am Broncho-Esophagol Assoc pp. 123–127, 1984
17. Yamashita K: Endonasal flexible fiberoptic endoscopy. Rhinology 21:233–237, 1983
18. Ward PH, Berci G, Calcaterra TC: Advances in endoscopic examination of the respiratory system. Ann Otol Rhinol Laryngol 83:754–760, 1974
19. Strong MS: Diagnosis of carcinoma of the larynx: A review of current methods. Laryngoscope 85:516–521, 1975
20. Andrews AH Jr, Gould WJ: Laryngeal and nasopharyngeal indirect telescope. Ann Otol Rhinol Laryngol 86:627, 1977
21. Berci G: Analysis of new optical systems in bronchoesophagology. Ann Otol Rhinol Laryngol 87:451–460, 1978
22. Gould WJ, Kojima H, Lambiase A: A technique for stroboscopic examination of the vocal folds using fiberoptics. Arch Otolaryngol 105:285, 1979
23. Saito S, Isogai Y, Fukuda H, et al: A newly developed curved laryngotelescope. J Jpn Bronchoesophagol Soc 32:328–331, 1981
24. Yanagisawa E, Casuccio JR, Suzuki M: Video laryngoscopy using a rigid telescope and video home system color camera. A useful office procedure. Ann Otol Rhinol Laryngol 90:346–350, 1981
25. Konrad HR, Hopla DM, Bussen J, et al: Use of videotape in diagnosis and treatment of cancer of larynx. Ann Otol Rhinol Laryngol 90:398–400, 1981
26. Hirano M: Phonosurgery, basic and clinical investigations. Otologia (Fukuoka) 21(Suppl. 1):239–440, 1975
27. Yoshida Y, Hirano M, Nakajima T: A video-tape recording system for laryngo-stroboscopy. J Jpn Bronchoesophagol Soc 30:1–5, 1979
28. Yanagisawa E: Office telescopic photography of the larynx. Ann Otol Rhinol Laryngol 91:354–358, 1982
29. Aronson AE: Clinical Voice Disorders, an Interdisciplinary Approach. New York: Thieme-Stratton, 1980
30. Hirano M: Clinical Examination of Voice. Disorders of Communication. New York: Springer-Verlag, 1981
31. Yanagisawa E: Videolaryngoscopy using a low cost home video system color camera. J Biol Photogr 52:9–14, 1984
32. Yanagisawa E, Owens TW, Strothers G, et al: Videolaryngoscopy—A comparison of fiberscopic and telescopic documentation. Ann Otol Rhinol Laryngol 91:354–358, 1983
33. Yanagisawa K, Yanagisawa E: Copying CT scan with a reasonably priced video printer. J Biol Photogr 53:93–96, 1985

K. J. Lee
Raymond A. Gaito, Jr.

7

Instrumentation and Techniques of Office Removal of Foreign Bodies

Foreign bodies of the ear, nose, and throat are common entities presenting to the primary care physician. These calamities cause immense distress to the patient, but equally great rewards for the physician if they are expeditiously and safely removed in a simple office procedure. Not all foreign bodies lend themselves to office removal, by virtue of their location or the patient's inability to cooperate. Despite their simplicity, these procedures do carry a substantial risk with an uncooperative patient. Therefore, in any case where the age or constitution of the patient precludes cooperation, the procedures should be performed under general anesthesia.

Visualization and proper instruments are paramount to the success of any procedure. In procedures involving the ear, nose, or throat, the head mirror or headlight is indispensable, since most of the techniques described herein require that the operator's 2 hands be free. The head and neck regions of the body require some unique instruments, and these will be presented in a pictorial section following the narrative.

Foreign bodies of the nose are common in children and the mentally retarded. The symptoms are unilateral obstruction and irritation provoking pain and sneezing. A unilateral foul discharge is common; when such symptoms occur, foreign body should be suspected. Foreign bodies in the nose for protracted periods of time can form rhinoliths.

The removal of these objects requires good visualization afforded by a nasal speculum, head mirror, suction, and local vasoconstriction of the mucosa by such agents as cocaine flakes, ephedrine sulfate 3 percent, or epinephrine solution 1:10,000. Local anesthesia with cocaine or Pontocaine (Breon) 2 percent aids patient tolerance.

When removing objects from the nose, one must be cognizant of the possible danger of aspiration should the object be displaced posteriorly during attempts at extraction. Furthermore, the cribiform plate forms the roof of the nasal cavity and, if fractured, could produce a cerebral spinal fluid rhinorrhea with the possible sequelae of meningitis or frontal lobe abscess.

Patients should first be asked to "sneeze" while occluding the unobstructed nostril. If this is successful, removal of the object through the anterior nares can be attempted. Most objects lodge in the inferior meatus and can be grasped with bayonet forceps or Littauer forceps. Large objects can be crushed and the fragments removed. This should, however, be attempted only under general anesthesia or in another environment in which aspiration can be avoided. When the foreign body is too large to grasp, a right-angled hook or curved ring curette can be passed behind the object to pull it forward. Another technique is to pass a small-caliber Foley catheter to the nasopharynx and withdraw it after partially inflating the balloon. This technique could also be used to occlude the posterior nasal choanae when fully inflated, as a precaution against aspiration of the foreign body while attempting removal.

Some objects may be so posterior that mirror exam alone may disclose their presence. Objects that far posterior should best be removed under general anesthesia with the airway protected by an endotracheal tube.

Following removal of foreign bodies of the nose, patients should insufflate normal saline to moisturize the raw mucosa, and apply petrolatum to cut down on crusting. Antibiotic therapy may be required for sinusitis secondary to obstruction of the ostia.

EAR

Foreign bodies of the external auditory canal often present as a conductive hearing loss. Insects are particularly distressing to patients, as their wings or extremities irritate the exquisitely sensitive skin or tympanic membrane. Foreign bodies are removed to avoid external otitis and spreading cellulitis.

The greatest concern with procedures in the external auditory canal is the possibility of perforating the tympanic membrane and possibly disarticulating the ossicles. Poor visualization and abrupt movements of the patient's head are the most frequent causes. The patient's head should be supported by a headrest or by an assistant, if sitting. Children and less stoic patients should be supine with their arms at their sides and restrained if necessary. Visualization is provided by an otoscope with a surgical head or a head mirror. The largest aural speculum accommodated by the canal affords the best exposure.

When operating in the external auditory canal, the operator should hold the instruments with the small finger extended and resting against the patient's head, to stabilize the hand and act as a stop should the patient lurch abruptly towards the instrument. If suction is to be used, the patient must be forewarned of the loud noise to be expected. All live insects should be first drowned in alcohol, oil, or even antibiotic drops.

The simplest technique for removing foreign bodies is irrigation with tepid tap water. An irrigation syringe and basin to catch the irrigant are necessary. The patient and clothes should be protected with towels. Too warm or cold an irrigating solution can cause vertigo and should not be performed in cases of suspected perforations. Wax and soft objects not removed by irrigation can often be removed by suction with a Frazier tipsize 7 French or smaller. Hard wax can be softened with olive oil or commercial wax removers over several days prior to extraction. Softening should not be accomplished with vegetable matter because of its subsequent swelling and impaction in the canal.

Right-angled hooks and wax curettes can be passed behind foreign bodies to extract them. Fine grasping forceps such as the Littauer or Noyes type can also be used. When using any of the above instruments in the ear, one must take care not to push the object further into the canal, thus impacting it in the nondistensible bony canal or perforating the tympanic membrane.

The medial bony canal is exquisitely tender and very vascular. Even minor trauma can cause bleeding and can obscure vision in the narrow canal. This troublesome bleeding can be controlled with ephedrine 3 percent or epinephrine 1:10,000 applied topically.

Hemostasis and anesthesia of the ear canal can be obtained prior to the procedure with 1 percent lidocaine with epinephrine 1:100,000. This is injected with a 27- or 30-gauge needle in the 4 quandrants of the meatus. The bevel is aligned flush with the canal wall to avoid raising a bleb that obscures visualization. A total of 1 ml of solution is sufficient. Complications of the procedure occur when the solution dissects along the canal medially, entering the middle ear. Anesthesia of the facial nerve may ensue.

If the solution penetrates the round window, severe vertigo occurs, usually 45 minutes after injections. All patients should therefore be observed for 45 minutes after injection to avoid untoward reactions when the patient leaves to drive a car or work.

After removal of a foreign body from the external auditory canal, the tympanic membrane should be inspected for perforations. The patient should be treated as for an external otitis, with water precautions and otic drops.

THROAT

Foreign bodies in the oral and hypopharynx usually lodge in the crypts of the lingual or palatine tonsils, the vallecula, or the pyriform sinuses. The patients complain of a painful or tickling sensation poorly localized, except in the case of the pyriform sinuses, in which case the patient will indicate a point about the lateral thyroid cartilage. Most of these foreign bodies are not radiopaque, for example, fish or chicken bones and toothbrush bristles, which are the most common offenders.

Foreign bodies of the oral pharynx are visualized with a head mirror and tongue blade. Greunwald forceps are usually sufficient for extraction purposes. Examination of the lingual tonsil, vallecula, and pyriform sinuses requires indirect exam with the laryngeal mirror. Topical anesthesia provided by Pontocaine 2 percent is used. Wait for 5–10 minutes to allow the anesthetic to work. A curved Kelley forceps can be used to retrieve objects from the vallecula and lingual tonsil. The Fraenkel forceps are required when removing bodies from the pyriform sinuses.

Most patients will feel immediate relief after removal of the foreign body, but must be cautioned that continued symptoms of the foreign body presence are not uncommon due to the mucosal irritation. Not infrequently, no foreign body will be found on inspection or on plain films, despite the patient's bitter complaints to the contrary. A lateral neck x-ray can then be taken after the patient swallows a small piece of cotton soaked in barium. A foreign body may "catch" the cotton ball. Cine barium swallow is helpful at times. If these complaints continue beyond 36 hours despite reassurance, direct laryngoscopy and esophagoscopy may be required.

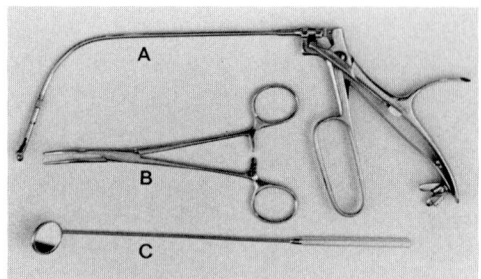

Fig. 7-1. Sample throat set. (A) Fraenkel forceps. (B) Kelly hemostat. (C) Laryngeal mirror.

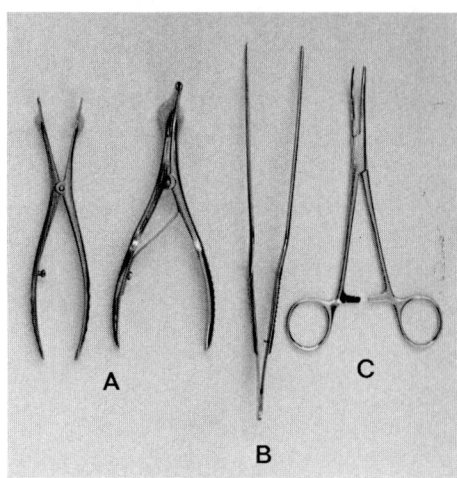

Fig. 7-2. Sample nose set. (A) Vienna nasal speculae. (B) Gruenwald bayonet forceps. (C) Kelly hemostat.

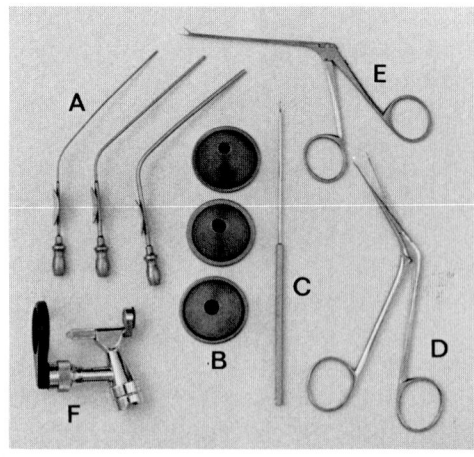

Fig. 7-3. Sample ear set. (A) Frazier tip suction numbers 3, 4, and 5. (B) Hartman ear speculae, various sizes. (C) Ring curette. (D) Hartmann forceps. (E) House forceps. (F) Operating otoscope head.

Removal of Foreign Bodies

INSTRUMENTS

The instruments illustrated in Figures 7-1–7-3 are available through most medical and surgical supply stores in metropolitan areas. Additional aid can be found at the nearest university department of otolaryngology, where information pertaining to area representatives for surgical supply companies can be sought.

Emil P. Liebman

8
Chemical Peel and Dermabrasion

Chemical peel and dermabrasion are procedures vastly different in technique but quite similar in their histologic results.[1] Both procedures produce a destruction of the epithelium and a superficial, controlled injury to the dermis. The skin surface is replaced by an epithelial outgrowth from the periphery of the wound and by epithelial proliferation from the skin adenexa (hair follicles and sebaceous glands).[2] Healing of the dermis involves the formation of a dermal scar. This scar produces a thickening of the treated skin. Healing of the epithelium is usually in 7–10 days, but the final improvement in skin appearance takes several months to occur. The amount of clinical improvement depends to a significant degree on the depth of the "injury." The depth of the injury by chemical peel depends, among other factors, on the type of chemical used. The depth of the dermabrasion injury is directly related to the mechanical depth of planing. This discussion will outline the indications, techniques of treatment, and complications of these procedures.

CHEMICAL PEEL

Various chemicals have been used for chemical peel treatments. The most common materials now used are trichloric acid in strengths of 35 and 50 percent and phenol.[3,4] The procedure which will be discussed here involves the use of phenol as it is contained in Baker's formula.[5]

Indications for Chemical Peel

Indications include acne scarring, hyperpigmentation, keratosis, and fine facial wrinkles.

Acne Scarring

Although chemical peel has been used in the treatment of acne scars, it is the author's feeling that dermabrasion is probably more effective for this type of condition.

Hyperpigmentation

The results of the use of chemical peel treatment for hyperpigmentation are somewhat unpredictable.[4]

Keratosis

Although keratotic lesions frequently improve after chemical peel, other treatments are available and are more effective.

Fine Wrinkles

Fine wrinkling of the skin of the face is the prime indication for the use of chemical peel treatments. It is the author's feeling that chemical peel is a more effective method of treating fine wrinkles than is dermabrasion. In addition, chemical peel can be used in areas such as the eyelids that would be extremely hazardous to treat with the spinning brush of the dermabrader.[5]

Patient Selection

The primary indication for the use of chemical peel is for patients with fine facial wrinkles.

Psychologic Evaluation

Careful screening of individuals for realistic expectations, as for any cosmetic procedure, must be carried out. The patient must be informed in detail of the difficult first several days following the chemical peel application. Photographs of treated patients showing the swelling and crusting that occurs during the first several days of treatment should be shown to the prospective patient. It is the appearance of the face rather than any significant pain or discomfort that causes the most anxiety in individuals receiving this treatment. Patients should also be prepared for the significant erythema of the skin which may last for several weeks or even months. Decrease in pigmentation must also be expected and the patient must avoid sunlight exposure for at least 4–6 months following the treatment. Some individuals may refuse to accept avoidance of sun exposure as it is an integral part of their lifestyle. If they refuse to avoid sun, it is the author's feeling that they should not be treated.

Skin Texture

Fine skin will have a smoother result and more uniform color when compared to oily skin.

Skin Pigmentation

Light-complected, blue-eyed individuals will have less skin color change after treatment and therefore less contrast between the treated and untreated areas than will darker complected individuals. Darker skin individuals show the bleaching effect of the peel to a greater degree.

Procedure

The technique discussed here involves the use of phenol as contained in Baker's Formula.[5] This formula contains: phenol 88 percent USP—3 cc; crotin oil—3 drops; liquid soap—8 drops; and distilled water—2 cc. This formula is a suspension and not a solution, and therefore it is important to mix the contents aggressively before each use.

Preoperative Preparation

Light sedation is used, since chemical peel is not particularly painful. Diazepam 5 mg and Merperidine (Wyeth) 50 mg given by mouth or I.M. about an hour prior to the procedure is sufficient for most individuals.

Technique

The skin should be washed thoroughly with soap and water. It should next be cleaned several times with acetone. This step is most important, since the acetone removes oil from the skin surface and allows uniform penetration of the Baker's Formula. As previously discussed, this formula must be mixed well prior to each application because it is a suspension and not a solution.

One or two cotton tip applicators are dipped into the chemical. Excess liquid is removed by rubbing the cotton tip applicator against the mouth of the bottle in which the mixture is contained. The formula is applied to the skin in a stroking motion. The skin will turn white within a few seconds and the patient will experience a stinging sensation which lasts about 30 seconds. After several minutes the skin turns a deep red color. The treated area, with the exception of the eyelids, is taped with a layer of waterproof Johnson and Johnson's tape. It is important that the tape extend just short of the full area treated, in order to allow a gradual transition from treated taped areas to treated nontaped areas to nontreated areas. This will facilitate "feathering of the edges" of the skin.

Full Face Peel

If a full face peel is being carried out, the forehead is done first. The mixture is carried onto the hairline and eyebrows in order to minimize the peel borders. Tape is then applied.

A minimum of 10–15 minutes must be allowed between applications to large areas of the face, in order to decrease the likelihood of cardiac arrhythmias.

The cheeks are done next. Peeling should carry over the edge of the mandible, approximately 1–2 cm onto the skin of the upper neck. The peeling is done more lightly at the periphery. Taping should be placed so that there is an irregular border along the mandible. This will "feather" the edges and minimize a demarcation line between peeled and nonpeeled areas (Figs. 8-1 and 8-2).

Again, 15–20 minutes is allowed before the opposite cheek is treated. The opposite cheek is then treated as previously described.

The perioral area is next done. When peeling the lips, the mixture should be applied 2–3 mm past the vermilion border onto the lip surface. Tape is applied.

The eyelid skin should be done last because it is the most painful. Great care must be exercised because of the potential for disaster if any of the mixture enters the eye. Eye irrigation solution should be readily available. A single semi-dry applicator is used. The eyes should be closed when the upper lid is peeled. Peeling should stop 2–3 mm above

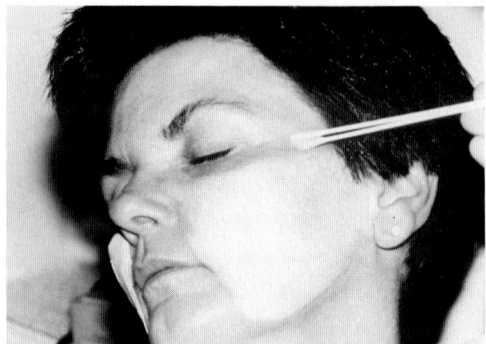

Fig. 8-1. Application of Baker's Formula to skin of left cheek. Note extension of peel past border of mandible.

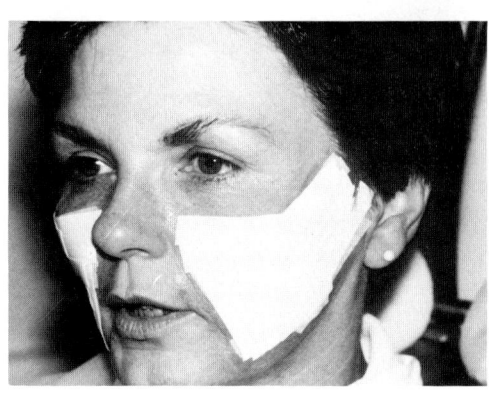

Fig. 8-2. Taping of left cheek. Note taping is done *short* of total area peeled.

the lid margin of the upper lid. When the lower lids are peeled, the eyes are open. The peel should stop 2–3 mm below the lower lid margin. Because of the acute stinging sensation, tearing may occur. It is important to remove any tears with a dry applicator or gauze before they run over the lid margin and onto the freshly peeled areas. The tears will dilute the peel mixture and produce a *deeper* burn. This deeper burn will produce an uneven result and can result in scarring. It is the authors' feeling that the eyelid skin should not be taped.

Regional Face Peel

If the entire face is not treated, the face should be peeled in aesthetic units to minimize the change in pigment from treated to nontreated areas. These units include the forehead, both cheeks, the eyelids—upper and/or lower lids can be used as separate subunits, and the lips—upper and lower lips can also be subdivided in two separate units (Fig. 8-3).

Peeling may be effectively combined with facelift only in the circumoral area. Skin which has been undermined should never be peeled at the same time as the surgical procedure because of the increased tendency for scarring.[6]

Post-peel Course

Pain will subside quickly after the peel suspension is applied. Pain returns within an hour or two and persists for the next 6–8 hours. It is controlled with analgesics and cold compresses. Crushed ice in small plastic zip-locked bags is suggested. These bags can be obtained in most grocery stores.

Chemical Peel and Dermabrasion

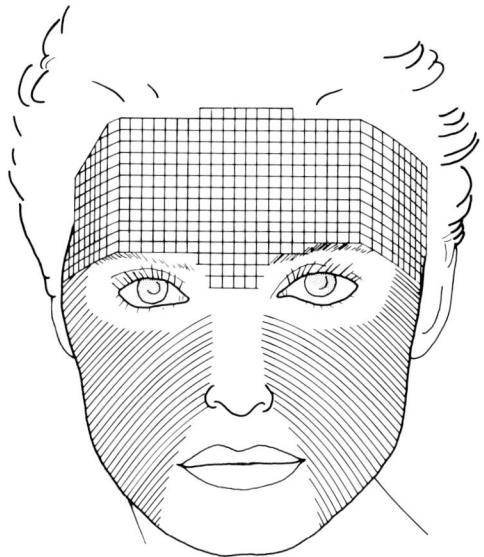

Fig. 8-3. Aesthetic units of the face.

Swelling

Swelling begins in approximately 4–6 hours and may be quite severe. Patients are asked to sleep with the head elevated for the first 48 hours. If there is no medical contraindication, oral steroids are prescribed for the first 3–4 days following the peel.

Tape Removal

Patients can usually remove the tape themselves at home in approximately 48 hours. A significant amount of serous exudate builds up under the tape by the second day. The patient is asked to stand in a warm shower and to allow the humidity to build up for several minutes. The combination of serous exudate and the humidity of the shower allows the tape to lift off with little effort. If the patient is reluctant to remove the tape at home it is done in the office (Fig. 8-4).

Following tape removal, the face is washed in warm water, using a soft cotton sponge or cotton balls. A washcloth is not suggested. The skin after washing should be covered

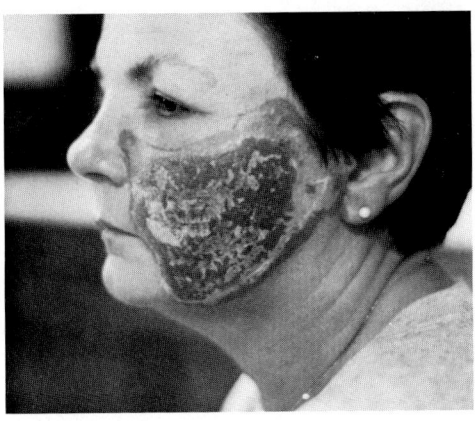

Fig. 8-4. Appearance of skin of left cheek 48 hours post-peel, immediately after tape removal.

with an ointment to prevent excess crusting. Crisco vegetable shortening is inexpensive and effective. The washing and application of ointment should be repeated 5–6 times daily.[7]

Patients are instructed never to pick at crusts or loose pieces of skin, since this will deepen the injury, prolong the healing process, and possibly lead to scar formation. After 7–10 days, the crusts have disappeared and the treated area is covered with an intact, thin, deep pink to red skin. The intensive color will remain for many weeks but can be covered with make-up. The new skin is quite delicate and should be treated gently. Patients are asked to wash with a gentle soap such as baby shampoo. Moisturizing creams should be applied frequently.

Direct sunlight should be avoided for several months. Sunscreens should always be used following chemical peel in order to avoid sun exposure which may lead to spotty hyperpigmentation.

The fine lines of the face may still be noted for the first several weeks after the swelling subsides. As the thickening of the dermis progresses, these lines will disappear, usually taking 1–3 months. The skin will then become smoother. It is important that the patient realize that several months are required for the optimum effects of the chemical peel to be noticed (Fig. 8-5).

It is the authors' feeling that a list of specific postoperative instructions to the patient is extremely important. The following are the postoperative instructions for chemical face peel that are issued to each patient.

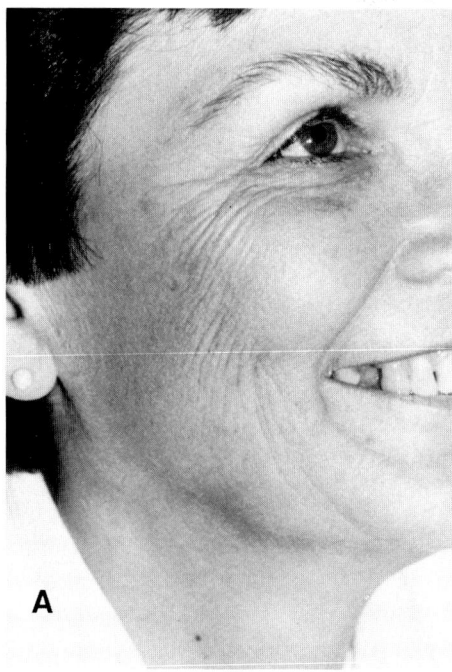 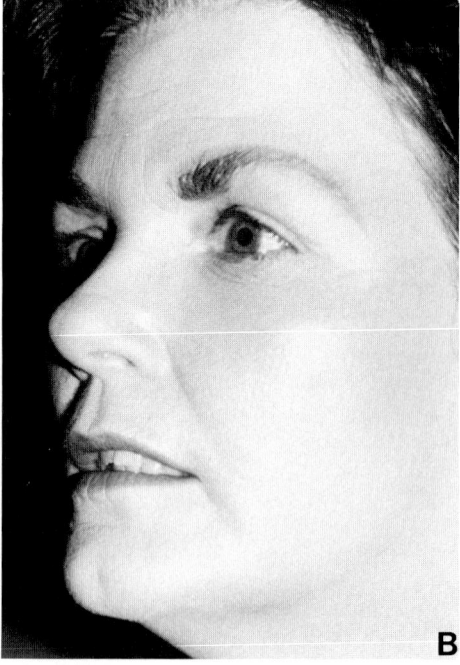

Fig. 8-5. Skin of left cheek 6 months post-peel (A), compared to skin of right cheek *pre*-peel (B).

Chemical Peel and Dermabrasion

Postoperative Instructions After Face Peeling

1. You will remember that upon initial application of the peel solution, there was a stinging pain for several seconds that soon disappeared. Later today you can expect 3 things:
    a. a recurrence of the stinging pain for 4–6 hours. (Take pain medication as necessary.)
    b. swelling—may be severe. (Keep head elevated at least 60° for 48 hours. Sleep in a recliner.
    c. possible fever. (Take Tylenol or aspirin.)
2. Use ice compresses or an ice bag (crushed ice in a small plastic zip-locked bag that can be obtained in most grocery stores).
3. Try not to move the peel area excessively. (Keep the lips stiff and avoid grimacing.)
4. Within 24–36 hours, you will notice that the peeled area resembles a deep sunburn, and you may notice serum exuding from the skin or through the tape; this is to be expected.
5. Approximately 24–48 hours following the procedure, gently remove all tape, gently wash the peeled area with tap water, and apply the A & D ointment, Crisco, or Bacitracin ointment. This procedure should be repeated 5 or 6 times a day; use a soft complexion sponge, cotton balls, or your hands, *not* a washcloth.
6. *Never pick at crusts or pieces of skin that do not loosen easily. Apply the ointment to them and they should come off easily with time.* (Usually 7 or 8 days after the procedure.)
7. After the crust has fallen off, you will have delicate new skin that must toughen during the next few weeks.
    a. Wash your face gently with mild soap twice daily. Johnson's Baby Shampoo works well.
    b. Keep moist by applying cold cream or moisturizing cream.
    c. You may begin using make-up 3 days after crust has fallen off. (Continuous Coverage by Clinique also has a sunscreen added.)
8. The intense pink color will fade rapidly, but a pink coloration will remain for 6–12 weeks. The skin will remain somewhat tense and smooth, with clearing of the finer wrinkles and the deep grooves much less evident.
9. Occasionally, small whiteheads may appear in the treated areas; these usually disappear in 2 or 3 weeks without specific treatment. *Do not pick these!*
10. Patients who are prone to develop fever blisters or cold sores occasionally have a flare-up of these lesions. If they should occur, call the office and we can prescribe treatment for them.
11. Try to avoid direct rays of the sun for at least 8 weeks (to avoid blotching). Minimize exposure for 6 months. Use a large-brimmed hat and sunscreen (Uval, PreSun, etc.).
12. Avoid excessive straining, lifting, bending, extreme cold or heat, or strong winds while you are healing.
13. Please make every attempt to keep all postoperative appointments, since it is vitally important that we monitor your healing.
14. *Do not take chances!* If any questions arise, do not hesitate to call us.

Complications

Milia

These are small inclusion cysts which appear within the first several weeks after the peel. Usually they are self-limiting. If persistent, milia can be treated by uncapping with an 18 gauge needle or a number 11 blade.

Hyperpigmentation.

This is usually ascribed to early sun exposure. It may also be due to uneven peeling technique causing an apparently darker area of skin next to a hypopigmented treated region. Sun exposure should be avoided and adequate sunscreen used. If hyperpigmentation occurs, 5 percent hydroquinone can be used to lighten the skin. If persistent, the hyperpigmented area can be re-peeled.[8,9]

Hypopigmentation

Post-peeled skin has a marked reduction in melanin-producing cells.[8] Decrease in pigmentation is most evident in darker complected individuals, and therefore proper patient selection is important. As was previously discussed, adequate feathering of the edges of the peeled area will decrease the demarcation from hypopigmented peeled areas to nonpeeled areas.

Scarring

Fortunately, the occurrence of scarring is rare. In most cases the cause is uncertain. Certain factors, however, are felt to play a part in possible scar formation. If tape is applied too tightly, especially around the lips, the motion of the lips during talking or eating can irritate the skin and produce a deepened injury.

Skin which is undermined surgically should never be peeled, as the incidence of scarring is markedly increased.

The skin of the neck and suprasternal areas should not be peeled because of the lesser number of skin appendages which promote the re-epithelialization of the skin.[9]

Should any scarring be noted, steroids applied topically or injected intralesionally usually control the problem.

Herpetic Infection

It is most important to obtain any history of herpetic eruptions of the lips or mouth. If the skin around the lips of such a patient is treated, exacerbations of the herpes may occur and extend to all areas treated. It is most important to seek immediate ophthalmologic consultation in such a patient, since the herpes eruption may involve the cornea as well as the skin of the peeled area. In most instances, the dermatologic problem clears without sequellae, although the healing process is significantly extended.

Cardiac Complications

The most effective means of preventing cardiac arrhythmias is the slow application of the phenol mixture. At least 15–20 minutes should be allowed between applications to aesthetic units. A total of $1^{1}/_{2}$–2 hours should be allowed for a full face peel. If a full face peel is carried out, cardiac monitoring is suggested. If less than 50 percent of the face is peeled, cardiac monitoring is probably not required.[10]

Summary

Chemical face peel is a highly successful procedure, particularly for the improvement of the fine lines of the aging face. Complications do occur. They can be serious and even life-threatening. Proper technique and adequate precautions are mandatory. Detailed instructions and explanations to the patient will allow for proper patient selection and will ease the difficult 5–7 days after the face peel has been carried out. Enthusiastic patient acceptance of the long-term results of this procedure is most gratifying.

DERMABRASION

Dermabrasion is a surgical procedure in which a rotating wire brush or diamond-impregnated burr is used to plane the skin and produce a smoother surface. The superficial surface of the skin is removed to the level of the dermis. Healing occurs by proliferation of the skin appendages (hair follicles and sebaceous glands). The healing process after dermabrasion is quite similar to that previously described with chemical peel. Full beneficial effects of dermabrasion, as with chemical peel, take several months to occur.

Indications

The most common indication for dermabrasion is to produce therapeutic improvement of facial scarring, especially those irregular scars resulting from acne. Planing lowers the level of the skin and smooths out the easily seen borders of these scars. Significant improvement in the facial skin can usually be obtained, but a perfectly smooth skin surface cannot result because the depressions in the skin are due to the pull of the scar tissue under the skin. Planing of the skin cannot be carried to the depth of the cicatrix without producing additional scarring. Deeper, "ice pick" scars respond better to excision with a hair transplant punch. The removed lesion is replaced by post-auricular skin removed with punch instruments.[11]

Fine Wrinkling

Fine wrinkling of the skin can be treated by dermabrasion, but it is the author's feeling that chemical peel is more effective.

Hyperpigmentation

Dermabrasion has been used in the treatment of areas of hyperpigmentation. The results, however, are unpredictable.

Keratosis

Dermabrasion has shown good results in treating patients with actinic or senile keratosis, especially in patients with sun-damaged skin.[12,13]

Procedure

The technique of dermabrasion requires training and practice. Planing too deeply will produce scarring. If done too superficially, minimal improvement will result. Most commonly, a rotating wire brush or diamond fraise is used. Various engines are available, but the Acrotorque (Robbins Instrument Company) hand engine has proven to be a reliable and quiet instrument with excellent speed and dependability.

Practice in the use of the dermabrasion instrument should be obtained prior to patient application. The skin of a grapefruit can be used to learn the touch of the instrument. Gradual deepening and creating various levels of depth on the grapefruit skin is most valuable.

A light touch on the skin is best. It is much better to dermabrade too lightly in the first few cases than to penetrate too deeply and produce scarring. One can always re-dermabrade at a later date. Patients will readily accept retreatment if they are prepared for this in advance.

General Precautions

When dermabrading around the lips, the rotating burr is brought towards the margin of the lips to avoid catching the lip margin. Do not dermabrade eyelid skin. Particular care must be used in freezing skin over bony prominces.

Preoperative Preparation

Sedation is carried out with diazepam 5 mg and Meperidine 50 mg given by mouth or intramuscularly one hour prior to the procedure.

The skin to be dermabraded must be changed from a soft, pliable state to a solid state for optimal results. This change is accomplished by using skin refrigerants which also produce local anesthesia. The effects of the refrigerants are improved if the skin is first cooled for 20-30 minutes using rubber gloves filled with ice water or ice chips. Various skin refrigerants can be used. These include Frigiderm, Floroethyl, Cryosthesia $-30°C$ and $-60°C$, Aerofreze, and Medifrig (A. H. Robins Co., Richmond, Virginia). Recent studies by Hanke et al.[14] indicate that Frigiderm and Floroethyl produce cooling temperatures which are in the safest range $-38°C$-$-42°C$. Cryosthesia $-30°C$ and $-60°C$, Aerofreze, and Medifrig produce skin temperatures which may be excessively low and therefore dangerous ($-50°C$-$-64°C$).

An area of 2-3 cm is frozen to a solid state. This area is then dermabraded. If the skin softens before the desired depth is achieved, the skin can be refrozen. Proper freezing of the skin also provides a bloodless field which allows identification of the depth of planing. Dermabrasion can be carried down to the papillary dermis. Deeper planing can result in scarring. Identification of the proper depth is made by observing the fine reticular cross-striations of the collagen fibers and capillary loops in this layer. It is best to start with the most dependent areas of the face, and move gradually to the more superior areas. It is important to treat only small areas, of 2-3 cm in diameter, since freezing a larger area will not allow time for proper, uniform planing.

The chin is treated first, then the cheeks and forehead. Once the area has been dermabraded, the skin warms and some oozing will occur. One can therefore work upward from an oozing area to a dry area, rather than having blood running into the working region. When dermabrading the lower cheeks and jaw line, the planing should be carried over the edge of the mandible lightly onto the neck for 1-2 cm. This is done to feather the edge of the treated skin and minimize any visible border between treated and nontreated regions. When dermabrading around the lips, the rotating burr is brought toward the margins of the lips to avoid catching the lip margin.

A word of caution must be included regarding planing the skin overlying bone. These areas include the skin over the mandible and zygoma as well as the forehead. There is less subcutaneous tissue in these areas then elsewhere and therefore less vascularity. This allows for a quicker, deeper, longer-lasting freeze. Additionally, the underlying bone offers resistance to the rotating instrument, and deeper layers of the skin are reached more quickly. Therefore, even greater care must be taken in areas overlying the bone to avoid scarring.

Periorbital

It is the author's feeling that eyelid skin should not be dermabraded.

Postoperative Course

Numerous studies have shown conclusively that wounds heal most quickly if kept moist.[15] Recent development in wound dressings allow the wound to remain moist but permit passage of excess tissue fluids through the wound covering. These dressings are nonadherant to wound surfaces and are therefore easily removed. Several of these membranes are available. The authors have been quite pleased with the results of the use of Vigilon (Bard Inc.). It is composed of 4 percent polyethylene oxide in 96 percent water in a colloidal suspension. The membrane is backed on both sides by an inert polyethylene film.[16]

After dermabrading, the wound is covered with the Vigilon dressing. One layer of the plastic covering of the Vigilon is removed and the moist layer is applied to the wound surface. This is covered with telfa and a light layer of adaptic-type roller gauze. If a small area is treated, the telfa can be held in place with tape strips. The dressing is removed in 24 hours. The wound is cleaned with peroxide solution. Vigilon is again applied to the wound and left in place for another 24–48 hours. The dressings are then removed and left off. The wound can then be cleaned with peroxide and kept moist with a covering of Vaseline or Crisco. The use of the moist dressing appears to greatly increase the speed of epithelialization and therefore quickens healing of the wound. Once the epithelialization is completed, the wound is covered by a thin layer of new skin. Treatment of the new skin is identical with treatment after chemical peel.

It is the author's feeling that a list of the specific postoperative instructions to the patient is extremely important. The following are the postoperative instructions for dermabrasion which are issued to each patient.

Postoperative Instructions After Dermabrasion

1. *Dressings.* Try to leave the dressing in place. You may trim the gauze carefully with scissors as it loosens, but do not pull the portions which are not loose.
2. Minimize crusting by keeping the dermabraded areas covered with a coat of ointment at all times. The ointments that can be used include Crisco, vegetable shortening, cold cream, or A & D ointment. After the dressings have been removed, the

skin can be washed with Lowila or Neutrogena soap, using your fingertips or cotton balls to wash very gently. Pat the area dry and apply a coat of cream or ointment to keep the skin moist. This should be repeated every morning and night for 7 days.
3. *Never pick at crusts or pieces of skin that do not loosen easily. Apply the ointment or creams to them and they should come off easily with time.* (Usually 7 or 8 days after the procedure.)
4. After the crust has fallen off, you will have delicate new skin which must toughen during the next few days.
   a. Wash your face gently with mild soap twice daily. Johnson's Baby Shampoo works well.
   b. Keep area moist by applying cold cream or moisturizing cream.
   c. You may begin using make-up 3 days after crust has fallen off. (Continuous Coverage by Clinique also has a sunscreen added.)
5. The intense pink color will fade rapidly but a pink coloration will remain for 6–12 weeks. The skin will remain somewhat tense and smooth, with clearing of the finer wrinkles and the deep grooves much less evident.
6. Occasionally, small whiteheads may appear in the treated areas; these usually disappear in 2–3 weeks without specific treatment. *Do not pick these!*
7. Patients who are prone to develop fever blisters or cold sores occasionally have a flare-up of these lesions. If they should occur, call the office and we can prescribe treatment for them.
8. Try to avoid direct rays of the sun for at least 8 weeks (to avoid blotching). Minimize exposure for 6 months. (Use a large-brimmed hat and sunscreen (Uval, PreSun, etc.).
9. Avoid excessive straining, lifting, bending, extreme cold or heat, or strong winds while you are healing.
10. Please make every attempt to keep all postoperative appointments, since it is vitally important that we monitor your healing.
11. *Do not take chances!* If any questions arise, do not hesitate to call us.

Complications

Milia

Milia can occur after dermabrasion as after chemical peel and are treated as previously described.

Hyperpigmentation

As with peel, hyperpigmentation is usually associated with early sun exposure and can be avoided by avoiding the sun and by use of adequate sunscreens.

Hypopigmentation

There is a decrease in melanin-producing cells after dermabrasion. The decrease in pigmentation, as with chemical peel, is most evident in darker complected individuals. Proper patient selection is important. Gradual transition from dermabraded areas to nontreated areas is also important.

Scarring

Probably the most serious complication of dermabrasion is scarring. Adequate technique and proper depth of planing is the most important factor in preventing scar formation. Any scarring which occurs can be treated with steroid injections. Obviously, the most important treatment is prevention.

Herpetic Infection

Herpetic infection can occur in dermabraded skin as with chemical peel. It is important to obtain an adequate history of herpetic eruptions in the past and to avoid treatment within 2–3 cm of the lips in patients.

Summary

Dermabrasion is a safe and effective treatment in smoothing the irregularities of facial scarring. This safety and effectiveness, however, is directly related to the training, experience, and technique of the operator. Unlike chemical peel, the technique of which is quite simple, the application of the whirling, diamond fraise or wire brush has a great potential for disaster. With practice and experience, however, the use of dermabrasion will produce significant and gratifying results.

REFERENCES

1. Stegman SJ: A study of dermabrasion and chemical peels in an animal model. J Dermatol Surg Oncol 6:490–497, 1980
2. Baker TJ, Gordon HL, Mosienko P et al: Long term histological study of skin after chemical face peeling. Plast Reconstr Surg 53:522, 1974
3. Stegman SJ: A comparative histologic study of the effects of three peeling agents and dermabrasion on normal and sun damaged skin. Aesthetic Plast Surg 6:123–135, 1982
4. Stegman SJ, Tromovitch TA: Cosmetic dermatologic surgery. Arch Dermatol 118:1013–1016, 1982
5. Baker TJ, Gordon HL: Chemical face peeling and dermabrasion. Surg Clin North Am 51:387–400, 1971
6. Baker TJ, Gordon HL: Chemical peeling as a practical method for removing rhitides of the upper lip. Ann Plast Surg 2:209,211, 1979
7. McCollough EG: Chemical face peel. Otolaryngol Clin North Am 13:353–365, 1980
8. Mosienko PM, Baker TJ: Chemical peel. Clin Plast Surg 5:79–96, 1978
9. Litton C, Trinidad G: Complications of chemical face peeling as evaluated by a questionnaire. Plast Reconstr Surg 67:738–742, 1981
10. Truppman ES, Ellenby JD: Major electrocardiographic changes during chemical face peeling. Plast Reconstr Surg 63:1, 1979
11. Hume B: Dermabrasion: An effective treatment for acne and its aftermath. Colo Med 78(4):115–116, 1981
12. Mechlin DC: Dermabrasion. Ear Nose Throat J 60:79–81, 1981
13. Salyer HL: Chemosurgery and dermabrasion. J Tenn Med Assoc 72:739–741, 1972
14. Hanke CW, O'Brien JJ, Solow EB: Laboratory evaluation of skin refrigerants used in dermabrasion. J Dermatol Surg Oncol 11:1, 1985
15. Kucan JO, Robson MC, Parsons RW: Amniotic membranes as dressings following facial dermabrasions. Ann Plast Surg 8:6, 1982
16. Mandy SH: A new primary wound dressing made of polyethylene oxide gel. J Dermatol Surg Oncol 9(2):153–155, 1983

Ronald H. Hirokawa
Richard C. Bryarly

9

Scar Revision and Facial Flaps

The facial plastic surgeon must continually be concerned about scars and scar formation. Scar tissue is a natural outcome of tissue healing. The development of scars may be planned, as in the excision of lesions or tumors of the face or in the correction of certain congenital deformities, or unplanned, as in traumatic lacerations, burns, abrasions, and so forth. The surgeon must be aware of the geography of the area, including the anatomy of the underlying tissue that will affect the eventual camouflaging of the scar. Placement of the scar lines within the relaxed skin tension lines (RSTL) (Fig. 9-1), as opposed to perpendicular to these lines, will result in the most desirable scar appearance.[1] Incisions should be planned, and, when feasible, should allow the resulting scar to be within a RSTL. Scars which fail to follow these concepts either by trauma or design may be revised at a later time. Several techniques will be discussed which will allow the surgeon to improve scars.

SCAR REVISION

During the primary closure of traumatic lacerations or of surgical excisions, several basic technical points which should be remembered involve the elimination of dead space, the close approximation of the dermis and epidermis, the level of the two surfaces which are being approximated, and the amount of trauma to the wound edges. One factor which may make a scar more obvious is the shadow which is cast either due to a depressed scar or because of a raised scar with shadowing of the neighboring tissue when exposed to indirect light. Careful attention should be paid to the closure of the dead space in the subcutaneous layer of tissue. The lack of careful suturing of the deep tissue may lead to the accumulation of a hematoma that will later liquefy and drain or become infected. As the area heals, the lack of deep, supporting tissue may later yield a depressed scar. Unequal thickness of the skin edges to be sutured will lead to a stepoff which will

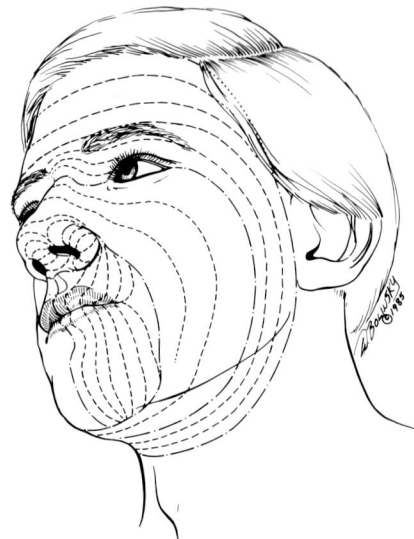

Fig. 9-1. Placement of the scar lines within the relaxed skin tension lines.

cause a shadow. Trauma to the skin edges by crushing with forceps or other instruments will likely lead to poor healing and increased scar formation. This concept is espoused by many surgeons, but often ignored as concern for other aspects of the procedure take precedence. Good soft-tissue technique, such as utilizing skin hooks and the proper suture, will lead to quite acceptable results. All too often, anticipation of the end of the procedure is often a deterrent to a successful outcome.

There is no substitute for good soft-tissue surgical technique. This includes the use of clean, sharp instruments to allow for accurate and clean incisions. Suture techniques should avoid wound edge inversion. Knots of the deep tissue should be buried. Foreign bodies which have become imbedded in the soft tissue and skin during trauma should be attended to during the primary repair. This will avoid future problems in dealing with the difficult tattooing of the skin.

The technique of a simple scar excision may be useful in those scars which lie parallel to a RSTL but are noticeable due to depression or elevation of the margins. Ideally, a scar should be no longer than 6 mm in one straight area; however, this does vary, depending upon the surrounding geography. The lip area, which is very visible, requires that straight scars be even less than 2–3 mm. On the other hand, a scar that lies near hair-bearing areas may be less noticeable despite its length. This point is useful to consider when trying to hide lengthy scars that may be near the scalp line.

The postoperative care of the revised scar will influence its outcome and is often as important as the technical aspects of the procedure itself. Keeping the area clean and avoiding crust formation can be accomplished by frequently coating the area with an antibiotic ointment. Systemic antibiotics are not routinely used; however, if there are circumstances which may increase the risk of infection, such as previous radiation exposure or contamination, one should consider perioperative use of antibiotics. A pressure dressing will often provide coverage of the incision and prevent undue swelling and possible bleeding and hematoma formation.

Tension of the healing incision line will aggravate the wound and promote widening of the scar. Tension has been implicated in the formation of a hypertrophic scar and a keloid scar. Other factors considered in the development of a keloid scar are infection and an autoimmune phenomenon. Ideally, skin sutures should be removed within 4–6 days following the procedure. Tension may be maintained after this period indefinitely with the use of sterile adhesive tapes. In general, scar revision requires meticulous observance.

Z-plasty

Z-plasty is a surgical technique used to improve a scar. By definition, it is the transposition of two interdigitating flaps, which when designed and transposed, form the appearance of the letter Z. The requirements are that the limbs of the Z equal its central member and therefore each other. The advantages of this technique are that the direction of the scar may be changed, length may be gained in the direction of the scar (thereby improving a contracture), and the scar will be broken up into shorter segments and be harder for an observer's eye to notice.

The technical aspects of the Z-plasty are as follows. The central member of the Z is usually the scar which is to be excised and revised. Two parallel lines are then drawn from each end of the central member in opposite directions, each equal in length to the central member. The flaps that are then formed are transposed and, in doing so, the central member lies perpendicular to its original position. The angle that is created at the junction of the central member and the limbs will not affect the final direction of the central member, nor the total increase in scar length. However, the distance between the ends of the original scar will be increased dependent upon the angle size. Theoretically, a 30° angle Z-plasty will lengthen the central member by 25 percent, a 45° angle will lengthen the central member by 50 percent, a 60° angle by 75 percent and so on (Fig. 9-2). A Z-plasty will thus lengthen a linear contracture scar. The increase is gained at the expense of the tissue at each side of the central member. The smaller the angle, the easier the flaps will be to transpose. The greatest angle theoretically possible is 90°; however, practically speaking, the largest angle used is about 60°.

This procedure may be used to improve a scar that crosses relaxed skin tension lines anywhere on the face. If the scar is lengthy, several Z-plasties may be combined in series to break up the scar and also to change the direction of its central member. One large Z-plasty might change the direction of the central member, but the result may not be as cosmetically acceptable as are multiple Z-plasties.

Contractures across creases are particularly amenable to correction by Z-plasty. An example of this might be a scar across the depression between the medial canthus and the nose. Such a scar could occur during blepharoplasty. Multiple Z-plasties would lengthen the scar and break it up to improve its appearance.

Another area that would benefit from multiple Z-plasty is the contracture of the upper lip following cleft lip repair or trauma. Generally, the scar of a cleft lip repair is vertical and therefore parallel to the facial favorable lines. Although the Z-plasty would change the direction of the scar and would be less favorable, the length gained and the symmetry between the two sides of the lip would make this procedure beneficial.

There are disadvantages to Z-plasty in certain situations. One must remember that by adding two limbs to an already present scar, the length of the scar is increased by 200 percent. Also, by lengthening the distance between the two ends of the original scar, one must shorten the distance between the ends of the legs of the Z. The soft tissue and skin with which the physician is dealing must be able to withstand this donation of skin and

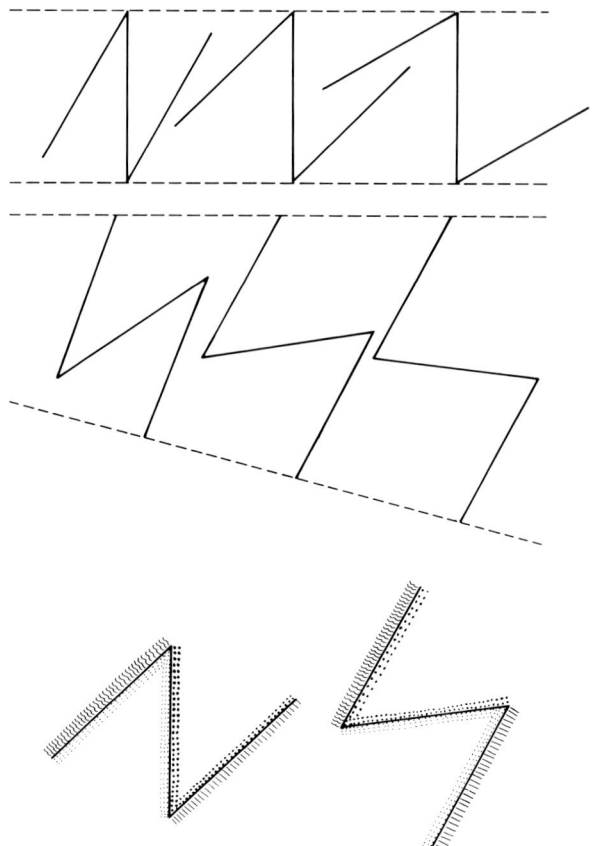

Fig. 9-2. 30° angle Z-plasty; 45° angle Z-plasty; and 60° angle Z-plasty.

length, otherwise there would be no benefit. In addition, when elevating and rotating flaps in this fashion, there may be damage to the hair follicles in the hair-bearing areas of skin. Those which are not damaged will display a change in direction by the nature of their transposition. Skin pigmentation may also be affected by the flaps of good soft-tissue surgical technique.

W-plasty

Another technique to camouflage of length scar is the W-plasty. This procedure follows the concept that the eye cannot track a short scar which is hidden in RSTL. As in the multiple Z-plasty technique, this transforms a linear or curvilinear scar into one with short segments which continually change direction. This is not intended to lengthen a scar in the sense of relieving a contracture. The running W-plasty, a term coined by Borges, combines several W-plasties.

The technical aspects of this procedure are that small triangles are removed from the side of a scar. On the opposite side a triangular projection is created. This produces interdigitating flaps that, when approximated, form a zigzag scar. This technique works especially well for curved scars and trapdoor scars. Should "dog-ears" develop at the ends of the excision, Burow's triangles should be removed to allow for a flat skin closure.

Broken Line Geometric Closure

An extension of the running W-plasty, but much more complex, is the broken line geometric closure as designed by Webster.[2] As with the running W-plasty, the broken line geometric closure is designed in a way which does not allow the observer to track or follow a scar. The running W-plasty occasionally can be picked up by the observer's eye and followed, but this is less true of the geometric closure. In this procedure, a series of rectangles, triangles, and squares are removed from one side of the scar at random, while the opposite side has the appropriate matching projection. The crossbars are lined up in the most favorable direction. Although technically somewhat more difficult and time-consuming than a W-plasty, this camouflages the scars quite well.

FACIAL FLAPS

Replacement of Skin Loss with Local Flaps

During the planning of the surgical excision of tumors and congenital deformities, and occasionally in closing a traumatic defect, facial flaps may need to be considered. Ideally, the first choice for closure would be to approximate the tissue with a primary direct closure. When the defect created requires more area coverage than the immediate tissue allows, one must consider the transposition of adjacent tissue to cover the defect. A skin flap by definition is a full-thickness mass of tissue for grafting, containing epidermis, dermis, and subcutaneous tissue, only partially removed from one part of the body so that it retains its own blood supply during its transfer to a new location. Facial flaps must be individually designed, taking into consideration the scarring that will result, the amount of tissue and skin that is available such that the donor site will be readily closed, the blood supply of the flap, the color match of the skin, and the thickness of the flap relative to the recipient skin.

A host of flaps have been devised and used for closure of a variety of facial defects. Just as no two lesions have identical characteristics, so also may designs for closure vary. The classification of facial flaps may be based on the movement of the flap (advancement, rotation, interpolation, transposition), shape (rhomboid, bilobed, flag, banner), anatomical area of the donor site (nasolabial, scalping, deltopectoral), and eponyms (Limberg, Juri, du Formental).

The success of a given flap will be based on several factors. The vascular supply must be adequate to continually support the flap until it is nourished by its new surrounding skin and subcutaneous tissues. The facial flaps are generally based on the dermal plexus of vessels and occasionally on a certain vessel. The second factor is the recipient site, which should have a good vascular supply to eventually nourish its recipient. Bone and cartilage devoid of their periosteum and perichondrium are poor recipient sites. Radiation, trauma, and infection reduce the potential for survival of the new flap. Hemostasis is important in that a hematoma may displace the flap and interrupt the blood supply from the base of the recipient area. A hematoma will also place tension on the flap and compromise the blood supply from the base of the flap. Tension at the suture line will cause ischemia of the flap at the suture line. Subcutaneous sutures are important to minimize the tension on the suture line.

The question of flap thickness is answered by evaluating the surrounding tissue. The skin of the temple and angle of the mandible are areas in which the underlying tissue contains many vital structures. Elevation of thick flaps should be avoided in these areas. Other areas generally allow for thicker flaps. If the flap developed is found to be too thick for its recipient area, the flap can be defatted. Caution should be taken not to thin the flap into the dermis and thus destroy the dermal plexus of vessels which supply the flap.

The following discussion will describe several basic flaps and concepts for flap development to assist the surgeon in handling different situations.

Advancement Flap

An advancement flap is a flap, usually rectangular in shape, designed to cover a defect of a similar shape by advancing the skin forward. Depending on the laxity of the tissue, Burow's triangles may need to be used at the base of the flap to allow the skin to advance. On occasion, a double advancement flap may be used to cover large defects which may not be adequately covered by advancing tissue from one side of the defect. These flaps are quite reliable as long as the ratio of width to length does not exceed 1:3. The disadvantage of these flaps is that the resulting cosmetic appearance may not always be acceptable.

Rotation Flap

A rotation flap is an advancement flap in which the advancement occurs on a rotational basis. This flap is reliable and simple in its technical considerations. The flap is an advancement of a semicircle at the expense of tissue at the opposite end of the curved incision. The flap is generally 4 times the area of the recipient site. The skin match is excellent, since the donor site is contiguous to the defect. Whenever possible, the arc of the flap should be placed in a natural skin crease such as the nasolabial fold (Fig. 9-3).

The disadvantage of this flap is in the length of the scar which is created. The scar is increased significantly due to the size of the flap necessary. Another problem is that the flap is curvilinear and may act as a trapdoor scar.

Nasolabial Flap

The nasolabial flap is a facial flap taken from the skin between the nose and cheek (Fig. 9-4). It is a vascular flap that may be based superiorly on the supraorbital and infraorbital vessels or inferiorly on the facial artery. It may be used effectively to cover

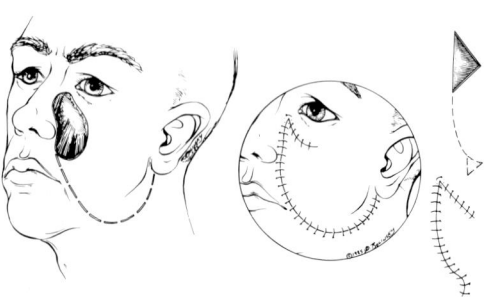

Fig. 9-3. Rotation flap placed in a natural skin crease such as the nasolabial fold.

Scar Revision and Facial Flaps

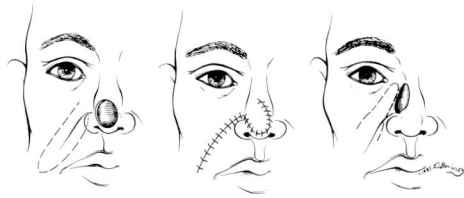

Fig. 9-4. Nasolabial flap incision placed in the nasofacial crease.

defects of the nose, cheek, and lip or may be brought into the mouth to cover a defect in the floor of the mouth. The secondary defect is closed primarily. Care should be taken to place the incision in the nasofacial crease, avoiding lateral placement on the cheek or too high a placement on the dorsum of the nose. One should also be aware of the hair-bearing areas and plan the flap accordingly. Occasionally, the flap is used in a staged procedure.

Bilobed Flap

The bilobe flap is a double rotational flap with the primary defect covered by an adjacent flap and the secondary defect covered by a flap adjacent to the first donor site (Fig. 9-5). The second donor flap site (tertiary defect) is closed primarily. This allows for movement of tissue from an area with lax skin capable of easily donating the skin to an area of limited skin mobility. Another way to consider this flap is as a single large rotation flap which is divided into 2 perpendicular limbs.

An example of this flap is on the nose. The primary defect on the nasal dorsum is filled by a flap from the lateral aspect of the nose. The second flap (tertiary defect) is derived from the glabellar area, which has loose enough skin to be advanced, and the tertiary defect is closed primarily. Skin texture may differ due to the coarseness and firmness of the nasal skin; however, this would be true of any donor skin when moved to this area.

Rhomboid Flap

A rhomboid flap is a transposition flap which can be transposed from several different sides of a defect (Fig. 9-6). This has also been known as a Limberg flap, after its designer, and the Du Formental flap, after a French surgeon who developed a modification of the flap to cover a defect forming an irregular parallelogram. The rhomboid has its opposite sides equal. The shorter diagonal of a rhomboid is equal to the length of its side.

The rhomboid flap is formed by extending the shorter diagonal a distance equal to its length. From the end of this line, another line is drawn parallel to the side of the rhomboid and equal to the length of the side. The defect is then covered by rotating the

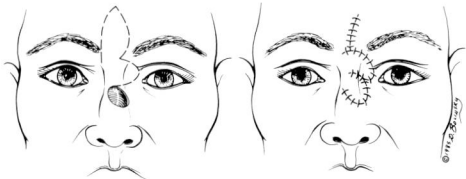

Fig. 9-5. Bilobe flap as shown is a double rotation flap.

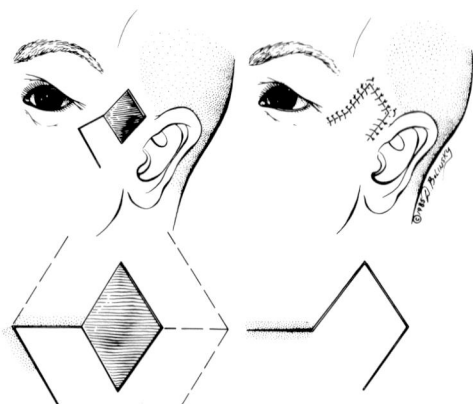

Fig. 9-6. The rhomboid flap, also known as Limberg flap and DuFormental flap, with equal opposite sides.

flap into position. The secondary defect created is covered by direct closure. Since this flap can be developed on either side of the rhomboid, four potential flaps are available to cover the same defect. This allows the surgeon four potential regions from which to obtain the transposed donor tissue.

This flap requires skin available to rotate into position and loose skin to close the secondary defect by primary closure. The lateral cheek and temple regions are common areas for use of this flap. Such a design would be a poor choice for the scalp, where the skin is not freely mobile.

O–Z Closure

The O to Z closure utilizes two rotational flaps to cover a defect (Fig. 9-7).[4] One flap is taken from each side of a circular or elliptical defect. The end result is a Z-like figure. This procedure would be considered in areas in which a primary closure might distort the appearance of an anatomical feature such as the eyebrow, eyelid, lip, hairline, or nose. In addition to approximating the structures to appear in continuity, the scar will be broken up and less noticeable than the primary closure.

Glabellar Flap

The glabellar flap deserves special note, for it is a very useful flap for closure of defects on the dorsum of the nose and to each side of the upper portion of the nose. This is a rotation flap based inferiorly on the supraorbital vessels utilizing the loose, non-hair-bearing skin of the glabellar region to swing over to cover the defect (Fig. 9-8). The

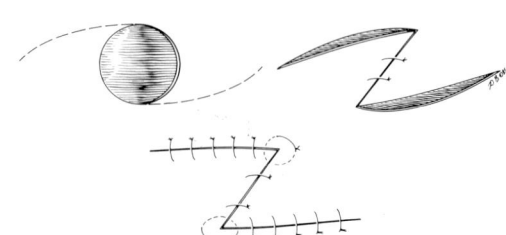

Fig. 9-7. O to Z closure utilizes two rotational flaps to cover a defect.

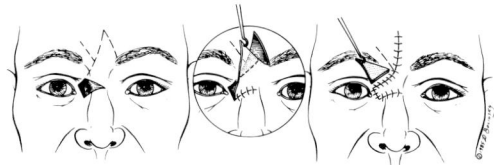

Fig. 9-8. Glabellar Flap is a very useful flap for closures of defects on the dorsum of the nose and to each side of the upper portion of the nose.

secondary defect is then closed primarily. The flap should be central and symmetrical. Should there be excess skin of the flap, this may be trimmed.

Difficulties may be found in individuals with hair growth between the eyebrows. Another problem may arise if the defect is too large for this flap to cover. In this case, one could develop a large flap and design a bilobe structure.

Midline Forehead Flap

The midline forehead flap is a finger-like flap taken from the midline of the forehead, based inferiorly on the glabellar region and extending up to the hairline (Fig. 9-9). Its vascular supply is from the supraorbital vessels. The base of the flap should be slightly angled to the side opposite the defect. This flap can reach to the tip of the nose and does quite well for lesions of the lateral aspect of the nose. The secondary defect is closed primarily and results in a quite acceptable scar.

Median Glabellar Flap

The median glabellar flap is an advancement flap of the glabellar skin which is based superiorly on the forehead approximately 1 cm above the level of the eyebrows (Fig. 9-10). With the appropriate laxity of glabellar skin, this flap may be advanced to cover the upper one-half of the nose. The vascular supply to this flap is based on the supraorbital vessels and also on the dermal plexus.

The problems with this flap are that the depression of the root of the nose may be obliterated due to the tenting effect of this flap as it stretches from the forehead to the dorsum of the nose. This is not cosmetically acceptable in many situations. In addition, the straight line scars which are produced along the lateral aspects of the nose may be apparent.

Island Flap

The island flap is a unique advancement flap in which the skin to be moved is connected to its base only by its vascular supply in the subcutaneous tissue.[2] The description of such flaps is somewhat more complicated than the scope of this chapter will allow, and the reader is referred to the bibliography for references.

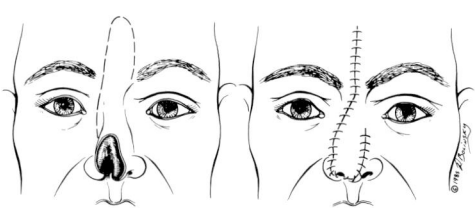

Fig. 9-9. Midline forehead flap.

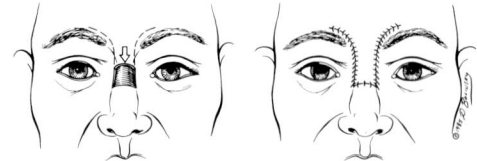

Fig. 9-10. Median Glabellar Flap.

As one can readily see, facial reconstruction utilizing flap technique can be quite challenging and one must be somewhat innovative. These flaps are quite numerous and the only limitations to their use are the imagination and technical skills of the surgeon.

In addition to the above-listed techniques of scar revision, one should consider dermabrasion and the use of injectible materials. Dermabrasion is helpful to plane the level of skin in situations in which the skin contains multiple scars of varying heights, such as in acne scars of the face. This tends to eliminate the shadows created by the different levels of the skin, thereby eliminating the features which call attention to the defect. Collagen injection attempts to do the same, but elevating the lower areas rather than planing down the ridges.

REFERENCES

1. Borges AF: Scar revision. Clin Plast Surg 4:165–319, 1977
2. Webster RC, Smith RC: Scar revision and camouflaging. Otolaryngol Clin North Am 15:55–68, 1982
3. McGregor IA: Local skin flaps in facial reconstruction. Otolaryngol Clin North Am 15:77–98, 1982
4. Stegman SJ, Tromovitch TA, Glogau RG: Basics of Dermatologic Surgery. Chicago: Yearbook Medical Publishers, pp. 73–90, 1982

Ronald C. Savin

10
Hair Transplant

Hair transplantation is a relatively simple surgical technique in which small full-thickness grafts of hair-bearing skin are removed from the hair-bearing donor area on the posterior rim of the scalp and implanted into the frontal and vertex areas of a bald scalp. Properly carried out with multiple staged procedures, hair transplants produce a moderate covering of hair which takes away the bald look and gives a more youthful definition to the face (Fig. 10-1).

Hair transplantation is by far the most common procedure for "correcting" male-pattern baldness. Though surgically easy, hair transplants require careful attention to anterior hairline planning, graft harvesting, and positioning of the hair-bearing grafts.

Well groomed and styled hair is of great importance in our society, as attested by the numbers of advertisements promoting hair products, as well as the millions spent on hair care. A full, normal head of hair is worth a fortune to those who are not so endowed. Hair transplants are a "partial" successful effort to achieve that effect.

Punch grafts were popularized in the late 1950s by Dr. Norman Orentrich.[1] He had been studying donor dominance in various skin diseases such as vitiligo and baldness. By exchanging small full-thickness skin grafts from hair-bearing to non-hair-bearing skin, and vice versa, he demonstrated that hair-bearing skin from the posterior and lateral rim of the scalp would "take" with complete healing and continued hair production by the transferred hair follicles. He went further and created fields of hair growth by repeatedly implanting numbers of "plugs" into the bald areas and in between previously planted plugs. Since then, others have further refined the procedure.[2-4] At the present time, hair transplantation in the properly selected patient produces a cosmetically pleasing, hair-covered scalp. It works (Fig. 10-2A&B).

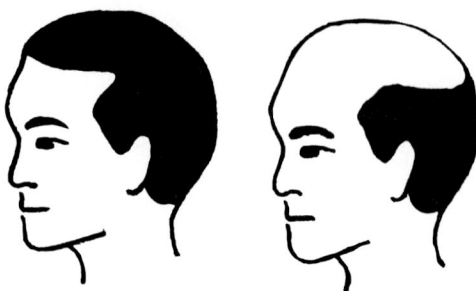

Fig. 10-1. Same facial features with and without hair. Note the elderly appearance without hair.

PATIENT SELECTION

Hair transplantation is not suitable for every person with male-pattern baldness. Selection of appropriate patients is dependent on several factors, including the quantity of existing hair and economic and psychological factors.

Obviously, the density of hair in the donor area is of prime importance. There should be sufficient hairs in each 4 mm punch area to produce good growth. The average 4 mm graft contains 12–16 hairs, and some of these hairs are lost due to the trauma of surgery and fine rim scarring. If the donor graft contains only half that amount, a thinner and probably inadequate covering of hair will be produced.

One only need examine the potential donor site in 10 men to get the feeling of what is adequate. Thicker hair looks better. More hair in each graft looks better. On the other hand, a sufficient, though larger, number of thinner hair plugs may still take away the bald look and be cosmetically pleasing. The only fixed rule is: Don't try to transplant patients with *very* thin hair in the donor site.

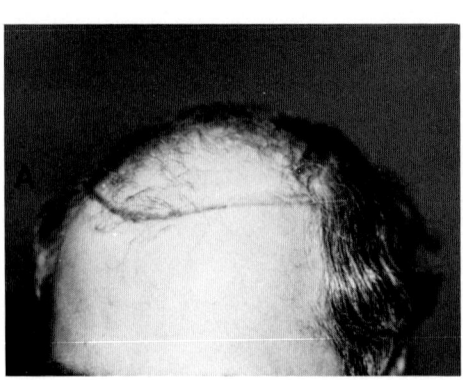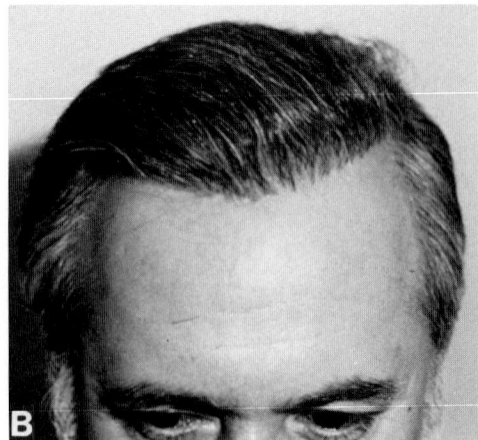

Fig. 10-2. Before (A) and after (B) 180 grafts in a 56-year-old man.

Hair Transplant

Candidates for hair transplantation must understand that the procedure will not produce a full head of hair like each one of them had at puberty. Rather, it merely redistributes the hair remaining on the surviving rim. It produces a moderate covering of hair which takes away the bald look. It grows and can be combed, brushed, permed, or whatever. Transplanted hair may be tufty in appearance, especially if the patient does not complete the planned number of procedures.

Careful combing and positioning of the transplanted hair is vital to a good visual result.

Patients who have extensive baldness and limited donor site are still candidates for surgery, though they must understand that only an anterior hairline may be created (Fig. 10-3—Patterns VI and VII). In some cases, a combination approach using scalp reduction is appropriate. An anterior hairline will take away the bald look and give age definition. In Figure 10-3, one sees identical facial features with and without an anterior hairline. The hair-bearing pate looks younger and looks better—though this latter impression may be a cultural factor.

The author is reluctant to transplant the young man with mild anterior baldness (Fig. 10-3—Patterns II and III) because the benefit gained by extending the hairline a mere centimeter or two is outweighed by the potential for scarring, tufting, and encouragement of more hair loss (in the surrounding hair) due to local surgical trauma. In addition, young men with little loss have great expectations. Their idea of an adequate result is the full head of hair, which they possessed only a few years before and that cannot be reproduced. By waiting a few years, those patients with progressive loss will become apparent, as will their need for transplants. Patients in need will prove to be the most satisfied patients. Men with little loss who are borderline candidates will often prove to resent their unnecessary surgery.

The most important first step in an initial transplantation is the placement of the anterior hairline. The hairline is always moderately high and rounded. Hair transplants look artificial and misplaced when inserted low on the forehead or when placed in a way that obstructs the temporal recession (Fig. 10-4).

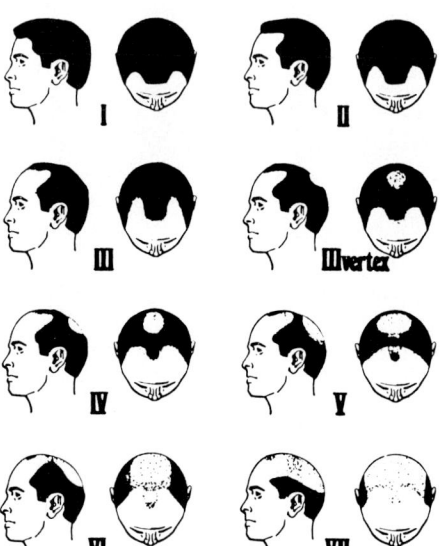

Fig. 10-3. Standards for classification of male-pattern baldness. From Norwood OT, Shell RC: Hair Transplant Surgery (2nd ed.). Springfield, IL: Charles C Thomas, p. 6, 1984. With permission.

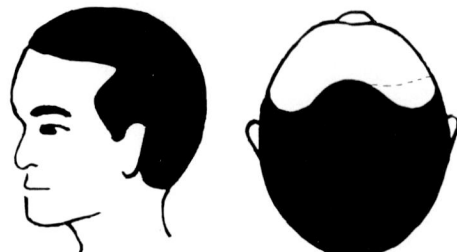

Fig. 10-4. Failure to maintain the temporal recession is an error. Placement of grafts along the dotted line is wrong.

It is impossible to re-create the patient's original hairline which was low and without a temporal recession. Hair transplants are most effective in creating a mature (high) hairline. Failure to observe this rule is the principle cause of poor results and a displeased patient.

The planned hairline is marked with a soft wax crayon (Fig. 10-5) and the patient is then ready for anesthesia. The patient is draped over his street clothes and positioned lying down on a table. Though it may be easier for the surgeon to have the patient sit in a chair, the frequency of syncope in a sitting position outweighs any advantage.

It is the author's habit to first place the patient in the supine position and trim (if permitted) fine unavoidable hair which may be in the way in the recipient area. The patient is then positioned prone (Fig. 10-6) and a 2 × 5 inch band of hair is clipped short with a scissors at the donor site (the hair-bearing rim at the back and sides of the scalp). Short hairs must be preserved in this area in order to allow identification of the angle at which the punch enters the skin. The area is cleaned of bits of hair with an alcohol-impregnated gauze.

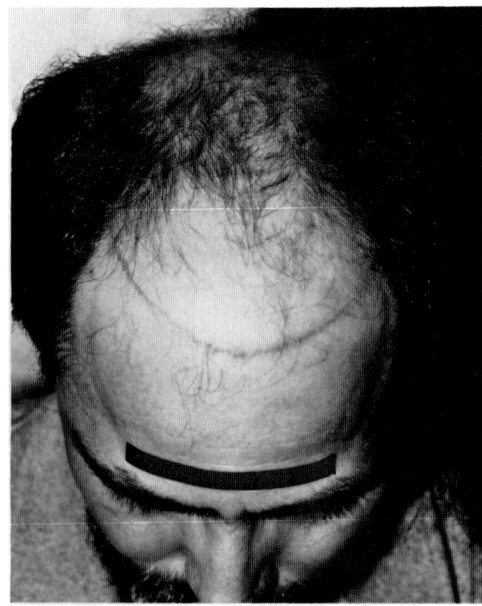

Fig. 10-5. A slightly high, semicircular hairline is aesthetically best.

Hair Transplant

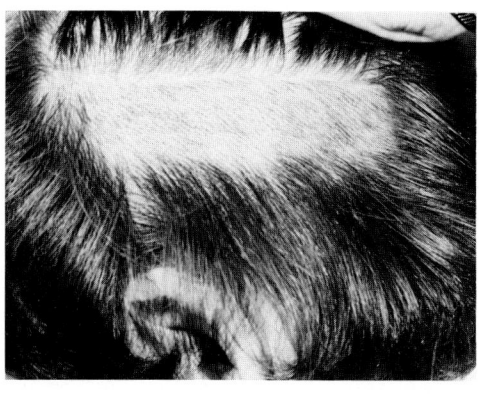

Fig. 10-6. Donor site clipped short (not shaved) prior to harvesting.

PREOPERATIVE TASKS

Prior to surgery, general medical history should be taken, including blood studies performed—including complete blood count (CBC), SMAC, urinalysis, and bleeding and clotting times. Hepatitis screening tests are required by some physicians. Bleeding is rarely a problem if the patient is properly sedated, calmly handled, and adequately bandaged only after all bleeding has stopped.

For 3 days prior to hair transplants, the patient is instructed to shampoo daily and take no aspirin. The patient may eat normally the day of surgery. No alcohol should be imbibed the day of surgery.

Preoperatively, the patient is given Valium (Roche) 5 mg P.O., as well as erythromycin 500 mg. The author prefers to use no other sedation, though others may use I.V. Valium or Penthrane (Abbott). Though apprehensive, especially at the first procedure, patients often drive home alone.

At this point, the author anesthetizes the donor and recipient sites with a total of 30 ml of lidocaine. This is really the only part of the procedure which is painful. The ideal anesthetic is 1 percent lidocaine with 1:100,000 epinephrine. The anesthetic effect lasts 2 hours, which is the length of the procedure. A bottle containing 50 ml is used and is not exceeded. Up to 50 ml of lidocaine is sufficient and quite safe. Without epinephrine, the bleeding is uncontrollable.

THE DONOR SITE

At the moment just prior to punching the donor site, the skin is rapidly injected with 3–6 cc of saline in order to tense and harden the skin so as to create a firm platform for the punch. This prevents folding of the skin and enhances straight cutting. By cutting a straight wall cylinder (Fig. 10-7), hairs on the periphery are preserved. The punch is angled parallel to the remaining hair stubs so as not to transect any roots. Attention to this positioning of the punch is vital. By examining the donor graft, one can check on the accuracy of the cutting angle. The saline dissipates in a moment and must be reinjected every 4–8 punches. The punch is inserted rapidly to the level of the vacuum hole, as the physician tries to avoid hitting the scalp.

Plugs are cut rapidly in the donor area from top to bottom. One-millimeter bridges

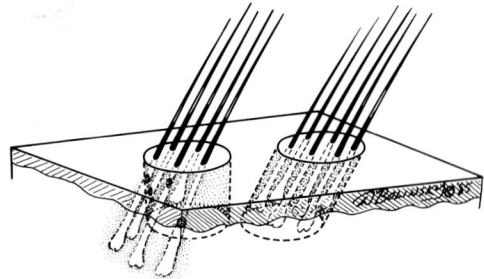

Fig. 10-7. Parallel positioning of the punch prevents cutting of the roots.

are left between holes (Fig. 10-8). Bleeding is controlled by the deft and experienced pressure of the surgical assistant. As a punch is advanced, the newly cut plugs are compressed to be harvested later. Within a few minutes, 60–80 plugs are cut. Following cutting, the plugs are lifted with forceps and the fatty loose stroma beneath cut with a scissors and placed in a Petri dish containing sterile saline. The saline need not be kept cold, though the author chooses to keep it so.

Most hair transplant surgeons do not suture the donor site except for arterial or venous bleeders. After complete hemostasis is achieved with pressure, the physician packs the area with Gelfoam (Sterile) Powder (Upjohn) covered with telfa and a 3 × 3 inch gauze. The area is then taped from temple posteriorly to temple (Fig. 10-9). The anterior forehead is left uncovered. In the past, rubber bandages and Coban were used, but they produce excessive pressure resulting in headaches and discomfort. The next day, the bandage is removed and the surrounding hair is combed over the donor site with excellent cosmetic results. Successful covering of the donor site is not a problem if the patient comes in with moderately long hair.

The donor area may be sutured with a simple running 3-0 suture. Some surgeons harvest very closely and then excise the bridges and suture the wound primarily. Pierce[5] has suggested simply cutting the bridge in a double row donor site and offsetting the holes and the skin bridge so that the skin comes together with a single suture line (Fig. 10-10). One must consider that primary closure of the donor site may act as a scalp reduction in reverse—increasing the bald area on the vertex. Though healing is fastest when the donor site is sutured, suturing holds no advantage in the long run.

The hair-bearing grafts are washed in Petri dishes containing sterile saline and trimmed of excess fat. Zealous trimming of the fat is to be avoided so as not to traumatize

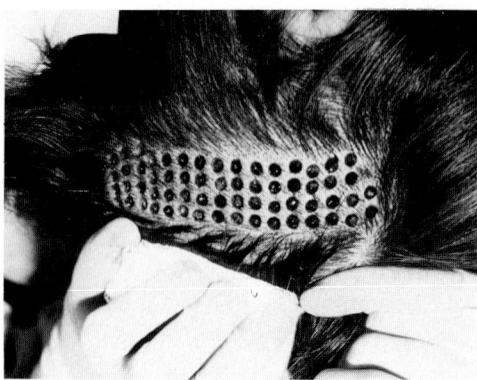

Fig. 10-8. One donor site after harvesting.

Hair Transplant

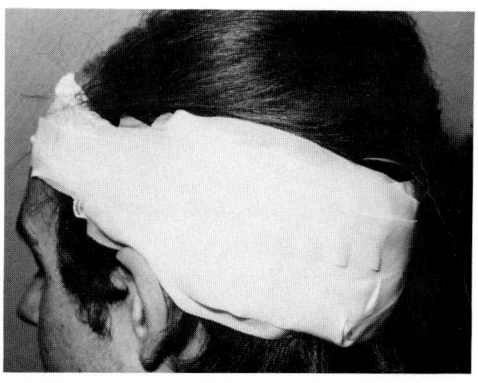

Fig. 10-9. Bandage over donor site.

the roots. They are then counted prior to making the recipient holes; it is nice to come out even.

The pattern of harvesting the donor area varies. The author prefers to harvest all the grafts from one 2 × 5 inch area of the hair-bearing scalp. Grafts are cut four down and 15 across. Others prefer to harvest bands only 2 plugs down and separated by a hair-bearing strip. Obviously, as much existing hair as possible is preserved in the donor area so as to be able to cover and mask the surgical site.

The author prefers to use an electrically driven punch and Australian double-beveled punches. The preferred manual punch is the Resnik-Lewis punch with a crosscut knurled handle. It is comfortable to initially perform hair transplants with the manual punch. When dexterity is gained, the power punch may be substituted.

The most popular motor is the Bell hand engine, though others may be equally good. The punch should rotate slowly (700 RPMs) so as to minimize frictional heat. The Australian punch probably yields more hairs than do single-beveled punches. The author prefers stainless steel, double-beveled punches, as the finish is preserved even when mishandled. Sharpening is difficult and the author recommends new punches or factory resharpened punches for each procedure.

Most hair transplant surgeons harvest with a 4 mm punch; the graft is inserted into a hole created with a 3.5 mm punch. Some surgeons use a 4.5 mm graft in a 4 mm hole, though the chances of dome-shaped objectionable scars in the donor area is thereby increased. A 4 mm graft may easily be placed in a 3.5 mm hole. The beginning hair transplanter should stay with 4 mm donor grafts into the 3.5 mm hole; experiment as your confidence builds.

Larger punches tend to heal with hairless scarring in a portion of the graft. This is also true of (and the problem with) full-thickness free strip grafting.

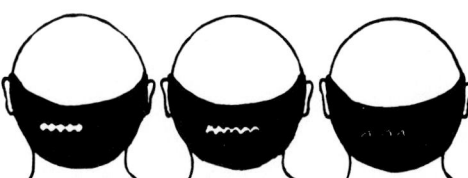

Fig. 10-10. Interdigitation and suturing of the donor site.

THE RECIPIENT SITE

The recipient holes are most easily cut with the patient in the supine position. Additional lidocaine is injected along the anterior edge, as this area is usually still sensitive. One must be careful not to erase the wax pencil line, at least in an initial hair transplant procedure, until the anterior line is cut. In the recipient area, the author usually uses a 3.5 mm punch, spacing the graft sites one punch width apart in both directions. The superior line of punches is offset or placed immediately above, depending on the selected plan of repeat fillings (Fig. 10-11). Manual punches work fine in the front. If using a motor-driven punch, no saline is needed. The graft receives its nutritional supply by diffusion from the surrounding intact skin; skin bridge must be preserved or the grafts will die.

The recipient hole must be punched deep enough so that there is sufficient room for the graft to sit deep and flush. There is a tendency with the motorized punch to grind against the skull; this is not a technical problem, but a source of wonder to the patient.

The angle at which the recipient hole is cut is also very important. The holes should be placed at a 90° angle to the head, much like the natural hairline—or the spokes in the head of the Statue of Liberty (Fig. 10-12). In addition, the holes should be angled low to the forehead so that the new hair growth will tend to cover whatever mild scarring, depigmentation, or tufting may occur. There are minor variations in recipient hole angles, though all are angled low to the forehead and at a 90° or slightly more anterior angle.

The pattern of the recipient grafts varies somewhat with the numbers of punches to be done, the number of procedures, the wish of the patient, and practical limitation. In general, the anterior hairline should be grafted tightly—wall to wall. Figure 10-11 shows various patterns to follow. They are theoretically ideal, but in practice the surgeon often gets off track and follows an individual variation. The goal is to plant hair-bearing grafts wall to wall.

The author prefers to plan procedures 6 weeks apart, allowing time for healing and collateralization of blood supply. Unger's research suggests that hair growth is maximized by not rushing subsequent procedures.[3]

After the recipient holes are cut, the non-hair-bearing plugs are lifted high with a forceps and deeply cut free. The purpose is to create a deep enough hole to easily accept the hair-bearing graft. The author removes all the hairless plugs, while controlling bleeding with pressure. The donor plugs are now inserted into the recipient holes, while the grafts are carefully angled so that the hairs point in an anterior-lateral position with a low angle to the forehead.

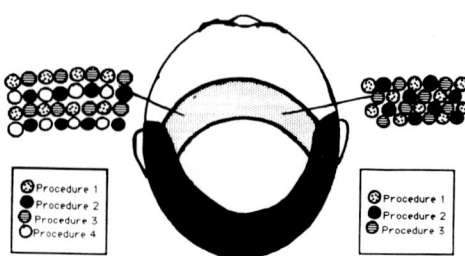

Fig. 10-11. Patterns of grafting the recipient site. Both 3- or 4-stage patterns are commonly utilized.

Hair Transplant

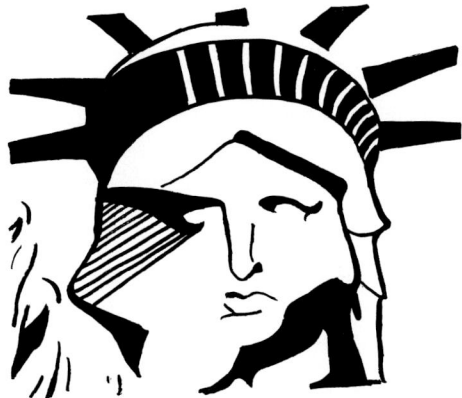

Fig. 10-12. Columbia.

The graft is grasped by the dermis with forceps; the author prefers Brown-Adson with multiple teeth. If the plug does not seat well, it should be turned until it does. Most of the final hair direction is achieved by the angle of the recipient hole that contains the graft, rather than by the graft itself. The plug should lie flat with the skin; the bandage will not push it down. If a plug will not sit properly in the hole, try pressing the graft with a cotton tipped applicator; try either end. If this fails, remove the graft and trim the fat, which is probably too long. After hemostasis, again turn the plugs as needed so as to align the hairs in a proper position.

In situations where the skin is thin or bound down due to scarring, the recipient hole needs to be enlarged by blunt undermining of the skin with a blunt probe such as a needle holder or hemostat. A pocket is, therefore, created which will accept the hair-bearing graft.[5]

As grafts are inserted, pressure is exerted over them by advancing gauze sponges; within minutes, bleeding is controlled. Arterial or venous bleeders in front rarely occur. The graft itself covers the wound and prevents bleeding.

The anterior scalp is now ready for bandaging. The author applies telfa over the grafts and surmounts a strip of adhesive-backed foam (Reston one-half inch), followed by a complete head wrap using 2 rolls of 3 inch Kling and Dermacel tape (Fig. 10-13).

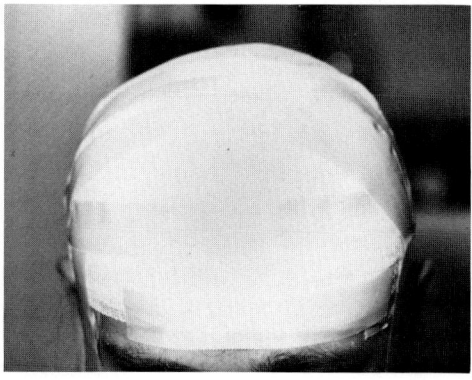

Fig. 10-13. Bandage is removed the next morning.

Others cover the grafts with antibiotic ointment before the telfa. Some use a light dressing, but the author prefers a heavy protective dressing that is removed the next morning.

Occasionally, the donor plugs are sutured in place, though the author sees no advantage. In fact, if limited numbers of grafts are done (30–40) no bandage is necessary. Nevertheless, the author prefers a large protective head wrap. This is always removed the next morning.

POSTOPERATIVE PROCEDURES

The patient is allowed to return home; he may even drive. Postoperative analgesia consists of either Tylenol (McNeil) or Percocet (Du Pont). That night, the scalp tends to ache but there is rarely severe pain. The next day there is little discomfort. Eighty-five percent of patients surveyed described no pain in the postoperative period.

Some patients feel fine until evening and delay filling their prescriptions; the author encourages filling of the pain prescription before the pharmacy closes—for the patient's comfort and to minimize unnecessary telephone calls.

The next morning, patients are encouraged to return to the office for bandage removal. Because the adhesive is not directly over the plugs, removal is easy. Occasionally, a few plugs have drifted and need to be reset; this usually means lifting them out and reinserting. The existing hair is brushed over the donor site and coverage is cosmetically effective. Combing is hazardous, as the teeth may lift a graft or dislodge a clot. The recipient site looks scabby and is covered with long side hair if available. The use of hair spray is encouraged. Otherwise, a light telfa (adhesive) dressing is put over the grafts.

One-third of the author's patients remove the bandage themselves at home. Postoperative bleeding is rare if the surgeon bandages only after hemostasis is complete. The author believes the Gelfoam powder is very important. Nevertheless, bleeding can occur, and when it does it is always about 4 hours after the procedure is over. This is probably related to the wearing off of the epinephrine. If the bandage is pink, no action is necessary. If the bandage is soaked, it must be removed, the bleeder tied, and the head rebandaged.

The patient may lightly shampoo his head on the third postoperative day and daily thereafter. The hair in the graft does not begin to grow for 12 weeks, as the surgery induces a resting stage for this period. Subsequent sessions are planned 6 weeks apart.

The author uses prophylactic antibiotics in the form of erythromycin, 1 g daily for 4 days. Though infection is rare, the author feels that he has encountered less problems with infection because of the antibiotics.

MINI GRAFTS

A new modification of grafting the anterior 3–5 cm of the scalp involves the use of mini graphs.[7] This is an evolving technique in which 4.5 mm donor grafts are quartered with cuts made parallel to the hair follicles so as not to transect the hair. These are inserted into 5 mm linear stab wounds created by a #15 blade (Fig. 10-14). The donor grafts should be trimmed of excess fat, otherwise they are difficult to implant. These are placed 2 mm apart like a picket fence and posterior rows are offset. The mini grafts are

Hair Transplant

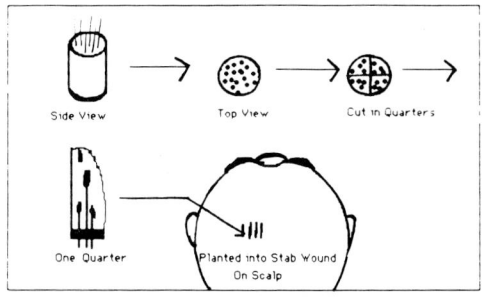

Fig. 10-14. The procedure for grafting mini plugs.

forced into the slash wound with a jeweler's forceps. Though many more total grafts are needed than when other graft procedures are used, the results are a thin covering of natural-looking hair. With subsequent procedures, thickness builds up. The posterior scalp is filled with the usual hair transplantation grafts.

The advantage to building an anterior hairline of mini grafts is the lack of tuftiness ("dolls' hairs"), even when the patient fails to return for further procedures. If the patient is only grafted once, the hair looks thin but natural. Mini grafts do not produce great density and they don't result in scarring or fibrosis. This innovation is exciting.

Mini grafts are commonly used to fill in between and in front of transplanted hair when prominent tuftiness has resulted. It is a most useful technique for "finishing" the anterior line.

SCALP REDUCTION

In bald patients (Fig. 10-3—Patterns VI and VII) with loose skin at the crown and vertex, this loose skin may be excised so as to reduce the area of baldness and to stretch up the lateral hair-bearing skin. Scalp reduction is probably useful in 20 percent of hair transplant patients (Fig. 10-15).

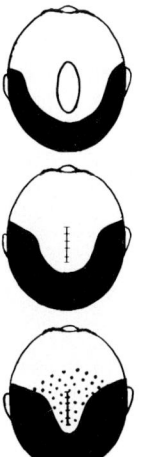

Fig. 10-15. Serial reductions can produce a marked diminution or absence of the bald crown.

The basic procedure is a long, midline, elliptical excision 2–3 cm wide and 15 cm long from the vertex to the crown. After wide undermining below the galea, the lax skin is excised and the galea and skin closed separately. Several procedures are often required, due to stretch-back of as much as 50 percent. The remaining bald scalp and scar line are then filled in with conventional hair transplants.

Scalp reduction causes elevation of the hairline. Careful planning must be done initially so that the position of the grafted hairline anticipates the elevation of that line by a scalp reduction.

An exciting innovation in posterior scalp reduction is the use of tissue expanders. Though there is a period of several weeks in which the patient develops a gradually enlarging head, the ability to easily remove the bald skin may prove worth the embarrassment.

RECONSTRUCTIVE SURGERY AFTER BURNS

Hair transplants take well and look good in burn scars and other traumatic injuries of the scalp.[6] In cases of severe facial injury, it is better to complete the facial surgery before hair transplantation to the scalp; otherwise, the hairline tends to shift as the forehead skin is disturbed with subsequent surgery (Fig. 10-16A&B).

COMPLICATIONS

Considering that hair transplant surgery is far from sterile, there are few complications apart from errors in surgical technique. Bleeding during surgery is minor and bleeders are easily tied. Postoperative bleeding can be minimized by waiting for complete

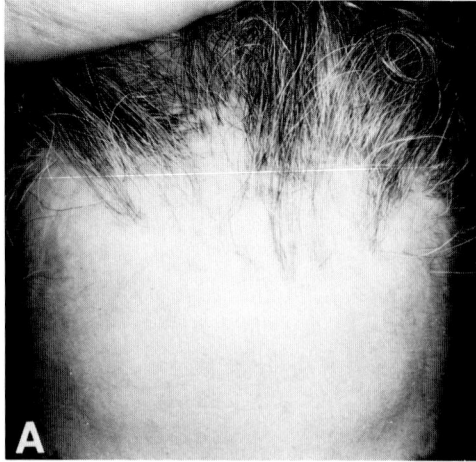 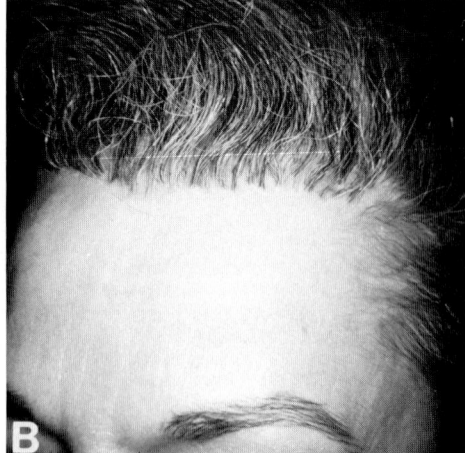

Fig. 10-16. Scarring of the anterior scalp due to boiling water before (A) and after (B) hair transplants.

hemostasis before bandaging, by tying all bleeders, and by using Gelfoam. Suturing of the donor site probably reduces postoperative bleeding.

Infection is rare and is managed with appropriate antibiotics. Many physicians use prophylactic antibiotics, but scientific support for this practice is lacking.

A major problem for the patient is embarrassment due to the presence of crusts and scabs at the recipient site. These may be covered by ingenious hair styles, hats, bandages, or hairpieces.

Two to three days following the first hair transplant of the anterior scalp, edema may develop in the forehead and over the following 3 days descends to the eyes and the nose and dissipates. It occurs in only 10 percent of patients (with over 40 plugs) and is a minor nuisance. Some surgeons combat the edema with systemic steroids, though the author finds that unnecessary.

The donor site may rarely develop arteriol-venous fistulas. Dome-shaped scars may occur with the taking of large grafts of 4.5–5.0 mm without suturing. Large donor sites should be sutured closed. In general, the donor site is well hidden by the surrounding hair and proves to be no problem.

Scarring always occurs to some extent, but it is rarely a problem. A slight palpable feeling to the graft must be expected, as is paleness of the graft. This latter problem tends to show only with a tan and is really not a significant problem. Prominent raised scars (cobblestoning) can occur and are not always due to poor technique. These can be treated in some cases by electrosurgical destruction of the elevated portion.

Failure of the grafted hair to grow in the expected amount probably occurs in 5 percent of patients. The causes include poor surgical technique, including performing too many grafts too often. Error such as cutting of the roots during trimming can be avoided. The author has operated on patients with poor yields per plug and has obtained good results. Yet, using this same good technique, the author has treated patients who yield poor growth. Obviously, other factors must occur, including unrecognized infection, inadequate nutritional supply, and God knows what.

Patients are upset with surgically created hairlines which are straight. Preserve the temporal recession or the anterior hairline will look unnatural. Resist filling the temporal recession even though the patient wants it; he doesn't understand.

Tufting may be corrected by inserting additional grafts and mini grafts. The surgeon is dependent on the patient to return for sufficient procedures to finish the job. Failure on the part of the patient to return is a common cause of tufting.

The anterior scalp tends to be numb for a year or longer after hair transplantation. This is due to the interruption of superficial nerves and their very slow repair.

Granulation tissue rarely occurs in the graft sites and resolves in 3–12 months; applications of silver nitrate may help granulomatous tissue to resolve. The presence of granulation tissue is difficult to explain and the patient requires support until resolution.

Several years ago, the author surveyed his patients who had had transplants more than 2 years before, regarding whether they thought the procedure was successful and worthwhile. The overwhelming answer was "yes."[8] Ninety-four percent said that if they were starting out fresh with the advantage of hindsight, they would go through it again. Twenty-five percent of patients were disappointed in not achieving more density, yet most of these men would still go through it again.

With proper patient selection and explanation, hair transplantation is an enormously successful cosmetic procedure (Fig. 10-17A1,A2,B1,B2,D1,&D2).

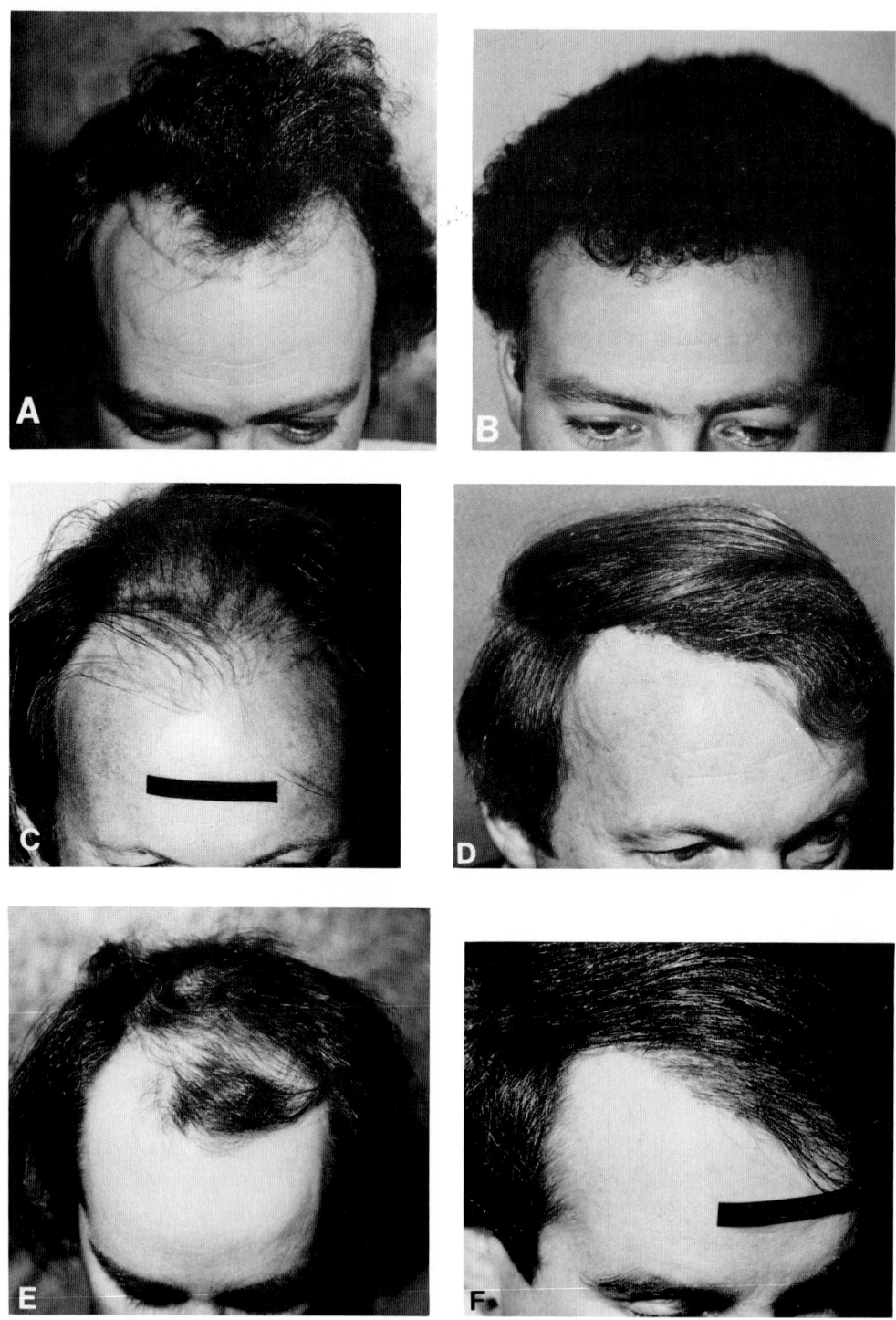

Fig. 10-17. Before (left) and after (right) hair transplantation.

Hair Transplant

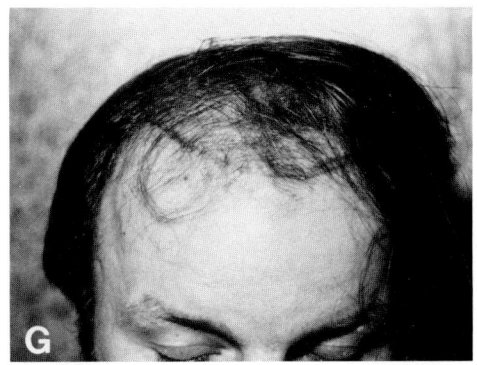 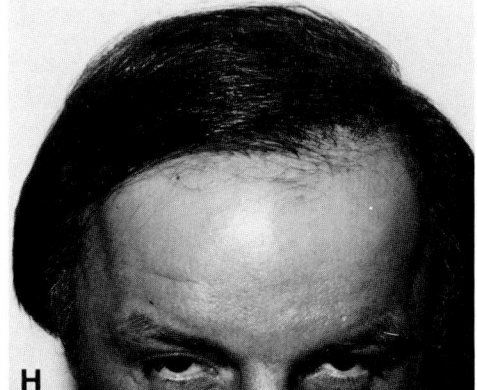

Fig. 10-17. Continued.

REFERENCES

1. Orentreich N: Autographs in alopecia's and other selected dermatologic conditions. Ann NY Acad Sci 83:463, 1959
2. Savin RC: Hair transplantation. Conn Med 33:47–51, 1969
3. Unger WP: Hair transplantation. New York City: Marcel Dekker, 1979
4. Norwood OT, Shell RC: Hair transplant surgery (2nd ed.). Springfield, IL: Charles C Thomas, 1984
5. Pierce HE: Improved method of closure of donor sites in hair transplantation. J Dermatol Surg Oncol 6:475–476, 1979
6. Bradshaw W: Personal communication, 1984
7. Savin RC: Hair transplants in burn scars and other alopecia's. Conn Med 37:501–503, 1973
8. Savin RC: Are hair transplants successful? Cutis 22:121–123, 1978

Douglas D. Dedo

11
Collagen Injection

Injectable collagen (Zyderm collagen implant—Collagen Corporation) is an effective material to correct facial cutaneous deformities of aging, surgery, trauma, disease, and atrophy. Roughly one-third of the body's structural protein is collagen. A zenograft collagen suitable for human injection has been prepared from bovine dermis. The major antigenic determinants are hydrolyzed to produce a hypoallergenic helical collagen molecule. Presently, two preparations are available commercially. Zyderm 1 is a pepsin-solubilized bovine dermal collagen suspended in buffered physiologic saline containing 0.3 percent lidocaine and 35 mg/ml of collagen. Zyderm II, introduced in 1983, contains 65 mg/ml of collagen.

MATERIALS

Collagen Corporation supplies the implant in 0.1 cc test syringes and the treatment syringes in larger volumes up to 2 cc. Thirty-gauge needles, patient information cards to interpret the test results, and a patient treatment record are also available from the company to facilitate recordkeeping. The collagen molecule will remain suspended at 0°C–5°C. When injected and heated to body temperature at 37°C, however, the fibrils and crosslinks form to convert the material from an opalescent gel to an opaque semi-solid. The saline resorbs in 24–48 hours. Over the next 2 weeks, as the implant stabilizes, there is a concomitant 65–75 percent gradual reduction in the volume of the implant.

PATIENT SELECTION

A complete medical history is taken to determine whether the patient has any autoimmune disease, rheumatoid arthritis, polymyositis, polyarteritis nodosa, scleroderma, Reiter's syndrome, lupus erythematosus, psoriatic arthritis, dermatomyositis,

Hashimoto's thyroiditis, Grave's disease, ulcerative colitis, Crohns's disease, Sjogren's syndrome, or mixed connective-tissue disease. Several contraindications have been changed since the material was first introduced commercially. Patients with a family history of autoimmune disease were formerly ineligible for treatment, as were patients who had received silicone injections. Both of these groups may now receive the collagen implant.

Patient satisfaction is directly proportional to the pretreatment counseling they receive. It is imperative that they understand that the treatment involves a skin test and series of injections, and that the cost will be proportional to the number of treatment sessions required to achieve the desired result. Perhaps more important is the fact that improvement will last from 3 to several months, depending upon the area treated, before a touch-up or further injections are required to maintain the result. An understatement as to the expected degree of improvement is safest for patient satisfaction.

The patient is tested with 0.1 cc of collagen injected in the volar aspect of the forearm. The site is observed for 4 weeks and the patient is instructed to note on the card any changes and to call the office if an adverse reaction is suspected. A positive test is defined as any localized erythema, induration, tenderness, or swelling at the test site, with or without pruritis, which persists for more than 6 hours, or appears more than 24 hours after the implantation. The onset of a rash, myalgia, or arthralgia is also considered a positive response. Approximately 3.5 percent of patients will have a positive skin test. If a test is equivocal, then the patient is retested in the oppositive arm 1 month later. Delayed hypersensitivity occurs in 1.3 percent of the patients. Four weeks after a negative test, treatment may begin.

IMPLANTATION TECHNIQUES

The crucial determinant in effecting a long-term result is the placement of the collagen in the superficial dermis. If the injection is deep in the fat or subcutaneous layers, it is quickly resorbed. A 30-gauge needle provides maximum control and the least discomfort. The skin is stretched or pinched (Fig. 11-1) to provide a firm surface for injection. Inserting the needle bevel down and beginning the injection just as the bevel disappears from view assures the most superficial placement of the collagen in the dermis. In some areas of the face where the skin is thicker, the bevel may be inserted up, allowing even more superficial placement. The angle of insertion should be between 30° and 45° with the skin. The hub of the needle rests on the forefinger or thumb (Fig. 11-2) and is rocked down against the fulcrum of the finger to allow even more superficial placement. Slowly inject into the papillary dermis and feel the resistance of the injection.

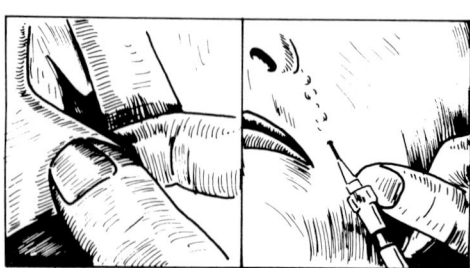

Fig. 11-1 Provide a firm surface.

Collagen Injection

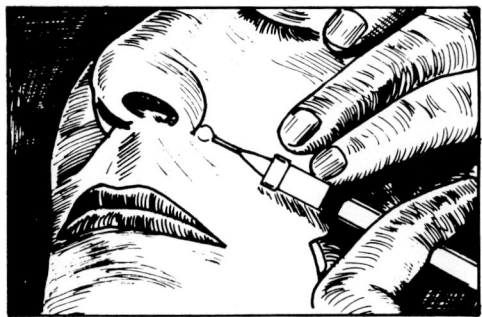

Fig. 11-2   Inject into superficial dermis.

There should be an immediate blanching of the skin and a wheal formation (Fig. 11-3). Lack of blanching indicates placement is too deep and sudden release of the pressure indicates the collagen is flowing freely into a deeper plane. The blanching will resolve in 10–20 minutes.

All depressions and defects are overcorrected by 100–200 percent (Fig. 11-4), since 70 percent of the injected volume is resorbed. The amount of overcorrection is somewhat self-limiting as to the distensibility of the scar or the proximity of pilosebaceous openings. If an area is overinjected, the epithelium will rupture and the material will extrude to the surface. If Zyderm II is being injected, less vigorous overcorrection is advised, since twice the volume of solid material is being injected and a longer period of time is necessary for assimilation of the material by the body. Cautious overcorrection is done in thin-skinned areas such as the periorbital area. After injection, the implant may be gently pressed or rolled with the finger to flatten the material and improve coalescence with adjacent injections.

The needle is usually inserted 3 mm from the edge of a depression such as an acne scar and advanced until the bevel lies beneath the scar. For long rhytids or grooves, the needle is placed directly in the defect and the serial puncture technique (Fig. 11-5 A & B) is preferred over the linear threading technique.

It is helpful to have the patient hold a mirror and check the areas that have been treated. When there is a small volume of material left in the syringe, ask the patient if there is one spot you've missed before using the entire syringe and discovering too late a depression you overlooked.

In one treatment session, the usual volume should not exceed two 2 cc. The patients are prepared from the preoperative counseling to return at 2-week intervals until the desired result has been achieved.

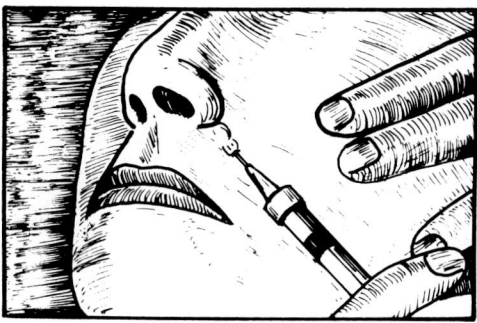

Fig. 11-3   Obtain Blanching and a wheal.

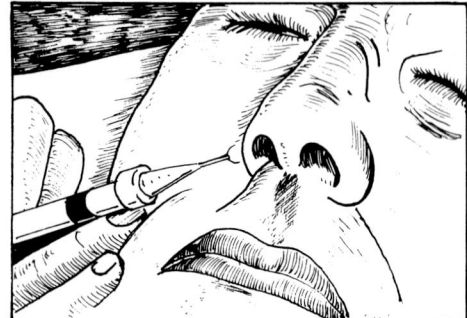

Fig. 11-4 Achieve overcorrection.

Immediately after the injection, the patient is reminded that the blanching and swelling will subside within a few hours and make-up may be applied in 4 hours. Rubbing or massaging of the treated areas will only hasten absorption of the implant. Exposure to sunlight should be avoided. Exercise and alcohol may cause mild swelling or redness at the injection sites in the weeks following treatment and restriction of these activities is advised if the skin so reacts.

CLINICAL EFFICACY OF INJECTABLE COLLAGEN

In general, soft, pliable, gently sloping edges and nonatrophic bases are the types of lesions most amenable to collagen injection. Success with acne scarring varies with the type of lesion, location, and pattern and state of the acne. Distensible acne lesions with relatively smooth margins that are quiescent afford optimal results (Fig. 11-6 A & B). Icepick acne scars are dilated gland orifices and do not respond to injectable collagen. Similarly, immature craters with dense scar bundles or atrophic bases are difficult to distend and frequently the material breaks through and leaks out.

Rhytids due to the vagaries of aging have provided the most dramatic response to injectable collagen. The duration of the improvement is directly related to the stresses that act upon the treatment site. Active muscular movement causes more rapid resorption of the implant. Horizontal forehead lines respond well to augmentation. Glabellar frown lines (Fig. 11-7 A & B) show a similar excellent result. The cheek-lip lines (nasolabial folds) distend quite nicely with collagen (Fig. 11-8 A & B). Care should be

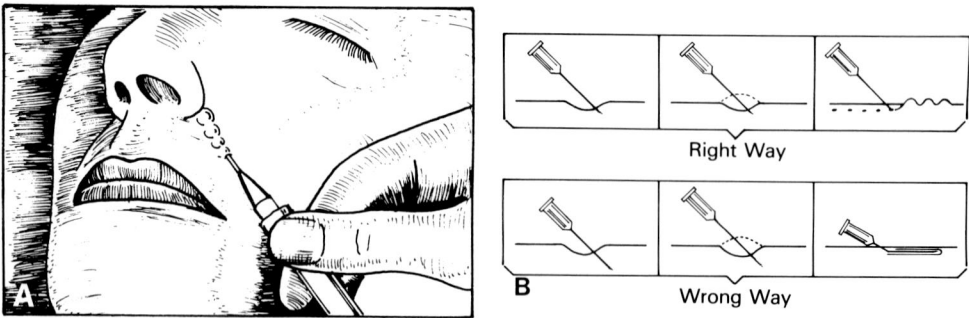

Fig. 11-5a and b Use serial placement technique.

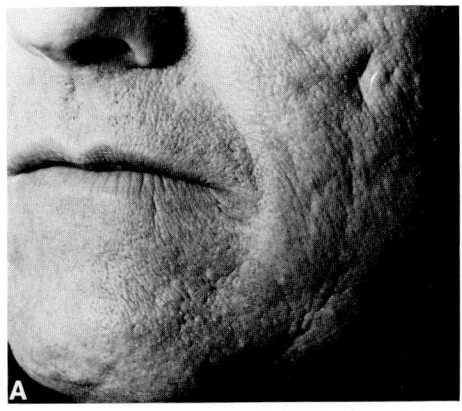
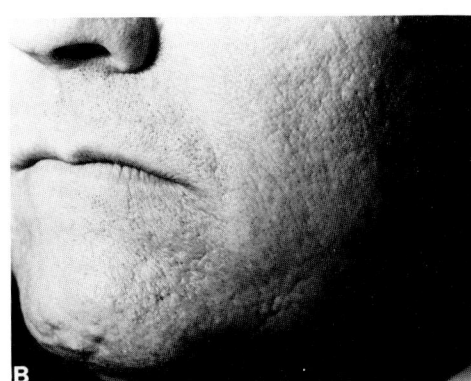

Fig. 11-6 (a) Acne scarring before ZYDERM® Collagen (b) Aging lines and scarring after ZYDERM® Collagen

taken to inject slightly medial to the fold. Periorbital lines, including the crow's feet, are judiciously injected without overcorrecting, since the skin is so thin. Circumoral rhytids require multiple injections. The lip is stabilized by pinching it, which also facilitates superficial placement of the implant. The transverse crease of the chin is stiff and does not distend well.

Post-traumatic soft linear scars obtain substantial improvement from injectable collagen. Areas of atrophy due to steroid injections similarly distend well. However, keloids, hypertrophic scars, and linear contracted scars that bridge contour concavities of the face do not lend themselves to correction.

Areas of atrophy from linear scleroderma are not treated until the disease becomes quiescent. Broad areas of atrophy requiring large volumes of material are best treated with other surgical techniques.

ADVERSE REACTION

Postinjection sequelae that are transient are bruising (sometimes turning almost black) that will resolve in 5–7 days, small pustules at the injection sites, erythema, and induration. Approximately 2–3 percent of the patients will develop an allergic response

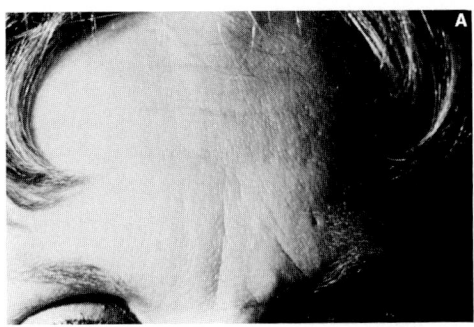
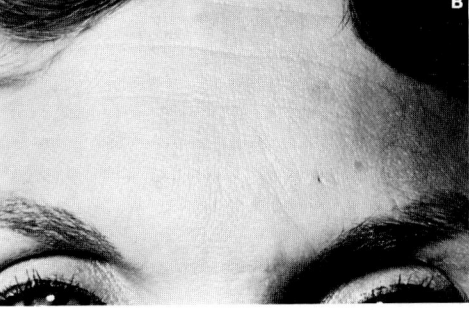

Fig. 11-7 (a) Frown line before ZYDERM® treatment (b) Frown line after ZYDERM® treatment.

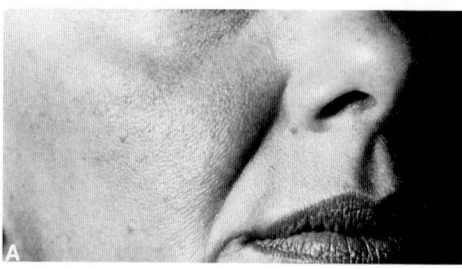 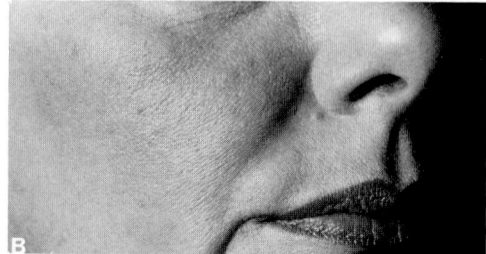

Fig. 11-8 (a) Aging lines before ZYDERM® treatment (b) Aging lines after ZYDERM® treatment.

to the collagen. Most of the time this response is a localized swelling with or without nodularity and erythema at the injection sites. These may develop after the first or second series of injections and can actually occur any time during treatment. The induration usually subsides in 2–4 months without serious sequelae. There have been no cases of permanent scarring. Topical systemic, or intralesional steroids have been tried with little success and the preferred treatment is supportive therapy. Systemic antihistamines provide some relief if pruritis is a problem. Ibuprofen (Motrin—Upjohn) 600 mgm 3 times a day and ice compresses applied for 20 minutes twice daily may reduce the local reaction. The most serious reported complication was one case of unilateral blindness following glabellar injection. A serum sickness type of reaction with intermittent episodes of arthralgia, myalgia, and fever has been reported and resolved in 6 months. During this time, patients are instructed to avoid beef, alcohol, caffeine, and prolonged exposure to heat and sunlight, since these may be inciting agents to continued adverse reaction.

CONCLUSION

The ideal candidate for collagen injection is a young patient with soft, premature wrinkles or lines who is eager for improvement but does not require facial surgery. For the older patient, injectable collagen is an adjunct to facial rejuvenation surgery to augment the surgical result. In all patients, the duration of the response is dependent upon superficial placement of the implant in the papillary dermis, and maintenance of the improvement requires patient compliance for repeat injections.

BIBLIOGRAPHY

Kamer F, Hunter D: "How I Do It": Head and neck & plastic surgery. Use of injectable collagen for cosmetic lines of the face: Preliminary report. Laryngoscope 93:950, 1983
Klein AW, Rish DC: Injectable collagen update. J Dermatol Surg Oncol 10:519–522, 1984
Stegman SJ, Tromovitch T: Implantation of collagen for depressed scars. Dermatol Surg Oncol 6:450–453, 1980
Tromovitch TA, Stegman J: Zyderm collagen: Implantation techniques. J Am Acad Dermatol 10:273–278, 1984
Webster RC, Kattner MD, Smith RC: Injectable collagen for augmentation of facial areas. Arch Otolaryngol 110:652–655, 1984

K. J. Lee
Nathan E. Nachlas

12
Otoplasty

Although a plethora of techniques for the correction of lop ear deformities has appeared in the literature over the past 40 years, two general approaches are evident. The first group consists of the procedures modeled after the horizontal mattress technique of Mustarde.[1-7] In this operation, the cartilage is not split, and the neoantihelix is created by the insertion of horizontal placement sutures. The degree of correction of the antihelical deformity is dependent upon the placement and tightness of the sutures.

The second group of techniques involves the incision and/or excision of auricular cartilage.[8-17] The neoantihelix is formed by direct sculpturing of the cartilage. Some auricular abnormalities are particularly suited to these techniques, especially severely cupped ears with firm, resistant cartilage.

Two alternative techniques for correction of the antihelical defect will be presented. The first procedure is derived from Mustarde and includes fish-scaling of the posterior layer of perichondrium and full thickness of cartilage, followed by the placement of horizontal mattress sutures.[18] It is the standard technique of the senior author. The second technique, the cartilage splitting otoplasty, was described in 1970 by Nachlas et al.,[14] and it involves the incision of the cartilage at the proposed site of the new antihelix. This is followed by sculpturing of the cartilage with a diamond burr or wire brush. The resulting neoantihelix is independent of the placement of holding sutures, and the resulting contour is smooth, natural appearing, and permanent. This continues to be the standard technique for correcting lop ear deformities in the Department of Otolaryngology/Head and Neck Surgery at the Johns Hopkins Hospital.

FISH-SCALING TECHNIQUE

This technique may be performed under local or general anesthesia. The latter is preferred in young children. Infiltration of 1 percent lidocaine with 1:100,000 epinephrine is done for hemostasis and to aid in the planes of dissection. Sufficient hair is shaved from around the auricle. Both ears may be prepped and draped simultaneously.

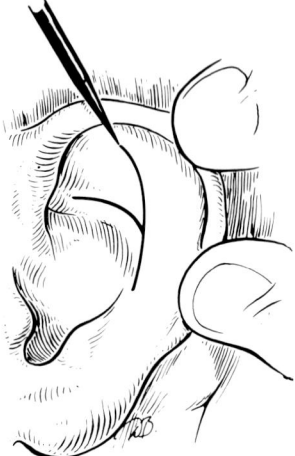

Fig. 12-1 Depressing the auricle posteriorly outlines the new antihelix. The center line of the antihelix as well as the superior and inferior crura can be penciled in with a surgical marker.

By depressing the auricle posteriorly, the new antihelix is demonstrated (Fig. 12-1). The center line of the antihelix, as well as the superior and inferior crura, are outlined with a surgical marking pen.

The anterior and posterior aspects of the auricle are then infiltrated with the local anesthesia (Figs. 12-2 and 12-3).

A dumbbell-shaped ellipse of skin measuring 0.5–1.5 cm is outlined and excised (Fig. 12-4). The posterior perichondrium remains intact. The width of the excision over the posterior aspect of the ear lobule is determined by the amount of preoperative bowing of the lobule. Similarly, the width of the dumbbell at the superior aspect of the auricle is dependent on the amount of protrusion in this area. In this manner, postoperative "telephone deformity" may be prevented.

The skin flaps are developed above the level of the perichondrium anterior to the helical rim and posterior to the junction of the concha and the mastoid (Fig. 12-5).

Using a sharp blade (no. 15 Bard-Parker blade; a Holmes' cartilage knife; or a Beaver 69 blade), fish-scaling of the posterior layer of perichondrium and full thickness of the cartilage is then done (Fig. 12-6). Great care is taken not to penetrate the anterior auricular skin. The fish-scaling is concentrated in the region of the new antihelix and the superior crus. This is then extended laterally or medially in order to achieve the desired

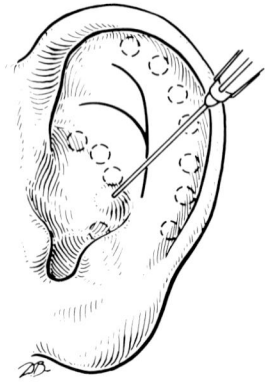

Fig 12-2 The anterior aspect of the auricle is infiltrated with 1% Xylocaine with epinephrine 1:100,000 concentration. This gives hemostasis and also dissects the skin away from the perichondrium.

Otoplasty

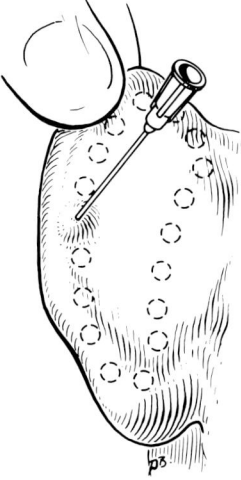

Fig. 12-3 The same is done on the posterior aspect of the auricle.

"break" of the existing cartilage spring. If the cartilage is still too resistant to folding, then a small section of posterior perichondrium is removed and the cartilage is subsequently thinned using a diamond burr.

Once the cartilage is sufficiently pliable, the placement of 3–5 mattress sutures is performed. These sutures are arranged in a radial fashion on the anterior aspect of the ear (Fig. 12-7). A 26-gauge needle is placed anteriorly to posteriorly, parallel to the proposed site of the new antihelix. The tip of the needle is touched with a cotton applicator soaked with a dye solution, such as brilliant green, prior to withdrawal. Further punctures are performed as demonstrated, in order that the position of the mattress sutures on the posterior aspect of the auricular cartilage be clearly demarcated. The most superior suture should be placed more in a superoanterior direction than in a straight superior direction, in order to avoid a postoperative "pointed ear" appearance.

A permanent, clear or white suture is used. Four-zero white mersilene, 4-0 clear nylon, or 4-0 white cotton is acceptable. A noncutting needle is preferred, in order to avoid damaging the cartilage. The needle is passed through the posterior perichondrium,

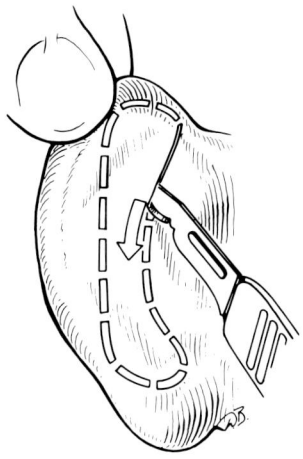

Fig. 12-4 A dumbbell-shaped ellipse of skin measuring 0.5–1.5 cm is outlined and excised. The skin and subcutaneous tissues are removed, leaving the posterior perichondrium intact. Hemostasis is achieved with cautery. The removal of the dumbbell-shaped skin enables the surgeon to bring back further the superior aspect of the auricle as well as the lobule to avoid a "telephone ear." In the case of excessive protrusion of the lobule on creating a new antihelix, wider excision of skin can be accomplished in the inferior portion of the incision. A W-plasty is helpful.

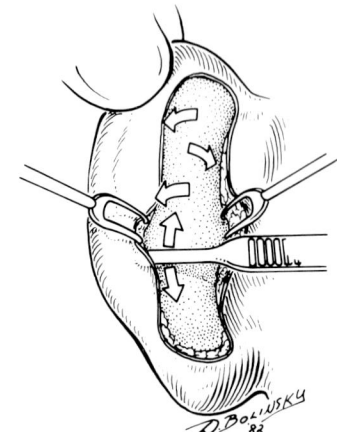

Fig. 12-5 The skin flaps are raised above the perichondrium anteriorly to the helical rim and posteriorly to the junction of the concha on the mastoid periosteum.

the full thickness of the cartilage, and the anterior perichondrium, avoiding the anterior auricular skin (Fig. 12-8). After it is advanced under the anterior auricular skin for 5–6 mm, it is brought back through these three layers. The second arm of the mattress suture is then placed in the opposite direction on the other side of the antihelical fold. Each suture is snugged down and inspected. If it provides the appropriate effect on the new antihelix, then the ends of the suture are temporarily held with a clamp while the remainder of the sutures are placed.

After all the sutures are placed, they are snugged down and the newly fashioned auricle is inspected. The cauda helicis may be partially removed at this stage if the lobule is protruding excessively. Beginning with the most inferior suture, the mattress sutures are tied (Fig. 12-9). The amount of tension with which each is tied depends upon the amount of auricular deformity present. A distance of 16–18 mm from the mastoid skin to the auricle is desired.

After meticulous hemostasis is achieved, the wound is closed with interrupted 5-0 nylon sutures. If necessary, a rubber drain may be used. Cotton impregnated with

Fig. 12.6 Fish-scaling of the posterior layer of perichondrium and full thickness of the cartilage done with a No. 15 Bard-Parker blade or a Holmes' cartilage knife. The Beaver blade also serves this purpose very well. It is important not to penetrate the anterior auricular skin. The area of fish-scaling should be centered around the centerline of the antihelix and the superior crus. The area of fish-scaling can be extended laterally or medially in order to achieve the desired "break" of the existing cartilage spring. If the cartilage is too thick or resistant to folding, a diamond burr may be used to thin the cartilage after a small section of the perichondrium has been stripped away.

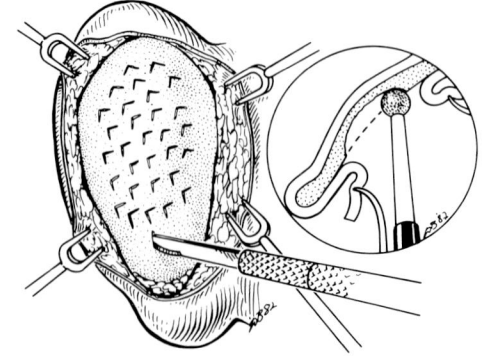

Otoplasty

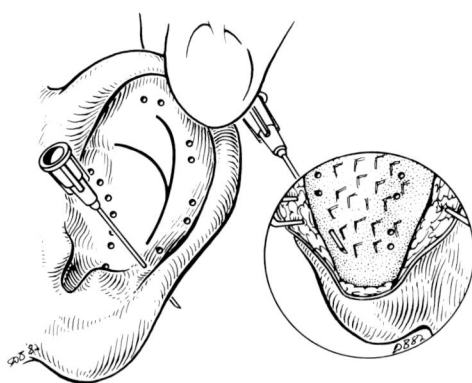

Fig. 12-7 The placement of three to five mattress sutures is planned. The position of the proposed mattress sutures is outlined in a radial fashion on the anterior aspect of the ear. With the use of a small No. 26 needle, through-and-through punctures are then made on either side of the centerline of the desired antihelical fold. The needle is introduced anteroposteriorly, passing through the anterior auricular skin, anterior perichondrium, cartilage, and posterior perichondrium. The tip of the needle is touched with a cotton applicator soaked with a dye solution prior to withdrawal. On withdrawal of the needle, the desired position for the mattress sutures is stained on the posterior perichondrium. When marking the position for the most superior suture, it is important to place it such that the curve of the newly created antihelix is more in a superoanterior direction rather than in a straight superior direction. This avoids a "pointed ear" appearance.

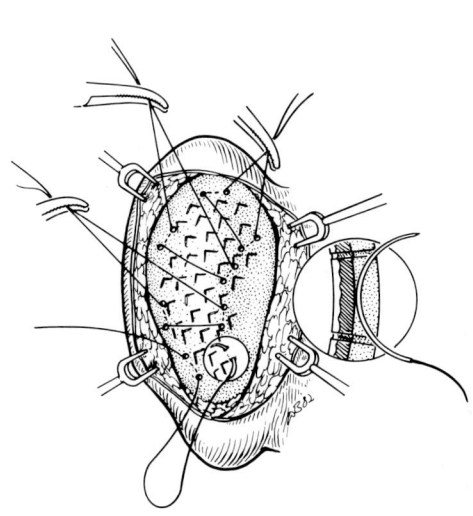

Fig. 12-8 Either 4-0 white mersilene, 4-0 clear nylon, or 4-0 white cotton can be used for these mattress sutures. A noncutting needle is preferred in order to avoid damaging the cartilage. The needle pierces the posterior perichondrium, the full thickness of the cartilage, and the anterior perichondrium, avoiding the anterior auricular skin. It is advanced underneath the anterior auricular skin for 5–6 mm and then passed through all the three layers again posteriorly. After this arm of the horizontal mattress suture is completed, the same motion is performed in the opposite direction on the other side of the antihelical fold guided by the correct dye indicator marks. As each mattress suture is placed, each should be temporarily snugged down to show its effect on the antihelix. An improperly placed suture should be removed at this time and replaced. When a mattress suture has been placed correctly, the ends of the suture are temporarily held with a mosquito clamp. It is important not to tie the sutures until all the sutures have been properly placed.

Fig. 12-9 By temporarily snugging down all the sutures, if it is felt that the lobule protrudes, the sutures are loosened and the caudal helix is dissected and partially removed. Partial or complete removal of the caudal helix will prevent protrusion of the lobule. When the surgeon is satisfied that the sutures are properly placed, beginning with the most inferior suture, they are tied with four to five square knots. The tension of the sutures vary depending on the deformity and the desired result. The auricle should be adjusted so that it lies 16–18 mm from the skin overlying the mastoid.

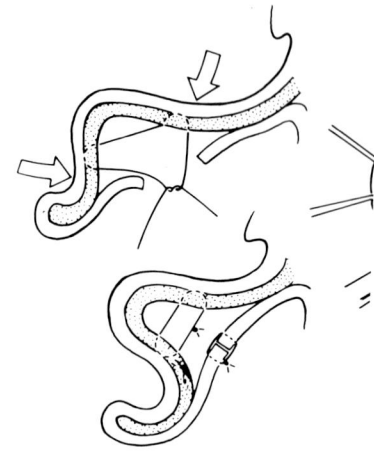

bacitracin is placed between the convolutions of the auricle, and a pressure dressing is applied. The ears are first inspected at 48 hours to check for hematoma formation. A similar pressure dressing is placed for an additional 7–10 days. An elastic headband is used to splint the ears for a total of 4–6 weeks. Prophylactic antibiotics are used for 1 week postoperatively.

CARTILAGE SPLITTING OTOPLASTY

Anesthesia, prepping, draping, and the administration of local anesthesia may be performed for cartilage splitting otoplasty as described for the fish-scaling technique.

The ear is folded into a normal position. If a large concha is present, then the inferior part of the fold is made through the conchal cartilage. Using 25-gauge needles,

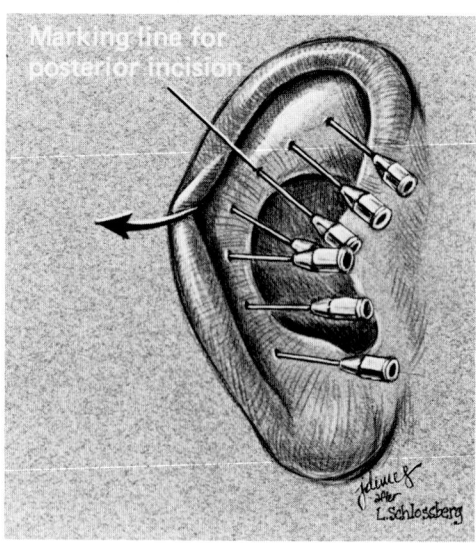

Fig. 12-10 Marking the position of proposed anti-helix.

Otoplasty

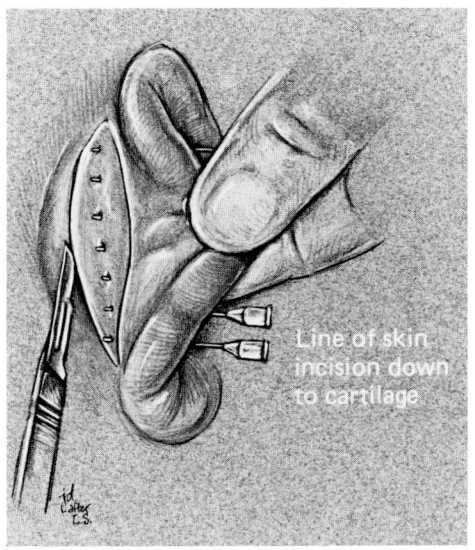

Fig. 12-11 Line of skin incision down to cartilage.

the apex of the antihelix is penetrated (Fig. 12-10). The ends of the needles are touched with marking dye and withdrawn. The site for excision of skin posteriorly is thus outlined (Fig. 12-11). An elliptical piece of skin is marked, approximately 1 cm in width. This may be adapted to an hourglass-shaped skin excision if there is a prominent ear lobe.

The cut is made through skin, subcutaneous tissues, and perichondrium, and the wedge of skin is removed. The skin and perichondrium are undermined to reveal the cauda helicis, fossa antihelicis scapha, and the conchal cartilage. An incision is then made with a Cottle knife through the posterior perichondrium and the full thickness of the cartilage along the previously demarcated neoantihelical line (Fig. 12-12). Care is taken to maintain the integrity of the anterior perichondrium. The superior end of the incision approaches, but does not encroach upon, the helix. Figure 13 demonstrates the relationship of this cut to the auricular cartilage landmarks.

The cauda helicis is removed. This helps to eliminate postoperative bowing of the lobule. Triangular wedges are removed perpendicular to the superior and inferior edges of the cut (Fig. 12-13).

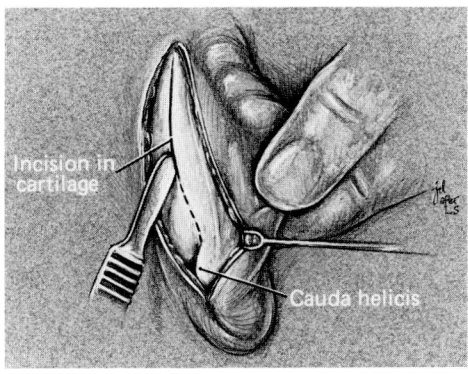

Fig. 12-12 Incision in cartilage exposing cauda helicis.

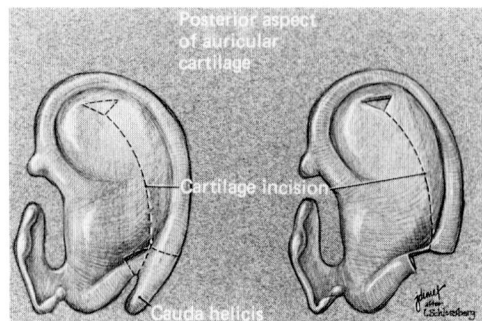

Fig. 12-13 Posterior aspect of auricular cartilage.

At this point, the lateral segment of cartilage is attached to its medial counterpart only at the superior rim. The perichondrium is dissected off of the anterior surface of the cartilage with an elevator for a distance of 1 cm (Fig. 12-14). The anterior surface of the medial cartilage is then beveled. This can be accomplished with a razor blade, a wire brush, or a diamond burr (Fig. 12-15). Beveling is continued until a round, smooth neoantihelix and superior crus are formed. Similarly, the anterior surface of the lateral cartilage is beveled. The medial beveled cartilage is placed anterior to the lateral cartilage, restoring the normal contour to the ear (Fig. 12-16).

No sutures are placed in the cartilage. The skin is closed with a running subcuticular layer of prolene or nylon. A pressure dressing is applied using wet cotton to form the desired contour, followed by cotton fluffs and cling gauze. This dressing is left in place for 2 days, at which time the ears are inspected. A second pressure dressing is applied for an additional 2 days. This is then removed, and an Ace bandage is left in place for a week.

Variations

In patients who have a deeply cupped concha, mattress sutures may be placed from the conchal perichondrium to the mastoid fascia. Three-zero clear or white permanent sutures are used for this. Care must be taken to prevent over-rotation of the concha anteriorly, with subsequent encroachment upon the external auditory canal. In the presence of an excessively large concha cartilage, a crescentric piece of cartilage may be removed anteromedially to the center line of the antihelix (Fig. 12-17). Burring of the cut edges with a diamond burr will prevent sharp edges postoperatively. The cartilage edges are then reapproximated.

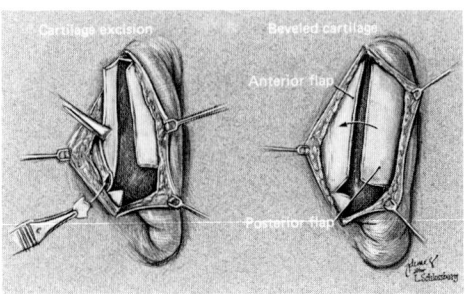

Fig. 12-14 Cartilage excision.

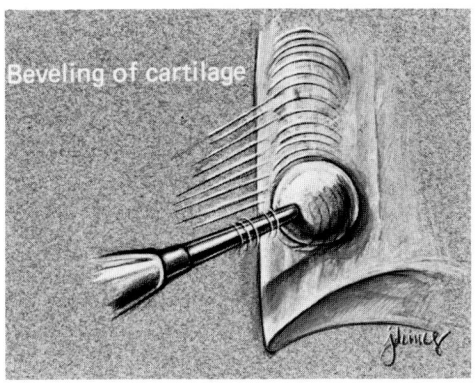

Fig. 12-15 Beveling of cartilage.

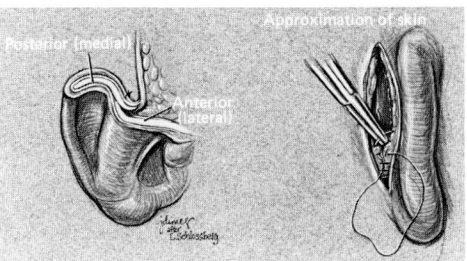

Fig. 12-16 Closing the incision.

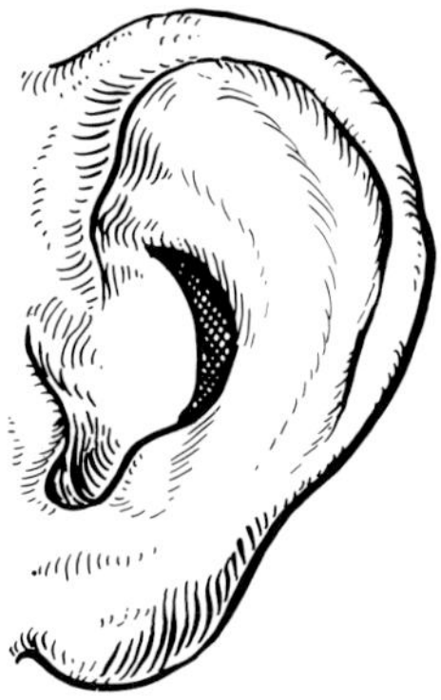

Fig. 12-17 In patients who have an excessively large concha cartilage, a crescent of concha cartilage can be removed. The crescent of the concha cartilage is to be removed from the area of the concha just anteromedial to the centerline of the antihelix. Whenever cartilage incisions are made, it is important to avoid producing sharp, unnatural edges. This can be minimized by proper cartilage thinning with the diamond burr, as well as meticulous approximation of the cartilage edges.

CONCLUSION

These techniques offer versatility and reliability in the correction of lop ear deformities. The fish-scaling technique produces weakening of the cartilage to the point of malleability in order that the mattress sutures may recreate the antihelix without tension. The cartilage splitting otoplasty is based upon the principle that by burring or beveling one surface of the cartilage, a smooth, round contour is gradually achieved. The latter result is independent of the placement of sutures, eliminating suture extrusion as a potential complication. One must always be concerned about hematoma formation when the anterior perichondrium is dissected off of the cartilage, but with careful dressing of the ears, this has not been a problem.

REFERENCES

1. Mustarde J: Correction of prominent ears using simple mattress sutures. Br J Plast Surg 16:170–179, 1963
2. Mustarde J: Correction of prominent ears using buried mattress sutures. Clin Plast Surg 5:459–464, 1978
3. Furnas D: Correction of prominent ears by concha-mastoid sutures. Plast Reconstr Surg 42:189–193, 1968
4. Spira M, McCrea R, Gerow F, et al: Correction of the principal deformities causing protruding ears. Plast Reconstr Surg 44:150–154, 1969
5. Tardy ME: Otoplasty. Otolaryngol Clin North Am 10:231–236, 1977
6. Tardy ME, Tenta L, Pastorek N: Mattress suture otoplasty: Indications and limitations. Laryngoscope 79:961–968, 1969
7. Templer J, Thomas JR, David W: Otoplasty. Ear Nose Throat J 60:97–101, 1981
8. Baumgartner P: A technical hint for the correction of prominent ears, based on the method of converse. Plast Reconstr Surg 37:66–68, 1966
9. Cloutier AM: Correction of outstanding ears. Plast Reconstr Surg 28:412–416, 1961
10. Dingman R, Peled I: Corrective cosmetic otoplasty: A simple and accurate technique. Ann Plast Surg 3:250–252, 1979
11. Manning B, Finger R, Dibbell D: Diamond burr otoplasty. Ann Plast Surg 11:114–120, 1983
12. McDowell A: Goals in otoplasty for protruding ears. Plast Reconstr Surg 47:17–27, 1968
13. Musgrave R: A variation on the correction of the congenital lop ear. Plast Reconstr Surg 37:394–398, 1966
14. Nachlas NE, Duncan D, Trail M: Otoplasty. Arch Otolaryngol 91:44–49, 1970
15. Stenstrom S, Heftner J: The Stenstrom otoplasty. Clin Plast Surg 5:465–470, 1978
16. Tanzer R, Bellucci R, Converse J, et al: Deformities of the auricle. In J Converse (Ed.): Reconstructive Plastic Surgery (vol. 3). Philadelphia: WB Saunders, pp. 1671–1773, 1977
17. Luckett W: A new operation for prominent ears based on the anatomy of the deformity. Surg Gynecol Obstet 10:635–637, 1910
18. Lee KJ, Hausfeld JN: Otoplasty. In Lee KJ (Ed.): Comprehensive Surgical Atlases in Otolaryngology and Head and Neck Surgery. New York City: Grune & Stratton, 1984

Ronald H. Hirokawa
Richard C. Bryarly

13
Blepharoplasty

Included in the repertoire of office or ambulatory surgical procedures are the facial cosmetic operations. As the cost of living has increased over the years, correspondent to this rise is the increased cost of medical care. The cost of cosmetic facial plastic procedures must generally be borne entirely by the patient. Fortunately, instrumentation, medications—such as anesthetics and sedatives—and the surgical procedures have improved to the extent that physicians can now perform many of these delicate procedures in an ambulatory care facility. This allows physicians to offer these procedures to patients who would benefit from them, and yet to maintain affordability, as well as optimal health care. As in most ambulatory care centers, the general good health of the patient is a primary prerequisite. Any underlying medical conditions should be well controlled preoperatively.

The preoperative evaluation of the patient is therefore of utmost importance to uncover any factors which may complicate the procedure, to evaluate the patient as to outlook and goal for the intended procedures, and to obtain an informed consent so that there will be no misunderstanding following these procedures. In outpatient or ambulatory surgery, the office visit is often the last encounter with the patient prior to the actual surgery.

Blepharoplasty, or plastic surgery of the eyelids, is a key procedure in restoring a more youthful appearance to the eyelids and face. Other factors which contribute to the aging of the face are eyebrow ptosis, furrowing of the skin, and jowl formation. Regarding the eyelids, two conditions that are considered to contribute to the aging process are blepharochalasis and dermatochalasis.

Blepharochalasis refers to the relaxation of the eyelids. This condition is found primarily in the young individual, usually female. It is a deficiency of, or relaxation of, the supporting structures of the eyelid secondary to recurrent edema. There may be orbital fat herniation. The condition is often found in members of the same family, and it primarily affects the upper eyelids.

Dermatochalasis, or laxity of the skin of the eyelids, is a disorder affecting the middle or older age individuals more commonly than does blepharochalasis. The eyelids are "baggy," with an abundance of skin. There may be a weakening of the orbital septum with herniation of fat. The process is seen in the upper and lower eyelids and is found in both males and females. Factors which may contribute to this problem are heredity, eyelid infections, thyroid disorders, and allergy.

ANATOMY

Anatomically, there is a combination of relaxed and redundant skin, as well as "herniated" or pseudoherniated orbital fat. The upper lid contains 3 areas of fat pockets. The medial pocket often contains fat which is slightly different from that in the remaining areas; the fat of the medial compartment is somewhat whiter and less vascular. The lateral pocket contains the lacrimal gland and caution should be taken when considering fat excision from this lateral pocket, due to the potential injury of the lacrimal apparatus. The lower eyelids contain 3 distinct areas of fat and these must be separately evaluated and approached.

PREOPERATIVE EVALUATION

In the process of evaluating the patient for possible facial cosmetic surgery and, specifically, eyelid procedures, one must not only determine the physical and technical concerns of the transformation, but must also evaluate the patient from the standpoint of emotional and medical candidacy. It is extremely important to determine the patient's expectations and relate the improvements which can be expected realistically. This will be valuable to the eventual satisfaction of both the patient and surgeon. One should investigate for underlying ophthalmologic problems: xerophthalmia (dry eye), previous ophthalmologic surgery, or orbital conditions, such as exophthalmos secondary to thyroid disease. It has been reported that a patient may be unaware of a visual disturbance prior to surgery and then become aware of such a disturbance after the procedure has been performed. This causes much concern for both surgeon and patient and has significant medico-legal implication. Should there be any concern as to the patient's visual function, an ophthalmologist should be consulted. Bleeding disorders, hypertension, and metabolic disorders which may lead to ophthalmologic disturbances should be evaluated. Preoperative photography is essential; this is helpful not only in determining what techniques should be utilized, but also for medico-legal purposes. One should also discuss with the patient the possibility of revisional surgery.

In addition, at the time of the preoperative evaluation, one should consider ancillary techniques that may be of benefit to the patient in attaining the goals that both the patient and the surgeon are striving to accomplish, such as brow lift for eyebrow ptosis, chemabrasion of furrows of facial skin, and facelift procedures.

EYEBROW PTOSIS AND EYELID PTOSIS

There are two associated deformities which should be mentioned in conjunction with upper eyelid blepharoplasty: eyebrow ptosis, which may be noted in conjunction with or separate from upper eyelid dermatochalasis; and eyelid ptosis. Eyebrow ptosis may easily be misinterpreted as blepharochalasis. The results of blepharoplasty alone in these cases will result in dissatisfaction to both the patient and surgeon. This problem can be approached by the excision of the suprabrow skin. This is generally removed by using a curvilinear elliptical pattern, with the widest resection at the lateralmost border (Fig. 13-1). The closure then elevates the eyebrow, primarily in the lateral aspect. The incision which is made along the upper cilia of the eyebrow should be angled or slanted in an upward direction parallel to the hair shafts to avoid transecting the hair follicles. Closure is performed by approximating the deep tissue with a nonabsorbable suture—this attaches the subcutaneous and muscular tissue. One should avoid direct attachment of the skin and eyebrow to the periosteum, as this will fix the eyebrow. The skin is approximated with the use of 6-0 nylon. This procedure, if performed in conjunction with temporal rhytidectomy or complete rhytidectomy, may be modified by removing the ellipse of skin in the temporal scalp instead of in the immediate suprabrow area. This avoids placing a scar in the visible forehead area. A technique of percutaneous suturing of the eyebrow to the superior frontal periosteum using a Keeth needle and nonabsorbable suture will provide the results desired and eliminate the forehead scar.

The second concern, which may be found in several patients, is eyelid ptosis, which should be noted preoperatively, and which generally presents as asymmetry of the upper eyelids. The etiology is generally a separation of the levator aponeurosis from the tarsus. The procedure for reapproximating the levator to the tarsus can be performed at the same time as blepharoplasty.

LOWER EYELID TONE

Lower eyelid tone should be evaluated during the preoperative assessment. This is achieved by pinching the lower eyelid and retracting it. Upon release, the lower lid should snap back into position against the globe. If the response is not immediate and complete, one should consider the lower lid tone poor. This is a dramatic finding in

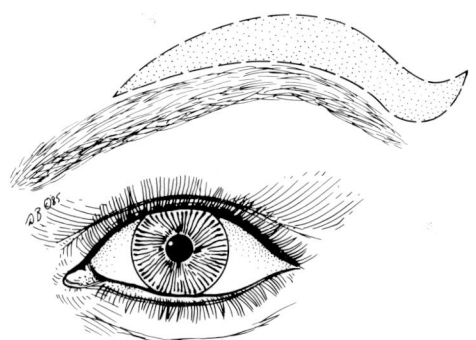

Fig. 13-1. Suprabrow curvilinear elliptical incision.

those patients with involutional ectropion and will be subtle in those patients with incipient ectropion.

The techniques used to correct this problem may be performed in conjunction with the blepharoplasty. One such procedure is the horizontal shortening procedure. In this procedure, after fat excision but prior to skin excision and closure, a vertical wedge of full-thickness lower lid is removed at the junction of the middle one-third and the lateral one-third of the lid. The first incision is made at the junction of the mid and lateral one-third of the lid. The medial segment is then grasped and retracted laterally. The overlap is then determined, with the excess excised. Closure is then performed with 6-0 silk in 3 positions: at the tarsal plate or grey line, at the mucocutaneous junction, and at the lash line. The sutures are left slightly long in order that they may be retracted anteriorly and tied under one of the skin sutures. This maneuver is to displace the suture ends anteriorly and away from the eye. The remaining incision is closed with 4-0 chromic or vicryl suture.

A variation of the horizontal lid shortening procedure is the excision of the lateral aspect of the lower lid (Fig. 13-2). The incision line in this case would be made as a continuation of the curvature of the upper lid, transecting the inferior portion of the lateral canthal tendon. After the excess skin, tarsus, and conjunctiva are excised, closure is performed by placing a nonabsorbable suture from the tarsus to a point on the medial aspect of the orbital rim approximately 4 mm behind the margin of the rim. This suture essentially replaces the transected lateral canthal tendon. Closure is then continued in the above-described fashion.

This procedure is designed to improve lower lid tension, avoid ectropion, and improve the problem of epiphora, all of which are associated with involutional ectropion.

ANESTHESIA

Anesthesia during facial cosmetic surgery may be local or general anesthesia, or a combination of local with intravenous sedation. There are many advantages to local anesthesia. The avoidance of endotracheal intubation eliminates the distortion of the oral area. Local anesthesia also avoids the risks of the general anesthetic, albeit small. The patient if awake is able to perform helpful movements which allow for the dynamic evaluation of the results of certain techniques.

Preoperative medications for patients having local anesthesia should include a sedative and a narcotic. Pentobarbital 100 mg given intramuscularly approximately 1½ hours prior to surgery is an excellent sedative, and meperidine 75 mg with hydroxyzine

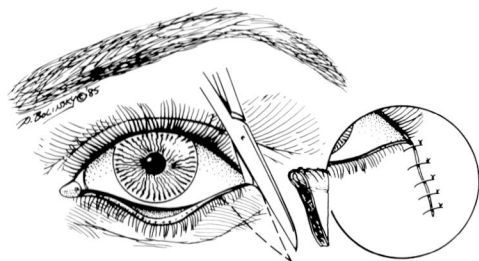

Fig. 13-2. Variation of the horizontal lid shortening procedure.

25 mg is a good narcotic-antiemetic combination. In addition, during the procedure, intravenous sedation may be continuously administered by the anesthesiologist.

Due to difficulties with the preparation of the skin at the time of surgery, it is the authors' routine to have the patient shower and shampoo with a bactericidal soap such as Hibiclens (Stuart), Betadine (Purdue Frederick), or pHisoHex (Winthrop), as part of the preoperative routine prior to going to the operating room.

SURGICAL TECHNIQUES

There are two basic techniques to be utilized depending on the patient's age and probable findings. It has been the authors' experience that, although age is a factor, the condition of the skin and the pseudoherniation of the orbital fat will determine which approach one will take. In performing a four-lid blepharoplasty, one would approach the upper lids first. This is to obtain symmetry of the upper lids and then judge what is needed to complement this procedure with the lower lid procedure.

UPPER LID BLEPHAROPLASTY

Upper eyelid blepharoplasty is approached in a similar fashion in the young person and the older individual, the variable being the amount of fat to be removed. The marking for excision of the upper lid skin is best done prior to the injection of local anesthetic for the most accurate marking of the skin (Fig. 13-3). The basic guideline is the lid crease, which should be approximately 8–10 mm above and parallel to the lash line. This should extend from the punctum, the medial border, to the lateral canthus, laterally. Should redundant skin be excessive, the medial margin may be extended superomedially and a small triangle removed; laterally, one would extend a curvilinear incision in a superolateral direction, attempting to stay within the margins of the orbital rim. A helpful technique in determining the crease line is to have the patient open and close the eyelids while slight tension is placed on the upper eyelid skin. The crease becomes evident as the patient opens and closes the eyes.

The upper border of the skin incision is determined by "pinching" the upper lid skin with a blunt forceps, placing one tine along the lid crease marking and the opposite tine superior to the crease in an attempt to approximate the two incision lines, bunching

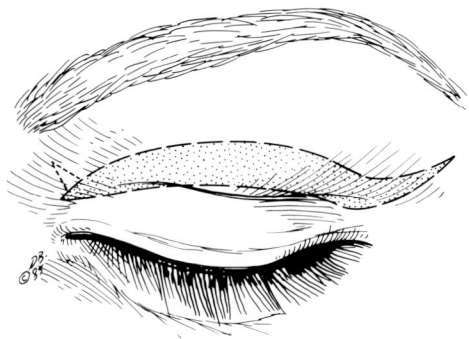

Fig. 13-3. Marking of upper lid incision.

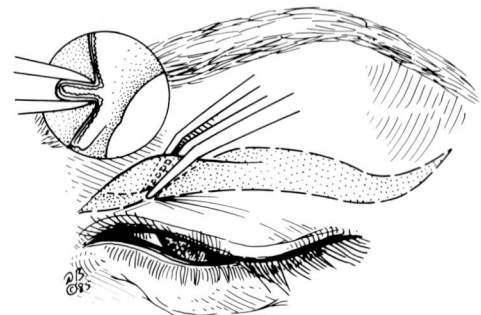

Fig. 13-4. The upper border of the skin incision is determined by "pinching" the upper lid skin with blunt forceps.

together the skin which is to be excised (Fig. 13-4). The patient should have approximately 1–2 mm of lagophthalmos with this maneuver while in the supine position.

Following the marking of the skin outline, injection is performed with approximately 1–1.5 cc of local anesthetic with 1:100,000 epinephrine. One should avoid injection of this anesthetic into the muscle in order to avoid hematoma formation. Injection of too large a volume of anesthetic will cause ballooning of the skin and distort the anatomy. After a period of about 10 minutes, the incision is made with a #15 scalpel blade. The skin is then elevated and dissected with the use of forceps and scalpel blade or sharp scissors. One should be cautious of inadvertent injury and resection of the muscle underlying the skin. In appropriate cases, one might consider removal of a narrow strip of orbicularis muscle to enhance the lid crease.

Hemostasis is obtained with battery-powered cautery or bipolar cautery at low setting. One should avoid indiscriminate use of the cautery, as this has been implicated in disturbance of visual acuity. If fat excision is considered appropriate, a small horizontal incision is made through the orbicularis muscle and the orbital septum and dissection performed with the iris scissors exposing the orbital fat. The "buttonhole" technique, which exposes small areas of fat by small, slit-like incisions in the orbital septum, is preferable to the "open sky" method, although the exposure is slightly more limited. (Fig. 13-5). The "open sky" method implies a horizontal incision made through the entire length of the orbital septum, exposing the orbital fat (Fig. 13-6). The orbital fat is then teased through the incision with the use of cotton tipped applicators and forceps while pressure is gently placed on the globe. The volume of fat to be excised is determined in part during the preoperative evaluation as well as during the intraoperative

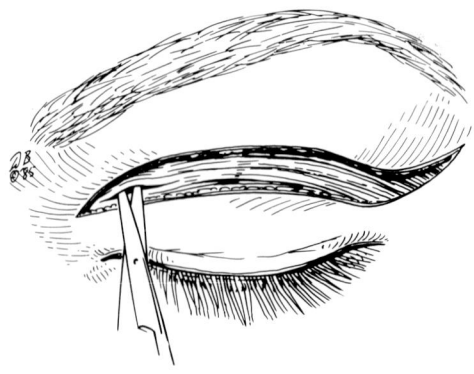

Fig. 13-5. The "buttonhole" technique exposes small areas of fat by small, slit-like incisions in the orbital septum.

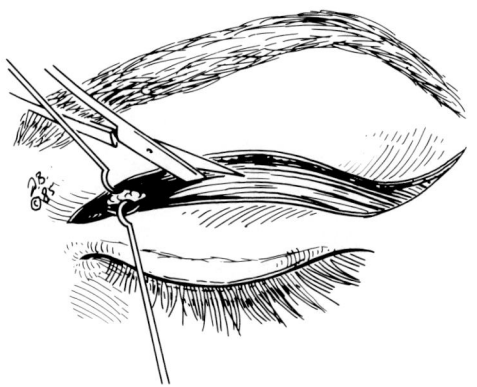

Fig. 13-6. The "open sky" method implies a horizontal incision made through the entire length of the orbital septum.

direct visualization of the bulging or pseudoherniation of the fat. The primary pockets from which the fat should be excised are the medial and middle. The lateral pocket should be avoided, due to the location of the lacrimal gland. Prominence in the lateral area may well be a ptotic lacrimal gland. The unwary surgeon could easily create a difficult situation by resecting or damaging this gland and thus interfering with tear production.

A hemostat can be used to clamp the fatty tissue and then the mass can be excised with cauterization at the base of the hemostat (Fig. 13-7). Many surgeons prefer to dissect the fat with forceps and scissors, thereby isolating the individual blood vessels and cauterizing them as the dissection progresses. This avoids the use of a hemostat and "blind" transection of vessels is kept at a minimum. Vessels may retract into the orbit and later bleed, causing increased orbital pressure.

Following the fat excision, should the lid crease require enhancement, a 3-4 mm strip of orbicularis muscle may be excised just superior to the lower incision (Fig. 13-8). The lower margin of the muscle can then be approximated to the levator aponeurosis, enhancing the lid crease. Following these procedures, a cottonoid soaked in the local anesthetic may be applied to the area while the opposite upper lid is operated upon.

Closure of the incision is then performed. Should supratarsal fixation be desired, this should be performed at this time, suturing through the skin and supratarsal tissues

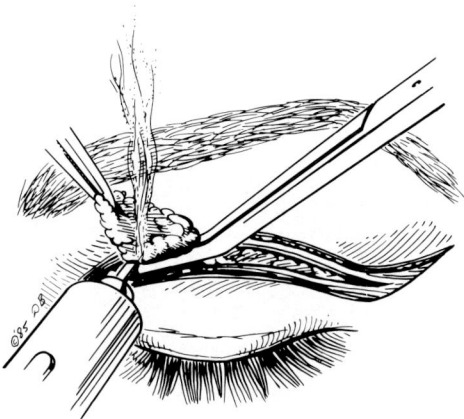

Fig. 13-7. A hemostat can be used to clamp the fatty tissue and the mass excised with cauterization at the surface of the hemostat.

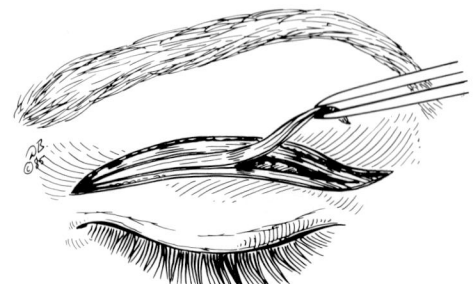

Fig. 13-8. A 3–4 mm strip of orbicularis muscle may be excised.

of the levator aponeurosis. One should avoid suturing to the orbital septum, for this may fix the eyelids in an open position. The skin is then approximated with interrupted 6:0 nylon in the lateral aspect of the upper lid incision. A subcuticular running monofilament 5-0 or 6-0 nylon may be used for the medial two-thirds of the incision (Fig. 13-9). Antibiotic ointment such as Bacitracin Ophthalmic (Upjohn) or Decadron (Merck Sharp & Dohme) ophthalmic ointment may then be applied. No dressing is required.

LOWER LID BLEPHAROPLASTY

Lower eyelid blepharoplasty is slightly more complex and difficult than the upper eyelid procedures, due to the fact that the orbicularis oculi muscle fibers insert directly into the fascia of the lower eyelid skin. There is a slight difference in approaching those patients whose primary problem is herniation of fat as opposed to redundant skin. In general, this can be thought of as the young patient versus the middle-aged and older-age patient, respectively. Young individuals require minimal skin excision.

The approach for removal of fat with minimal skin excision is the musculocutaneous flap. For situations in which there is a moderate amount of excess skin to be excised, the musculocutaneous flap may also be used; however, in addition, a skin flap dissection may be required to isolate and resect the excess skin.

The incision line is made 1–2 mm below the lash margin and parallel to it, with the medial extent being at the lower punctum (Fig. 13-10). Laterally, as one approaches the canthal angle, one may vary the extent of the incision, depending upon the amount of skin to be excised. Those with excessive skin require that the lateral aspect of the incision be angled in an inferior direction, parallel to or within one of the laugh lines or "crow's feet" for approximately 1 cm in length.

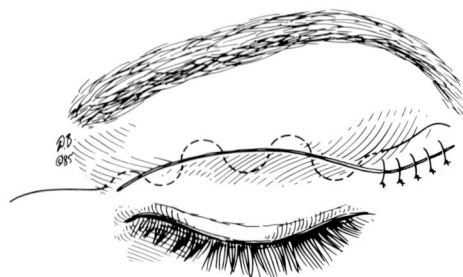

Fig. 13-9. Skin closure.

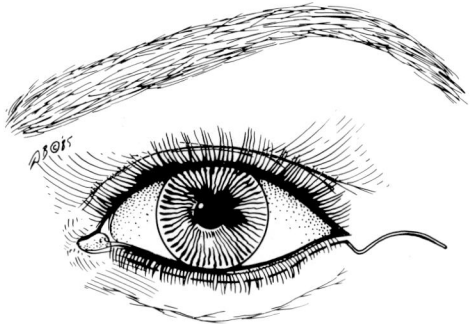

Fig. 13-10. Lower lid incision.

Following the outline, the lower eyelid is injected with the local anesthetic, with a small amount to be injected into the infraorbital neurovascular bundle. A stab incision is then made through the skin with a #15 scalpel blade in the lateral aspect over the orbital rim. Using a sharp, straight scissors, such as an iris scissors, the incision is made by placing one blade under the skin with the other blade above the skin (Fig. 13-11). As the scissors are advanced, the skin is dissected in the subcutaneous plane and incised. Caution should be taken to avoid cutting the eyelashes. It is technically difficult to use a scalpel blade to perform this incision, due to the pliability of the skin being incised, and the concern for the globe beneath the lid.

Following the completion of the incision, attention is again turned to the stab incision which was performed laterally over the orbital rim. Small, blunt scissors are then used to dissect just superficial to the periosteum of the inferior orbital rim (Fig. 13-12). Thus, this tunnel is created under the orbicularis oculi muscle and superficial to the orbital septum. With double-pronged skin hooks to retract the skin margin in an inferior direction, blunt scissors are used to connect the tunnel with the skin incision (Fig. 13-13). This maneuver is most simply performed by placing one blade of the scissors into the tunnel, while the opposite blade follows along the skin incision. The skin-muscle (musculocutaneous) flap is thus created. Hemostasis is obtained with the cautery. At this point, the fat pockets are exposed. The fat excision is then performed in a fashion similar to that used for the upper lid. The majority of fat excised from the lower lid is in the lateral compartment, with smaller amounts in the middle and medial pockets.

To determine the amount of skin to be excised, one should retract the skin-muscle flap with a slight amount of tension in a superior and lateral direction. At this point, the patient is asked to open the mouth and gaze in an upward direction. This causes slight

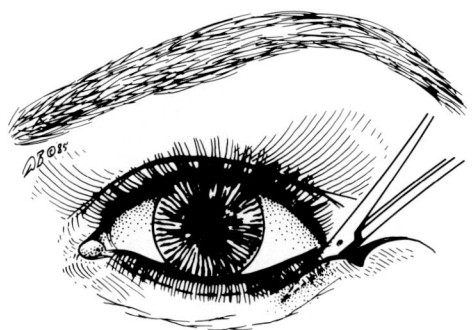

Fig. 13-11. The skin is incised in the subcutaneous plane as the scissors are advanced.

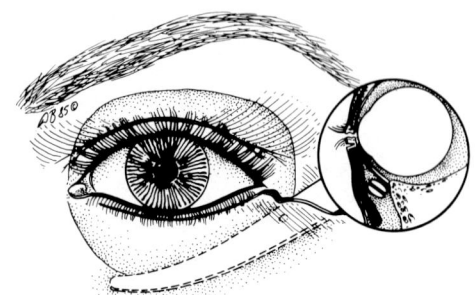

Fig. 13-12. Small blunt scissors are used to dissect just superficial to the periosteum of the inferior orbital rim, following completion of the incision.

countertraction on the flap in an inferior direction. The amount of skin overlap still remaining can safely be excised without significant concern of excising too much skin (Fig. 13-14). The skin is then excised in 2 triangles: a long, narrow triangle under the lash line with its base facing the lateral canthus, and a smaller triangle at the lateral aspect of the incision.

One may note at this point that the margin of the skin flap may now appear quite thick relative to the skin of the lash side of the incision. This is due to the increasing muscle thickness of the beveled edge of the inferior flap. In order to correct this discrepancy, the muscle along the margin should be trimmed in a gently angled fashion. The skin edges should now be of similar thickness to avoid the appearance of a step-up or roll.

To begin closure, a key suture is placed at the lateral canthus. This will hold the inferior medial margin in close approximation. Often, the medial aspect of the incision will not require sutures. The lateral aspect of the incision is then closed with interrupted 6-0 nylon sutures (Fig. 13-15).

As a general rule, the width of the skin excised in the lower lid should be no more than 5–6 mm, and often one will not require any skin excision.

POSTOPERATIVE CARE

Postoperatively, the patients are placed at bedrest at home for 48 hours. The head is kept in an elevated position at an angle of approximately 30°. Visual acuity is checked periodically. Antitussives and antiemetics are used to control coughing and nausea and vomiting. The incision lines are coated with an antibiotic ophthalmic ointment. This minimizes crust formation and reduces the development of blepharitis. No dressing is required, although some surgeons use a light dressing of eyepads.

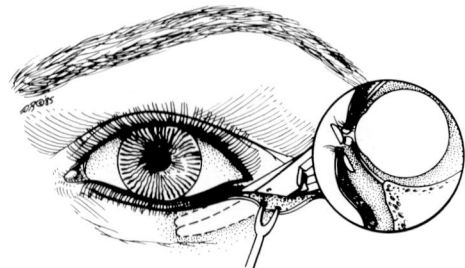

Fig. 13-13. Double-prong skin hooks are used to retract the skin margin in an inferior direction, blunt scissors are used to connect the tunnel with the skin incision.

Blepharoplasty

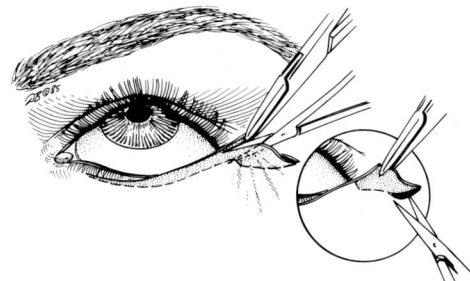

Fig. 13-14. The skin is excised in 2 triangles: a long, narrow triangle under the lash line with its base facing the lateral canthus, and a smaller triangle at the lateral aspect of the incision.

The interrupted sutures are removed on the third or fourth postoperative day and the subcuticular sutures removed on the fifth or sixth postoperative day. At this time, sterile adhesive strips may be used to maintain tension on the lateral suture line.

COMPLICATIONS

As in any surgical procedure, there is a risk of an undesirable event or result which is considered a complication. The complications that are common to all surgical procedures are anesthetic drug reactions, infection, and bleeding. Infection is a relatively uncommon complication of blepharoplasty, due to the good blood supply of the face and the periorbital region. Drug reactions are unpredictable in most cases and one must be continually aware of their potential occurrence and be prepared for their treatment.

Hemorrhage from the wound edges and hematoma formation are known to occur and are best treated preventively by good hemostasis during surgery. Should bleeding be active in the immediate postoperative period, one should consider reopening the incisions and locating and cauterizing the bleeding point. A hematoma, if it is first noted during the postoperative period, is best observed. After several days, the clot will liquefy. This is the time it may be readily drained.

Orbital or retro-orbital hemorrhage may cause increased orbital pressure and, if the pressure is uncontrolled, may lead to blindness due to arterial or venous compression with obstruction of the vascular supply to the retina.

Careful investigation should be made in the preoperative evaluation for a bleeding diathesis. This would include knowledge of medications used, such as aspirin and anticoagulants. Hypertension should be investigated and controlled. Routine preoperative testing should include a platelet estimate, a PT (prothrombin time), and a PTT (partial thromboplastin time).

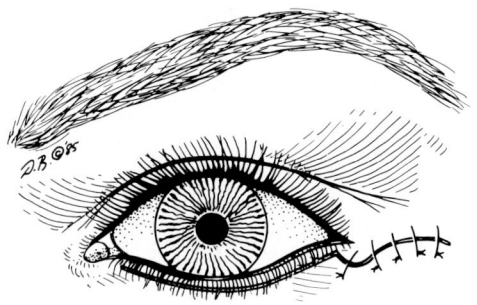

Fig. 13-15. The lateral aspect of the incision is closed with interrupted 6-0 nylon sutures.

The etiology of retro-orbital bleeding would include laceration of a vessel during deep injection and transection or laceration of a vessel during the dissection and excision of orbital fat, with resultant retraction of the vessel into the retro-orbital space, with continued bleedings. The initial treatment is pressure, followed by localizing and cauterizing the vessels. One should be concerned about the patient who complains about deep orbital and ocular pain. Evaluation of visual acuity, and inspection for proptosis, ecchymosis, chemosis, pupil reactivity, and ocular pressures should continue into the postoperative period. An ophthalmologist should be consulted should any question arise regarding increased orbital pressure.

Management should include reopening of the incision and the septum orbitale to inspect for the bleeding vessel and to evacuate a hematoma. Acetazolamide should be administered 500 mg orally and 500 mg intravenously with mannitol 20 percent intravenously at 2 gm/kg body weight over 20 minutes. A lateral canthotomy may be performed by placing a hemostat on the lateral canthal tendon and incising the tendon horizontally with scissors. This will allow the orbital contents to be displaced forward.

An occasional sequela of orbital hematoma is blindness. This dramatic and tragic situation has been known to occur in blepharoplasty. Although rare, blindness has been reported in association with blepharoplasty and without any known causal relationship to other sequelae. One factor which is considered important is the dissection of orbital fat. With this fact in mind, one should avoid pulling or vigorously teasing the fat and obtain meticulous hemostasis. Most surgeons perform a careful preoperative visual acuity evaluation, as some patients may be unaware of a visual disturbance, or may be reluctant to volunteer such information for fear of being turned down from having the surgery. If this information is then made known during the postoperative period, it may be of serious concern to the unprepared surgeon.

Xerophthalmia has been known to occur following blepharoplasty. During the preoperative evaluation, the interview should include questioning about tear function and eye irritation. If there is doubt about tear function, tear production should be assessed by testing using something such as a Shirmer test. Corneal irritation is the primary concern of reduced tear formation. In addition to tear function, lower lid tone and ectropion would also play a role in this form of corneal irritation. This would lead to poor eye coverage and allow for increased exposure with drying. Treatment initially should be conservative, with eye lubricants and taping of the eye closed, especially at night.

Epiphora is also known to occur, especially in the immediate postoperative period. This is usually secondary to lid edema and obstruction of the nasolacrimal apparatus. This should resolve spontaneously over the ensuing 2–3 days. Should this problem persist, one should evaluate the lower lid tone and canaliculus. Ectropion will cause the tears to overflow over the lower lid rather than to be directed into the inferior canaliculus.

Corneal abrasion may occur intraoperatively secondary to drying, especially when general anesthesia is used. An eye shield may be used. It is understood that care should be taken to avoid any direct corneal trauma. In the postoperative period, abrasion may occur from adhesive dressings. Prolonged exposure must be avoided.

Enophthalmos has been seen if too much fat is removed during the procedure. If this is noted at the time of surgery, the fat can be replaced into the orbital space through the septum orbitale. In the postoperative period, this is a very difficult problem to correct.

Wrinkling of the skin is another aspect of this surgery that is very difficult to predict and correct; one should be cautious during the preoperative discussion. Should this be noted as a problem following the surgery, chemabrasion or dermabrasion may be the best alternative method of treatment.

Postoperative ectropion may be temporary or permanent. A discussion of this problem can be found in the preceding discussion regarding the surgical technique and lower lid tone. In the immediate postoperative period, a temporary form of ectropion may be secondary to chemosis. This may be quite effectively treated with topical steroids. Temporary paresis of the orbicularis oculi muscle may also present as ectropion and will later improve as recovery ensues. A more serious and permanent ectropion may be caused by the excision of too much skin: cicatrical ectopion. Should this occur and be noted at the time of surgery, one should replace a portion of the skin that was excised in the form of a full-thickness skin graft. In the postoperative period, one should be conservative in the management. This would include taping of the lower lids in an upward direction, skin massage, and lubricants. If the defect does not respond and appears to be permanent, the incision should be reincised, the flaps undermined, scar bands released, and a full-thickness skin graft applied. Donor sites for lower eyelid skin in their order of preference would include the postauricular skin, the skin from the upper eyelid, the skin from the supraclavicular area or the skin from the inner arm.

Poor lower eyelid tone may contribute to the cicatrical ectropion. In this situation, lower lid tone should be evaluated in the preoperative period and treatment planned during the blepharoplasty. A discussion of this is given above in the section on surgical technique. If this was not appreciated preoperatively, a horizontal shortening procedure may be performed as a second procedure.

Webbing can occur at the ends of the incisions, specifically at the medial and lateral aspects of the upper eyelid. Several precautions that should be observed during an upper eyelid blepharoplasty are that the incision should be no closer than 5-6 mm from the lateral canthus, and that the lower lid incision should be no closer than 3-4 mm to the lateral canthus. Thus, the upper and lower incision should be no closer together than 8–10 mm. If lateral canthal webbing occurs, conservative treatment is again the choice. Observation should be continued for 4-6 months. If the webbing does not improve during this period of time, a Y-to-V plasty should be considered.

At the medial canthus, webbing may occur if the incision is extended beyond the inferior canaliculus and crosses the nasocanthal depression. If this problem does not correct itself after a period of observation, a Z-pasty may be required to correct the problem.

BIBLIOGRAPHY

Beekhuis GJ: Blepharoplasty. Otolaryngol Clin North Am 15:179-194, 1982
Beyer-Machule CK: Plastic and Reconstructive Surgery of the Eyelids. New York City: Thieme-Stratton, pp. 114-132, 1982
Castanares S: Complications in blepharoplasty. Clin Plast Surg 5:139-165, 1978
Patipa M: Cosmetic Blepharoplasty. The Atlas of Aesthetic Facial Surgery. New York City: Grune & Stratton, pp. 75-120, 1984
Rees TD: Blepharoplasty. Aesthetic Plastic Surgery. Philadelphia: W.B. Saunders Company, pp. 459-580, 1980
Smith JW: Cosmetic surgery of the aging face. In Grabb WC, Smith JW (Eds.): Plastic Surgery, a Concise Guide to Clinical Practice (2nd ed.). Boston: Little, Brown and Co., pp 555-570, 1973
Spira M: Blepharoplasty. Clin Plast Surg 5:121-137, 1978

Julius Newman
Abram Nguyen

14

Cervical-facial Lipo-suction

Eradication of fatty accumulation in the face and neck has been a major concern for the facial plastic surgeon. Abnormal fat deposits are frequently seen in the melolabial mound, the cheek itself (buccal fat pad), and in the submandibular (jowls) and the submental areas. It is generally agreed that facial and cervical fat pads are more or less difficult to manage by sharp dissection methods.

Since the first description of submental fat excision by Maliniak[1] in 1932, many surgical techniques have been reported to correct the classical fat deposition in the neck-chin region. Different procedures, such as submental lipectomy, platysma muscle plication, and excision of skin with Z-plasty, W-plasty, or TZ-plasty closure, have been advocated. On the other hand, the purpose of facial cosmetic surgery is to achieve satisfactory reduction of abnormal fat deposits and restoration of the cervicomental angle without making long, obvious incisions together with extensive dissection that may cause unsightly scars which were frequently disliked and difficult to revise.

Following experience with the body suction lipectomy advocated and popularized by French surgeons, the senior author developed facial and cervical lipo-suction[2] to remove fat accumulation, and incorporated it into facial profileplasty methods to create a more pleasing contour for the lower face and neck. Since its inception, the technique and instrumentation have evolved to become an important adjunct to facial cosmetic procedures.

Fischer,[3] in 1977, conceptualized a technique of removing fat through a small suction curette using 3 basic principles: liquefying the fat lobules by a rotating instrument, vacuuming the liquid by suction, and achieving hemostasis by thermocautery, topical coagulants, or pressure dressings. Other European surgeons, especially Josef Schrudde[4] of West Germany and Ulrich Kesselring[5] of Switzerland, experimented with similar methods of removing body fat, but it was Yves-Gerard Illouz[6] of Paris who made the concept popular by using a lipolytic solution composed of normal saline, water, and hyaluronidase, then vacuum-suctioning out the fat cells by a blunt cannula. This technique was presented by Illouz in a paper entitled "Suction Technique for the Treatment of Cellulite and Fat Deposits" before the American Board of Cosmetic Surgery Annual Scientific Meeting in January, 1982 at Los Angeles.

The senior author began to explore facial lipo-suction procedures with an emphasis on the protection of important anatomical structures of the face and the camouflage of incision sites. The instrumentation has evolved from the use of a plastic abortion extractor that was shortly replaced by a cannula derived from the body suction counterpart. Finally, the construction was perfected by the development of a flat, spatula-shaped-tip cannula. To date, facial lipo-suction has been employed to extract fat in the submandibular and submental areas, the buccal space, the malar sad pad, and the nasolabial folds. It is now used in conjunction with rhytidoplasty and becomes a necessity for this procedure.

SUPERFICIAL ANATOMY OF THE FACE AND NECK

Major structures such as facial nerve branches and blood vessels are covered by deep cervical fascia consisting of a true parotid fascia and its continuity to platysma muscle.[7] This deep fascia embeds the paratod gland superiorly and the submandibular gland inferiorly. This layer is separated from the subcutaneous fat by a superficial muscular aponeurotic system frequently called SMAS layer.[8] In the cervical region, the anterior and external jugular veins with their tributaries and the marginal mandibular nerve are covered by the superficial layer of the deep fascia and the platysma muscle. The sternocleidomastoid muscle passes obliquely down across the side of the neck and divides it into 2 triangles: anterior and posterior. Superficial to the sternocleidomastoid are thin fibers of the platysma, scanty but dense subcutaneous fatty tissue, and skin. Under the thin platysma layer in this area are found the external jugular vein and the great auricular and transverse cervical nerves.

The superficial cervical fascia is a thin lamina investing the platysma and may contain considerable amounts of adipose tissue, usually to a greater extent in the female than in the male. It may vary significantly in its development and adherence to the deep fascia. The most adherent zones are the pretragal, submandibular, and malar prominence. In addition, dense subcutaneous tissue is found in the region of the sternocleidomastoid and posterior triangle of the neck. The superficial cervical fascia is connected to the skin by a network of loose connective tissue septa which divide the subcutaneous adipose tissue into lobules and contain blood vessels, lymphatics, and nerve endings.

STRUCTURE OF FATTY TISSUE

It has been known that after puberty, the number of adipocytes in human adipose tissue is fixed[9] in the amount of approximately 25 billion cells. Each cell is capable of changing its size by incorporation of oil droplets consisting of triglycerides under hormonal influences. Abnormality of lipoid distribution is termed local adiposity. It is found to be stable and cannot be reduced by dieting. Studies in a group of obese adults sustaining weight loss showed that the adipocytes had shrunk by 45 percent in size but that there was relatively little change in cell number. Therefore, the only method of extracting fat deposits is by surgical means.

NATURE OF CERVICO-FACIAL CHANGES

The face is described as a complex morphological unit which undergoes a number of anatomical changes related to fatty deposit or the aging process. Local adiposity is seen above the superficial cervical fascia in the areas around the jowls and below the chin. Excessive fat accumulation in the buccal space gives rise to a bulky cheek appearance. As part of the aging process, combined fat deposit, even in a small amount, in the cheek rolls and pulling action of facial muscles may create deep folds in the melolabial mound of certain people.

Beyond the fifth decade of life, the muscle tone is relaxed and the SMAS has become an inelastic sheet of tissue. At this stage, it does not contribute to the amplification of the contraction of the muscles of facial expression. Loosened interplane tissue causes slippage of the platysma-SMAS unit on a stronger core of the deep cervical fascia. This results in wrinkled, hanging skin over the jowls and mentum associated with platysma muscle folds and bands of the neck.[10]

CONCEPTS OF CERVICO-FACIAL LIPO-SUCTION

The difference between body lipo-suction and facial lipo-suction is that body suction is based on the principle of fatty tissue collapsing whereas the endpoint of facial lipo-suction is complete removal of excess fat and, in case of loose hanging tissue, creation of a skin flap to be subsequently redraped over the core cervico-facial structures. The facial skin has a rich blood supply and lymphatic drainage as compared with poorly circulated skin of the body or extremities. Necrosis of facelift skin flap rarely occurs. Hence, the concept of concomitant suction and preservation of connective tissue septa to maintain dermal blood supply does not apply to the face. To achieve satisfactory results with minimal morbidity, the principles to be followed are (1) prevention of injury to the dermis; (2) preservation of subdermal fat layer which is necessary to maintain cutaneous lymphatic drainage, skin sensation, tonicity, and trophicity; and (3) prevention of injury to deep tissue. These are the basis for the development and perfection of the facial lipo-suction cannula.

The construction of the cannula has evolved from the use of a plastic abortion cannula that caused excessive bleeding and unsatisfactory results. This was replaced with a small metal cannula that had round, bullet-type tip, which was mainly designed for body lipo-suction surgery. The bullet-shaped extractor had an aperture opening that extended from one side of the cannula to the other (Fig. 14-1), thus facilitating inadvertent currette injury to the dermis by the side edges.

The newly designed cannula for facial suction has the tip modified to a spatula shape (Fig. 14-1), which significantly decreases the tissue resistance. Consequently, it is easier for the operative surgeon to control and manipulate the suction cannula over the thin and delicate cervico-facial skin. The tunnel passages created by a flat tip are much smaller than are those created by a round tip, thus resulting in less tissue trauma and a smoother scarring process. The edges of the aperture are protected by the side surface of the cannula (Fig. 14-2), therefore curetting effect of the cannula on the dermis is avoided.

Theoretically, a blunt cannula with dull aperture edges does not damage the fibrous tissue, such as connective septa, the adventitia of the blood vessels, and the perineural tissue. By direct observation during open lipo-suction, the authors have often found that

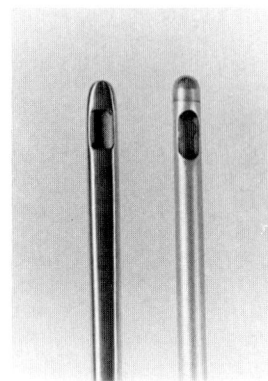

Fig. 14-1. Cut-away aperture on the rounded tip cannula as compared with fully protected aperture on the flat, spatula-shaped tip.

the blood vessels were left intact. The authors had intentionally suctioned over the course of the great auricular nerve and found no residual sensory damage postoperatively.

EQUIPMENT

The currently used facial suction cannulas are constructed of stainless surgical steel with a straight body, highly polished to decrease the contact resistance to the surrounding tissue. They all have flat, spatula-shaped tips with a dull aperture opening near the tip. All cannulas are of the same length and are made straight. The curved cannula was found to be unnecessary in facial lipo-suction. The cannula length is sufficient to reach the sternocleidomastoid muscle from an incision below the mentum and the midline from the earlobe. The cannula set is available in 5 sizes as related to the width of the tip: 4, 5, 6, 8, and 10 mm, with an opening near the tip varying from 3 to 10 mm, accordingly (Fig. 14-3).

The suction machine is a one-half horsepower, double diaphragm unit (Fig. 14-4) that generates one atmosphere of negative pressure, which it reaches in 5–6 seconds. The

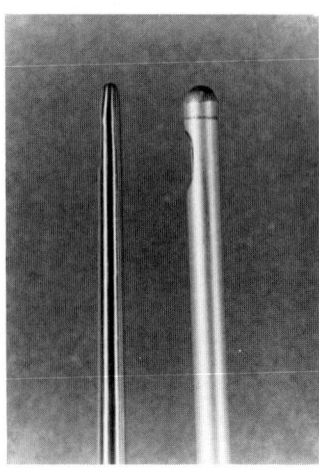

Fig. 14-2. Side view of the rounded and flat tip cannulas.

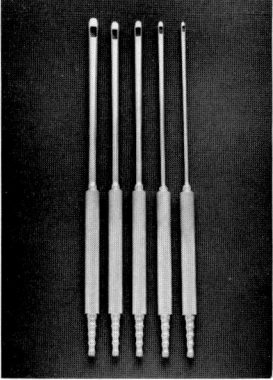

Fig. 14-3. Newman facial extractors. Cannula sizes from left to right: 10 mm, 8 mm, 6 mm, 5 mm, and 4 mm.

machine is capable of retaining high residual suction pressure for fat extraction from an open wound.

The tubing connecting the cannula to the suction machine is made of rigid, transparent, and non-collapsible plastic that is essential to maintain constant suction pressure (Fig. 14-5).

PREOPERATIVE CONSULTATION

Choosing patients for the appropriate procedure in order to assure satisfactory aesthetic results is a very selective process. During the initial office consultation, the patient is examined with regard to clinical presentation of the facial skin (tone, elasticity,

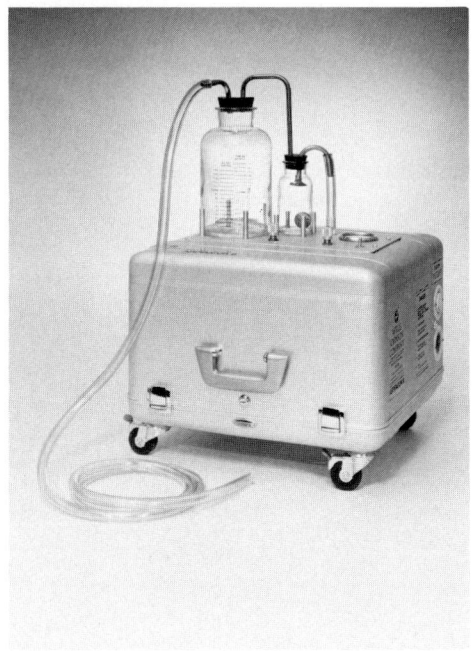

Fig. 14-4. Lipo-suction machine with tubing.

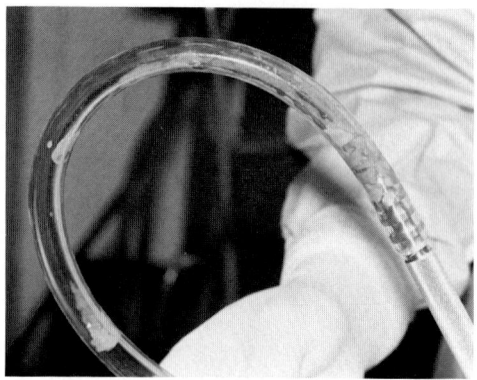

Fig. 14-5. Rigid, non-collapsible plastic tubing.

redundancy), location and amount of subcutaneous fat, to determine if that patient is a good candidate for the procedure. Age is not a contraindication for cervico-facial liposuction, but is an important factor involving the skin tone and elasticity.

The midface is evaluated to determine the appearance of the melolabial mound with or without deep smile lines and sad pads. The cheek contour is examined for the coordination of cheek bone prominence superiorly and buccal fat pad inferiorly.

In the lower face and neck, the majority of patients who were not satisfied with liposuction alone were in the advanced age group and presented, in the authors' practice,

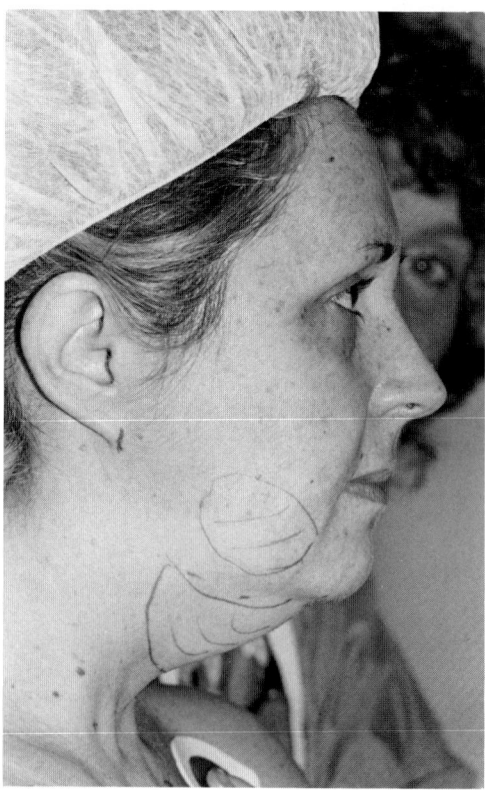

Fig. 14-6. Marking while the patient is in a sitting position.

Cervical-Facial Lipo-Suction

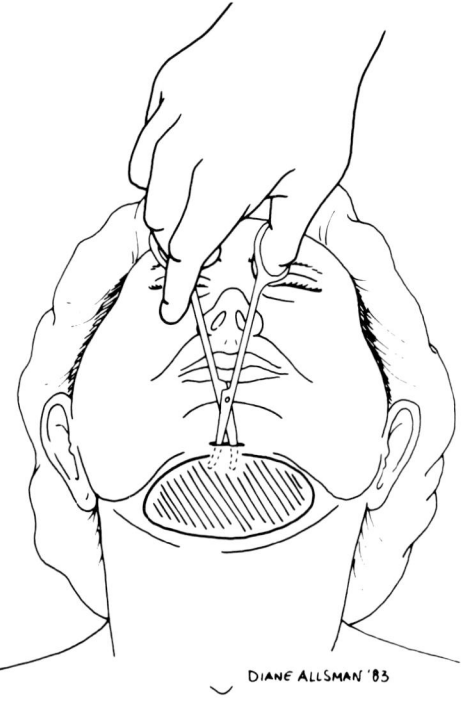

Fig. 14-7. Entrance into the submental fat.

with loose, redundant skin without true submental fat, combined with poor skin tone. The authors have concluded that it is primarily the tone and condition of the skin that dictates which patients are best suited for the appropriate procedure.

Generally, for younger patients with good skin tone and isolated fat accumulation, lipo-suction can be performed alone with good results. In the older age group, platysma

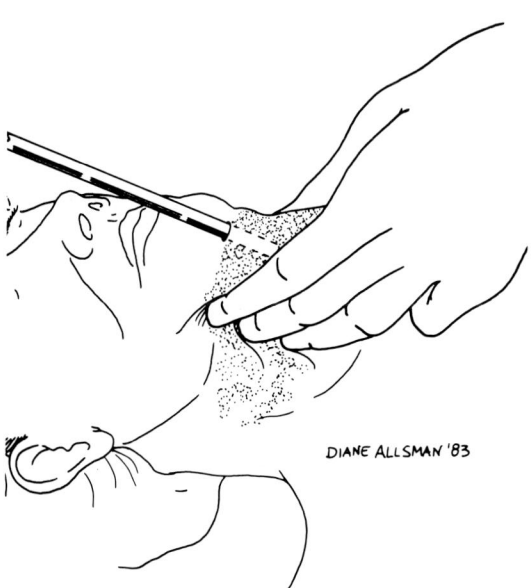

Fig. 14-8. Insertion of the fat extractor.

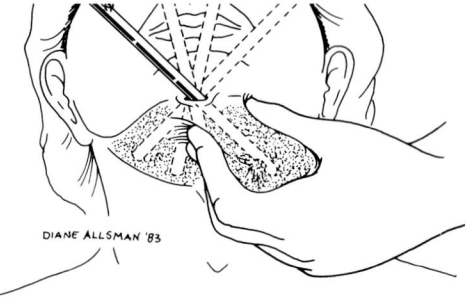

Fig. 14-9. Cannula directions, guided by the operator's thumb and index finger.

bands, so-called "turkey neck," and sagging neck and jowls appear and worsen with age. Depending on the redundancy and inelasticity of the skin, a total neck suction and flap redraping or a combined rhytidectomy and facial lipo-suction is indicated. For the combined procedure, initially the closed method of lipo-suction is performed; after the flap is raised, the open technique is used to remove the remaining fat over the platysma muscle and the facial flap.

Preoperative evaluation also focuses on the position of the chin and the cheek bones in relation to the patient's facial profile. A fat neck and a recessive chin could undoubtedly form an unpleasing look to the face. In many instances, the neck almost comes to the edge of the recessive chin line. As an adjunct to lipo-suction, a hard acrylic chin augmentation is performed to restore the neck-chin angle. Similarly, reduction of the buccal fat pad in the lower cheek, combined with augmentation malarplasty, is necessary to achieve better definition of the midface.

PREOPERATIVE PREPARATION

The head and neck areas are washed with a disinfectant soap prior to the procedure. While the patient is in a sitting position, the areas of abnormal fat deposit and all possible incision lines are marked with an indelible pen (Fig. 14-6). Either general anesthesia or local standby is used, depending on the extent of surgery, the surgeon's preference, and the equipment and staffing of the surgical suite.

The deformed area is infiltrated with a solution of 2 percent xylocaine and 1:100,000 epinephrine to achieve good hemostasis. The infiltration is usually extended 2–3 cm beyond the fat bulge, since it is necessary to feather the cannula into the normal surrounding fatty tissue in order to eliminate a stepladder effect on the overlying skin.

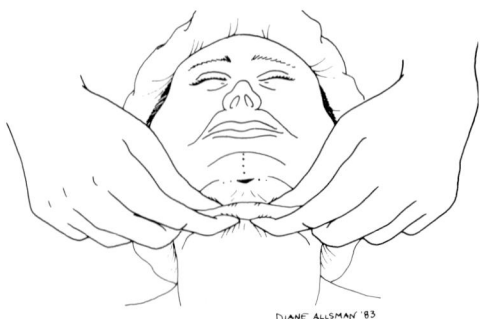

Fig. 14-10. The "pinch" test.

Cervical-Facial Lipo-Suction

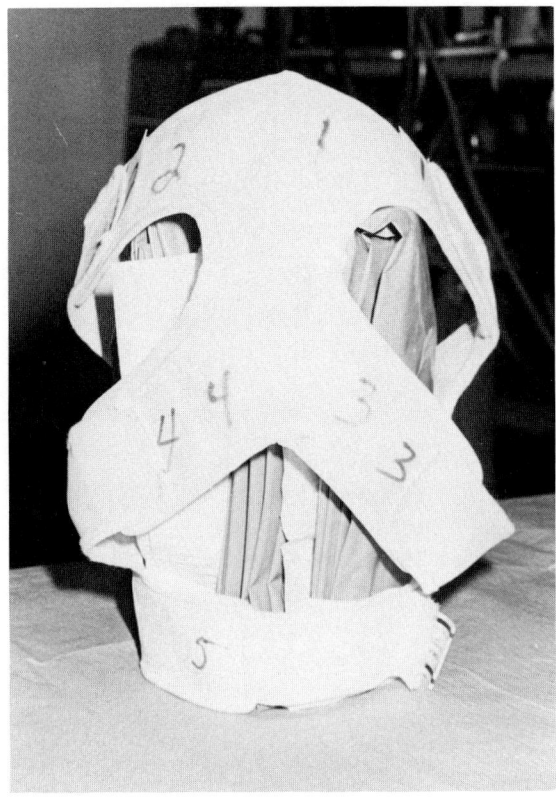

Fig. 14-11. Back view of head garment with adjustable elastic straps.

TECHNIQUES

Submental Fat Pad

Indications

1. Restoration of the neck-chin angle
2. Young age group (not an absolute factor)

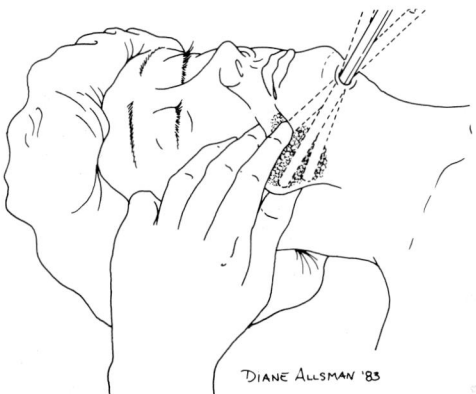

Fig. 14-12. Approach to the jowl from submental incision.

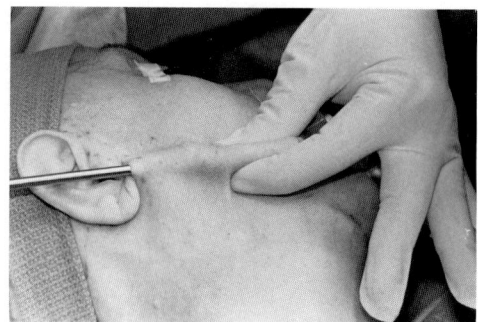

Fig. 14-13. Approach to the jowl from incision below the earlobe.

3. Good skin tone and elasticity
4. Isolated fat accumulation below the mentum

Preoperative preparation

The fat bulk and submental incision are marked while the patient is in a sitting position. Infiltration is done within the fat deposit and extended only 2 or 3 cm beyond its boundary.

Step-by-step Technique

A small half-centimeter incision is made in the submental crease.

A narrow subcutaneous plane, approximately 1 cm deep to the skin is created using a blunt scissor to start a small tunnel over the fat layer (Fig. 14-7). A 6 mm facial fat extractor is inserted into the tunnel (Figure 14-8). Using the thumb and forefinger as a guide, the extractor is advanced and maneuvered within the abnormal fat layer in a radial fashion, with back and forth motions to rupture and remove the fat lobules (Fig. 14-9). In persons with thin skin, the opening of the extractor is placed down toward the fascia plane. In the heavily fat, bull-necked and thick-skinned patients, the aperture of the extractor is sometimes placed against the skin to allow cleaning of the skin flap, with care taken not to injure the dermis.

During suction, the subcutaneous tissue is constantly palpated by gently pinching the skin between two fingers to determine the uniform thickness of the treated area (Fig. 14-10). The results are not only usually determined by the amount of fat extracted, but are also dictated by the amount and distribution of fat left behind, which remains and constitutes the new integument layer.

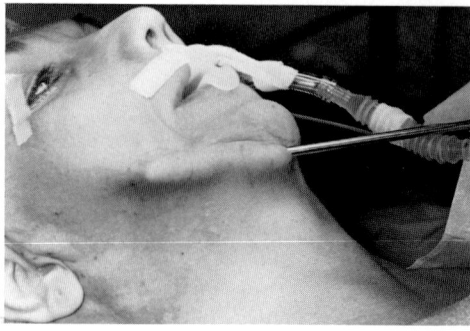

Fig. 14-14. The cannula is aimed toward the skin.

Cervical-Facial Lipo-Suction

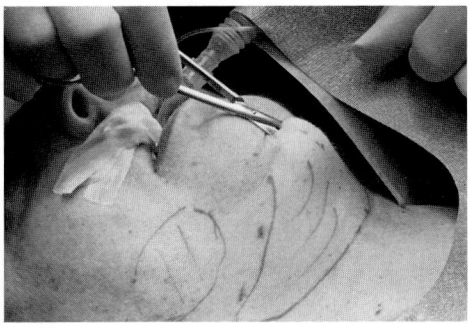

Fig. 14-15. Entrance into the submental fat.

The cannula should undermine 2 or 3 cm beyond the field of fat extraction in order to achieve smooth transition on the skin surface.

The skin incision is closed with one or two simple sutures, using 5-0 nylon. They are removed after 4 or 5 days.

Dressings

The submental area is covered with a fluff dressing, which is held in place by an elastic bandage placed in one piece from one side of the mandible to the other (Fig. 14-25). A head garment (Fig. 14-11) is placed and adjusted to provide appropriate compression (Fig. 14-26). Duration of pressure dressing is about 5 days.

Jowl Fat Pad

Indications

1. Good skin tone and elasticity
2. Isolated fat accumulation in the jowls or combined with submental fat

Preoperative Preparation

Areas of abnormal fat deposit and incision sites (beneath the earlobe or below the mentum) are marked while the patient is in a sitting position. Infiltration is done at the incision sites, along the margins of the mandible, and in the abnormal fat layer.

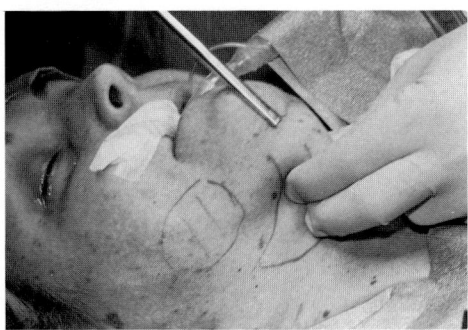

Fig. 14-16. Insertion of the facial extractor.

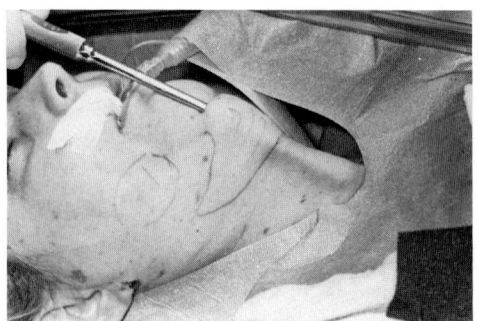

Fig. 14-17. Wide cannula undermining in the neck.

Step-by-step Technique

There are two approaches to the jowls: from the submental or infralobule incision. If there is associated submental fat pad, the submental suction is performed following the steps described in the previous section. From the submental incision, the cannula can be extended toward the submandibular area in either side to extract the jowl fat (Fig. 14-12).

A stab wound incision is made below the earlobe, through which a small 4 mm extractor is inserted and advanced toward the inferior margin of the mandible (Fig. 14-15). It is important that the tip of the extractor be palpated beneath the mandibular skin, guided by the operator's thumb and index finger (Fig. 14-13). The extractor must ride over the mandible and not deep to it. If the extractor remains in the subcutaneous tissue and superficial to the platysma, danger to important structures of the sudmandibular area can be avoided.

The extractor must be aimed toward the skin, with the aperture down as it approaches the lower edge of the mandible (Fig. 14-14). Any deep penetration in this region would result in injury of the platysma muscle, the submandibular branch of the facial nerve, major blood vessels, and the submandibular gland.

To preserve the mandibular contour, the opening of the extractor is never allowed to present itself against the dermis. It must be placed down toward the SMAS layer. Too vigorous maneuvering of the skin in this area may give rise to areas of skin retraction and puckering.

The skin incisions are closed with one or two simple 5-0 nylon sutures.

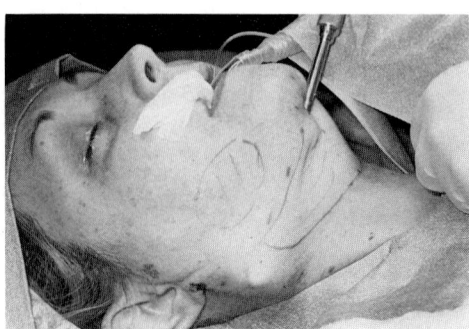

Fig. 14-18. Cannula undermining in the submandibular area.

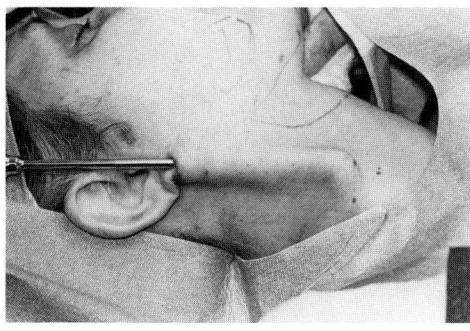

Fig. 14-19. Cannula direction from an infralobule incision.

Dressings

Fluff dressings are placed under the mentum and the jowls, held by one piece of elastic bandage (Fig. 14-25). Appropriate pressure and molding are achieved by use of an adjustable head garment that is kept on for 5 days (Fig. 14-26).

Total Neck Extraction

Purpose

Total neck extraction or combined wide submental and submandibular lipo-suction is employed to remove abnormal fat accumulation and separate the rather loosened skin flap and redrape it over the dense core of the deep cervical fascia.

Indications

1. Fair skin tone and elasticity
2. Mild degree of skin redundancy; condition of skin not poor enough to warrant a facelift

Preoperative Preparation

With the patient in a sitting position, the neck and jowls are marked. Infiltration is done widely extending to the thyroid cartilage inferiorly and the sternocleidomastoid laterally.

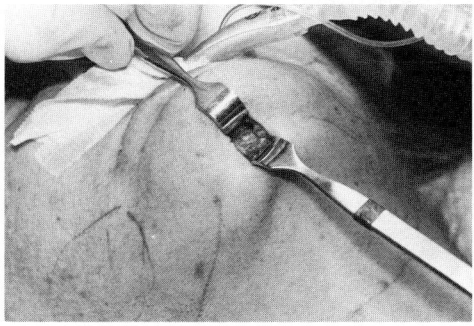

Fig. 14-20. The submental incision is retracted to mandibular rim and continued to the periosteum of the anterior mandible.

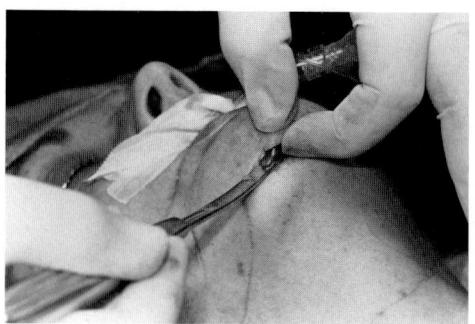

Fig. 14-21. Insertion of the hard chin implant in shoehorn fashion.

Step-by-step Technique

A subcutaneous tunnel is created through a small skin incision made below the mentum (Fig. 14-15). A 6 mm cannula is inserted (Fig. 14-16). The cannula is maneuvered widely across the entire neck in a radial fashion, one tunnel passage next to another from the thyroid cartilage anteriorly to the sternocleidomastoid laterally (Fig. 14-17).

The cannula is directed toward the submandibular area to extract fat and separate the hanging jowl skin from the fascia (Fig. 14-18). To create criss-crossed tunneling, the cannula is inserted into an incision beneath the earlobe and advanced along the sternocleidomastoid toward the lower neck, laterally and anteriorly (Fig. 14-19).

Remaining tissue webs between tunnels are broken down as much as possible by sweeping motions of the spatula-shaped cannula over the jowls and neck. Sweeping motions bluntly separate the cervico-facial skin flap and break up vertical platysma bands. This is necessary for the management of sagging jowls and a neck with flaccid "neck folds" appearance. Once separated, the flap can be redraped over the strong deep cervical fascia to achieve a better neck-chin contour line.

Skin incision is closed with one or two simple sutures using 5-0 nylon.

Dressings

The method of dressings is similar to that used for the submental and jowls extraction.

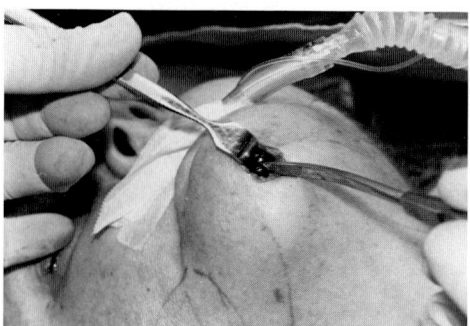

Fig. 14-22. The small center notch of the implant is positioned into the midline.

Cervical-Facial Lipo-Suction

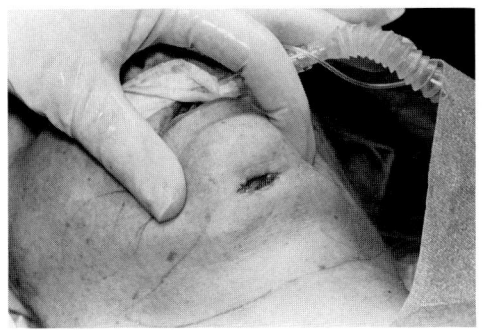

Fig. 14-23. The implant is palpated for symmetrical position.

Cervico-facial Extraction with Combined Augmentation Mentoplasty

Indications

Indications for this procedure involve a combination of submental submandibular fat and a recessive chin, which obliterates the neck-chin contour. Augmentation of the chin projection is necessary for restoration of the cervicomental angle.

Preoperative Preparation

In addition to markings of the fat pads and skin incision, the midline of the chin is marked with a dotted line. Infiltration is done in the fat pads and around the chin, on the anterior surface of the mandible.

Step-by-step Technique

Following suction extraction of the cervico-facial region, the chin augmentation procedure is performed. The submental incision is continued through the periosteum of the anterior aspect of the mandible (Fig. 14-20). The periosteum is elevated using a specially designed Rish-Newman periosteal suction elevator with crosshatched grooving to create a pocket, large enough to permit a hard acrylic chin implant to be inserted.

The pocket is made larger on the left side than on the right, in order to allow the

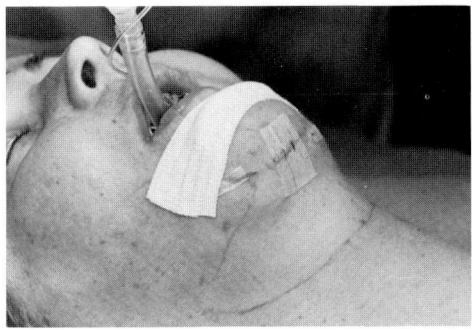

Fig. 14-24. Bolster dressing to keep the chin implant in place.

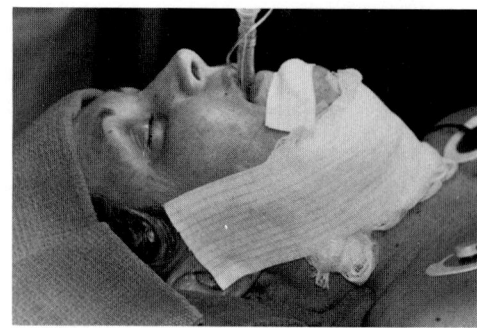

Fig. 14-25. Method of dressing.

initial insertion of the left portion of the implant through the skin incision. Using the thumb of the right hand, the body of the implant is pushed laterally toward the left mandible until only a small portion of the right edge of the implant is seen.

The suction elevator is applied beneath the implant and, in a shoehorn fashion, exerted on the right side; the implant is placed into the pocket (Fig. 14-21). The periosteal elevator is engaged in the small center notch of the implant to position it into the midline of the mandible (Fig. 14-22). The chin is finally inspected and palpated for symmetrical position of the implant (Fig. 14-23).

Closure of the submental incision is done in 2 layers. The subcutaneous tissue is closed using 000 chromic catgut. The skin is approximated using subcuticular suture, which is removed after 5 days.

Dressings

A bolster made of a role of 2 x 2 gauze is placed in the sulcus between the lower lip and the implant in order to lock the implant in place. The bolster dressing is taped down to the skin using a 1-inch strip of elastic bandage (Fig. 14-24).

The area of cervico-facial suction is supported with a fluff dressing, held in place by a strip of elastic bandage (Fig. 14-25). A head garment is placed to provide appropriate compression and skin molding (Fig. 14-26). The entire complement of dressings is removed after 5 days.

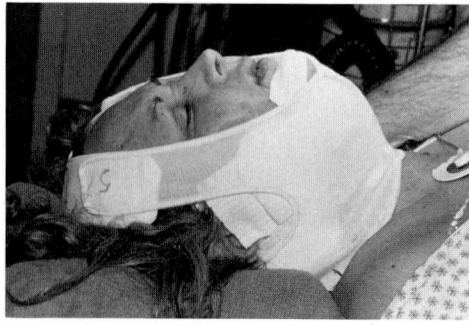

Fig. 14-26. Head garment in place.

Cervical-Facial Lipo-Suction

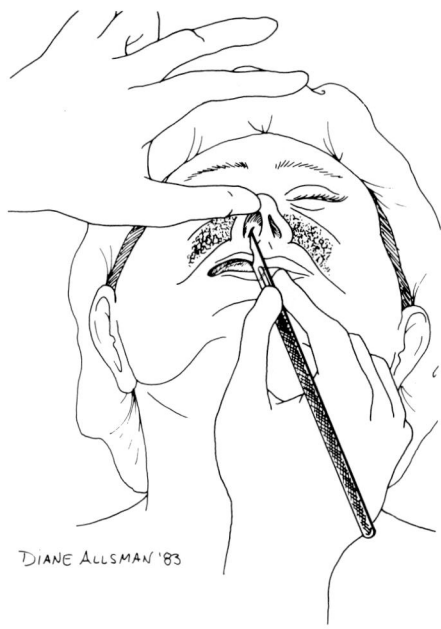

Fig. 14-27. Lateral osteotomy incision.

Melolabial Mound Extraction

General Principles

The authors' experience of lipo-suction in the melolabial mound showed that the amount of fat removed is often negligible. It is probably the breaking up of connective tissue attachments to the skin by a blunt extractor that induces the depression of the

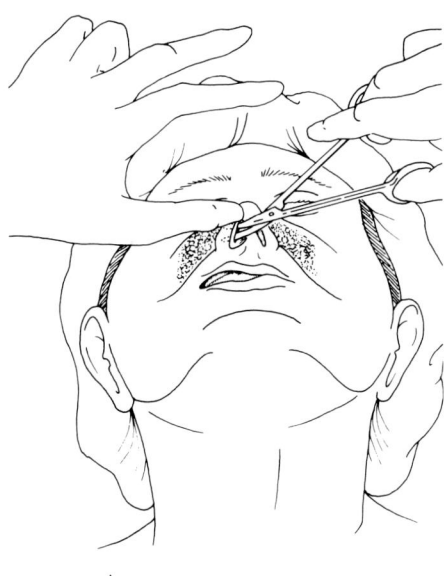

Fig. 14-28. Tunnel into the melolabial mound.

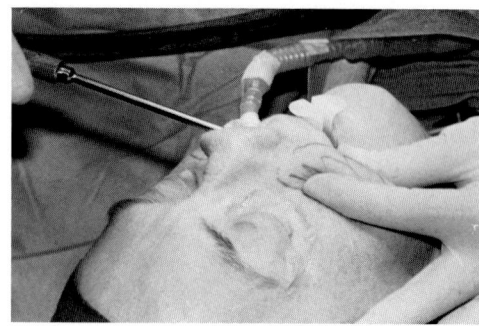

Fig. 14-29. Insertion of the 4 mm extractor.

cheek rolls by subcutaneous scarring effect. Prominent cheek rolls are seen in all age groups.

Preoperative Preparation

Prominent melolabial mound is marked beyond the crease line. Infiltration includes the intranasal vestibules.

Step-by-step Technique

A stab wound incision is made at the nasal aperture in the vestibule, which is similar to a lateral osteotomy incision (Fig. 14-27). A subcutaneous tunnel is created by a blunt scissor (Fig. 14-28).

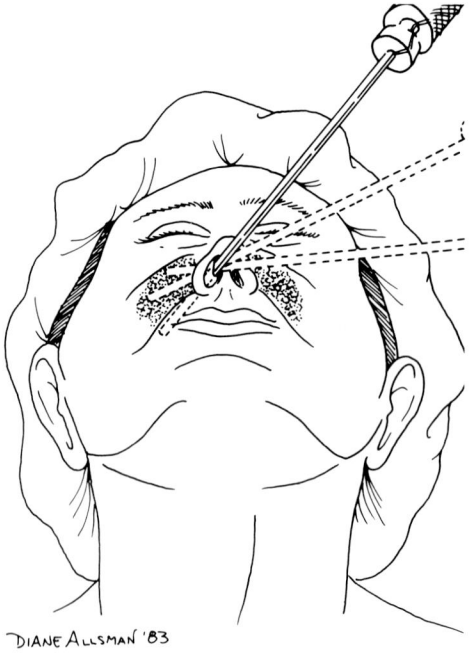

Fig. 14-30. Radial tunneling.

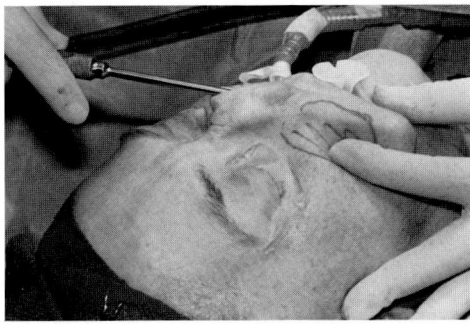

Fig. 14-31. The extractor is advanced beyond the crease line.

The 4 mm extractor is always used first (Fig. 14-29) to create radial tunneling into the cheek with side-by-side passages (Fig. 14-30). The extractor must be maneuvered beyond the crease line of the melolabial mound (Fig. 14-31). The opening of the extractor must always be placed down and never be turned up toward the dermis; this will avoid linear scarring from dermal injury.

After the flap is created with the 4 mm extractor, the 5 mm is inserted to remove some of the larger fat lobules that did not go through the narrow 4 mm lumen. There is immediate flattening of the melolabial mound and the amount of fat removed is often negligible (Fig. 14-32).

The intranasal stab wound is left open and no dressing is applied.

Buccal Fat Pad

Anatomy of the Buccal Space

The cheeks form the side of the face and are continued anteriorly with the lips. Externally, cheeks are covered by facial integument and separated internally from the

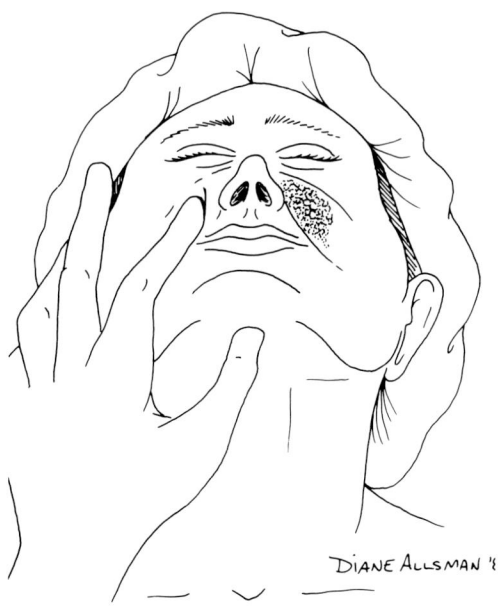

Fig. 14-32. Flattening of melolabial mound.

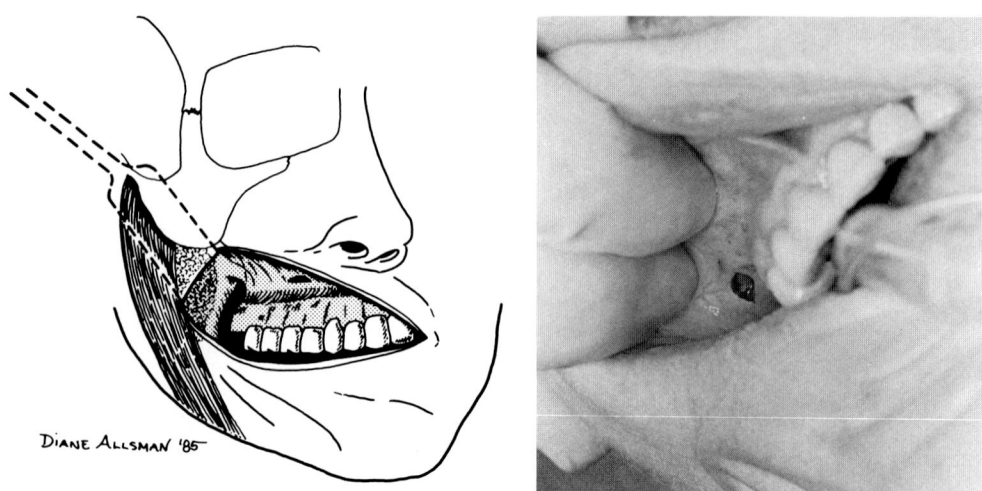

Figs. 14-33 and 14-34. Stab wound incision to enter the buccal space.

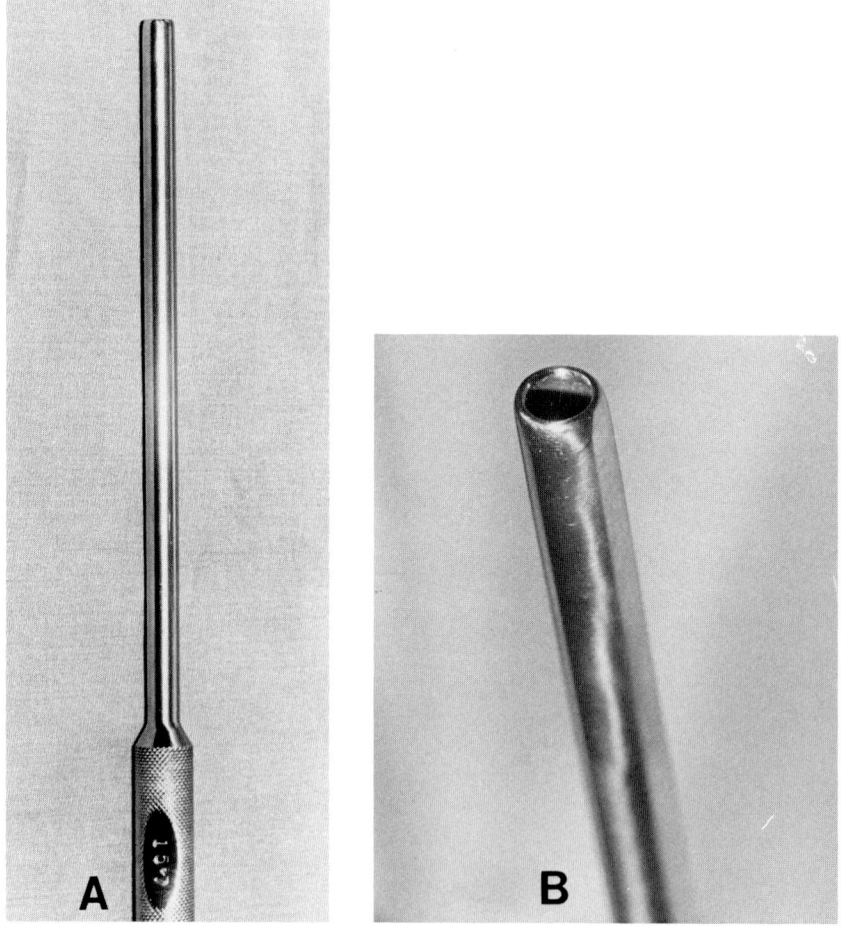

Fig. 14-35. (A and B) Newman buccal extractor with blunt rounded end at the tip.

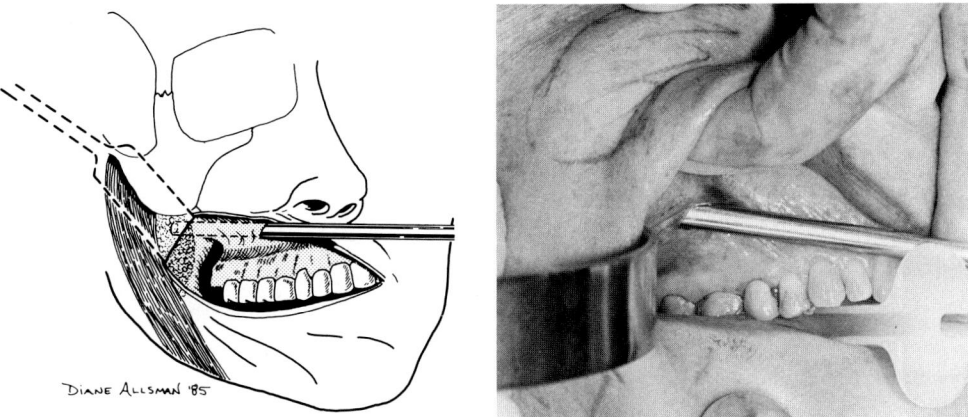

Figs. 14-36 and 14-37. Insertion of buccal extractor into buccal space.

mouth by mucous membrane. The buccal space is situated between 2 muscular layers: the inner layer is formed by the buccinator and the outer layer is formed by the anterior border of the masseter muscle. Important structures in the buccal space include the parotid duct, which perforates the buccinator and enters the mouth opposite to the second upper molar tooth. Lying between the buccinator and mucous membrane are several buccal glands. They are similar in structure to the labial glands, but are smaller. Some of the larger glands are found between the masseter and buccinator muscles around the distal portion of the parotid duct. Their ducts open in the mouth opposite to the last upper molar tooth. The transverse facial artery and vein, after crossing the superior portion of the masseter muscle, anastomose with the anterior facial artery and vein along the anterior border of this muscle. The buccal fat pad is located between the parotid duct anteriorly and the masseter muscle posteriorly.

Indications

1. Fat bulky lower cheek in patients of all age groups
2. In patients with flat malar bones and bulky lower cheeks, buccal fat extraction is done in conjunction with augmentation malarplasty to accentuate the cheek bone prominence.

Preoperative Preparation

No marking is necessary, since the buccal fat pad is a deep structure. Infiltration is done only at the incision site on the buccogingival sulcus.

Step-by-step Technique

Isolated buccal fat extraction. Approach to the buccal fat pad is best achieved through the mouth by a 5 mm incision made on the conventional Caldwell-Luc incision at a distance about one-half cm from the buccogingival sulcus (Figs. 14-33 and 14-34). A specially made buccal extractor (Fig. 14-35) with an open, rounded end is inserted (Figs. 14-36 and 14-37). The buccal fat pad is pulled into the cannula by negative suction pressure and brought out to the wound.

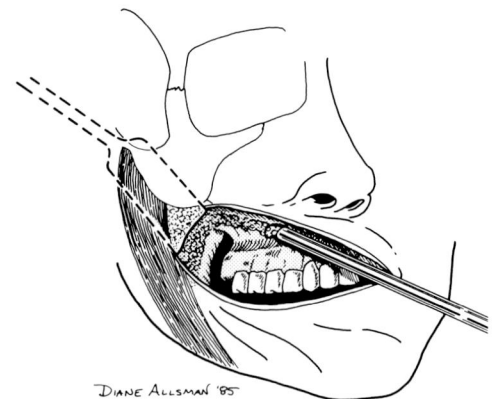

Fig. 14-38. The buccal fat pad is being teased out and extracted.

With gentle teasing of the fat pad by a smooth DeBakey forceps (Fig. 14-38), the fat lobules are broken down and suctioned out. Direct observation shows a dry field with intact connective tissue septa in the fat pad. There are no major blood vessels visible in the space anterior to the masseter muscle.

The cannula is not maneuvered in any direction in this buccal space because of the presence of important structures such as the parotid duct and anastomosing branches of the transverse and anterior facial blood vessels. An immediate flattening of the lower cheek is noted.

The incision on the buccal mucosa is closed with 1 or 2 000 chromic sutures. No dressing is required.

Combined buccal fat extraction and augmentation malarplasty. After a Caldwell-Luc incision is made for the malarplasty procedure, the buccal fat pad is seen under the

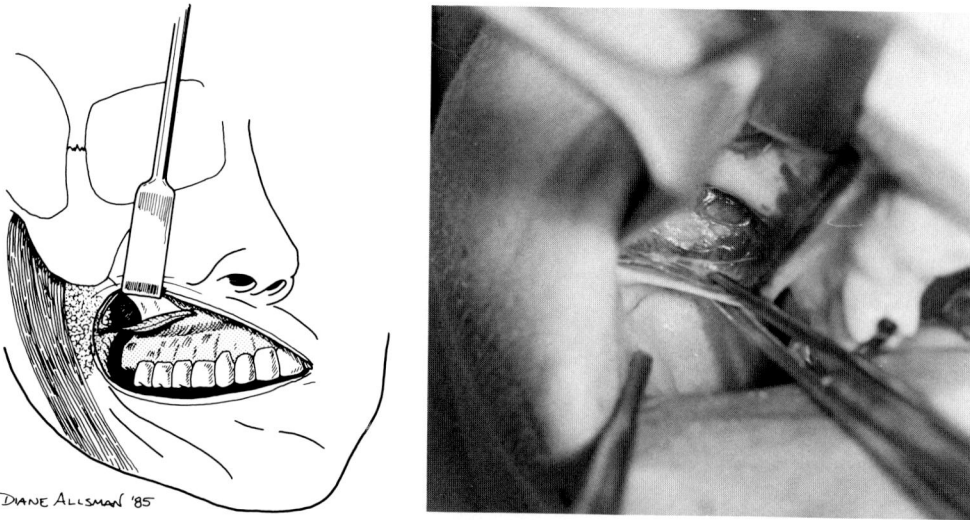

Figs. 14-39 and 14-40. Caldwell-Luc incision exposing the inferior rim of the maxilla and the buccal fat pad.

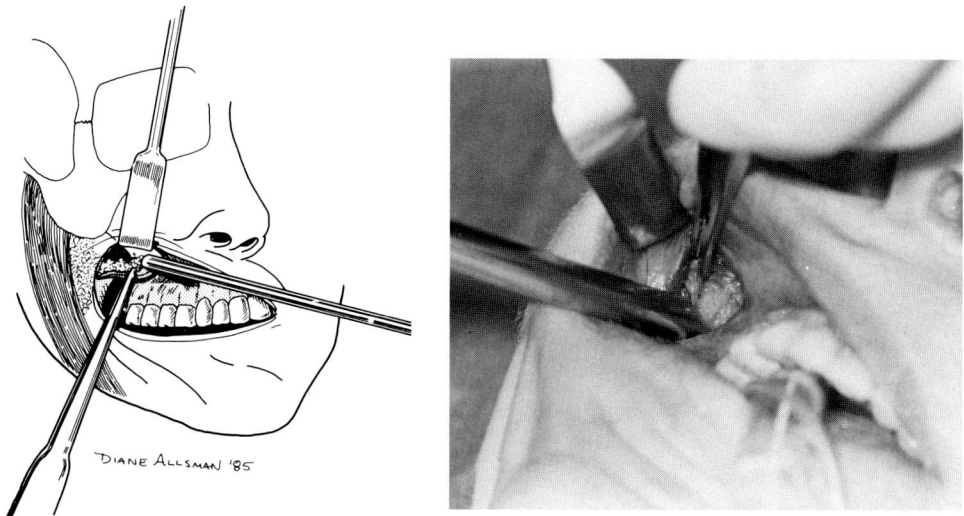

Figs. 14-41 and 14-42. Open suction removal of the buccal fat.

inferior margin of the maxilla (Figs. 14-39 and 14-40). The fat pad is picked up by the buccal extractor, and is teased out and removed by suction pressure (Figs. 14-41 and 14-42). The extractor is not advanced deep into the buccal space. When suction is accomplished, the malarplasty is carried out in a routine manner.

Sad Pad

General Principles

As part of the aging process, combined fat accumulation and sagging skin is seen on the gravitational line of the malar region. Effect of gravity on loose, poorly toned skin is probably the mechanism of sad pad formation. It cannot be corrected by conventional facelift procedure.

Preoperative Preparation

The sad pads are marked while the patient is in a sitting position. Infiltration is done in the subcutaneous plane and at the incision site.

Step-by-step Technique

A stab wound is made on the orbital rim near the lateral canthus of the lower eyelid, in the direction of the crow's feet lines.

A small subcutaneous tunnel is made, through which a 4 mm cannula is inserted and gently advanced throughout the malar region (Figs. 14-43, 14-44, and 14-45). The cannula tip must be constantly palpated under the skin to prevent deep penetration which could injure the infraorbital nerve and anastomosing ramification of the zygomatic and buccal branches of the facial nerve.

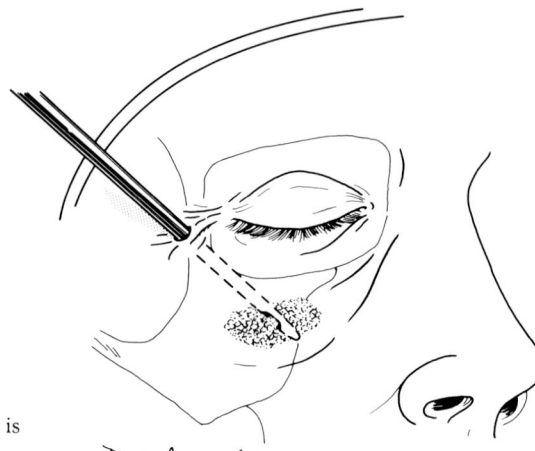

Fig. 14-43. Incision for sad pad suction is made on the crow's feet line.

Subcutaneous scarring and adhesion will cause flattening of the sad pad and prevent gravitational pulling on the malar skin.

The stab wound incision is closed with one or two simple sutures using 6-0 nylon. No dressing is required.

Cervico-facial Lipo-suction in Conjunction with Rhytidectomy

This procedure is selected for those in the older age group having loose, redundant skin and poor skin tone, with the appearance of so-called platysma bands and sagging "turkey neck". Generally, beyond age 50, the SMAS layer becomes inelastic and stretched out in its anterior to posterior dimension. Together with the relaxed facial muscles, it forms with the platysma a sliding plane over the dense, strong deep cervical fascia. Fat extraction alone does not correct this anatomical defect. Plication of the SMAS layer by rhytidectomy is necessary[10] to restore the dimension and tension of this amplification system. Lipo-suction in this age group is designed to assist the rhytidec-

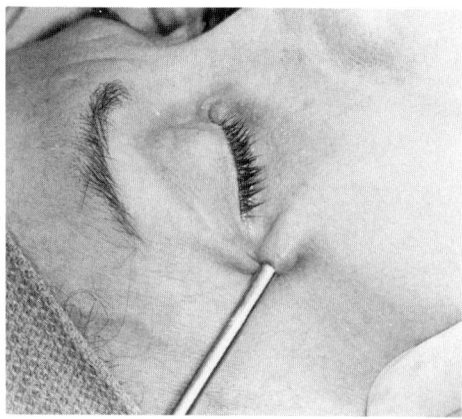 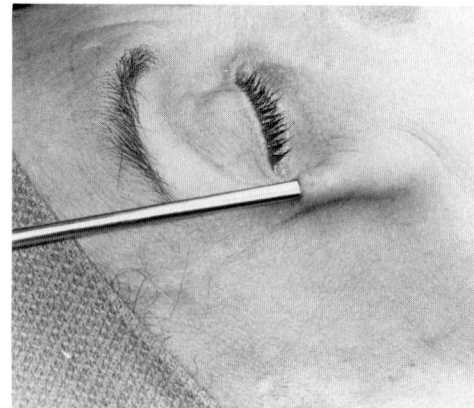

Figs. 14-44 and 14-45. Direction of the cannula in the sad pad area.

Cervical-Facial Lipo-Suction

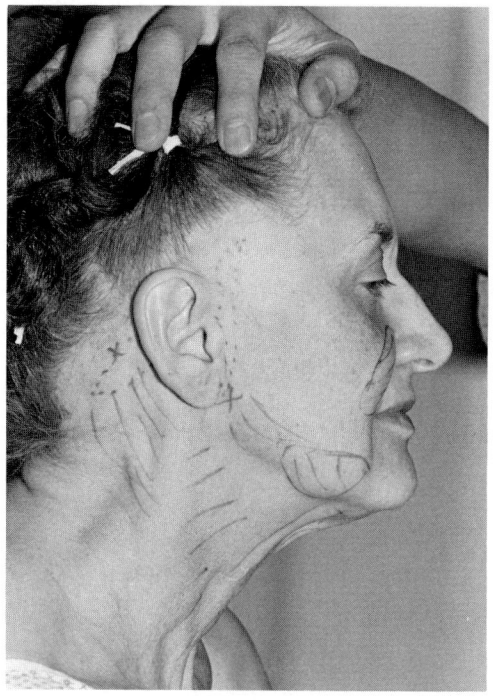

Fig. 14-46. Areas of cervico-facial suction and facelift incision are marked.

tomy procedure. It includes closed suction dissection of the submental, submandibular, posterior cervical and pretragal areas. Open lipo-suction is performed when the flap has been raised.

Preoperative preparation

With the patient in the sitting position, the areas of loose hanging skin and fat are marked. Incision for the facelift is also outlined (Fig. 14-46). Infiltration of the entire face, neck and posterior cervical area is done with a solution of 0.5% xylocaine and 1:200,000 epinephrine.

Step-by-step Technique

Closed lipo-suction. From the submental incision, a 6 mm cannula is maneuvered inferiorly, passed the thyroid cartilage (Fig. 14-47). It separates the skin folds from the

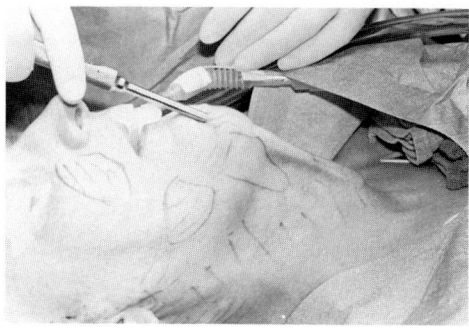

Fig. 14-47. The facial extractor is advanced toward the lower neck.

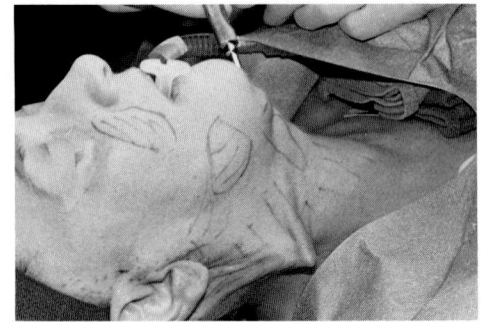

Fig. 14-48. The extractor is directed laterally.

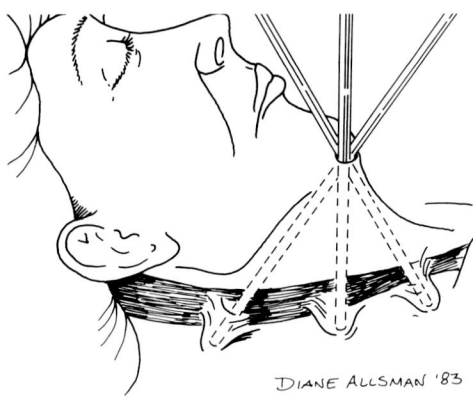

Fig. 14-49. Radial direction of the extractor in the lateral neck.

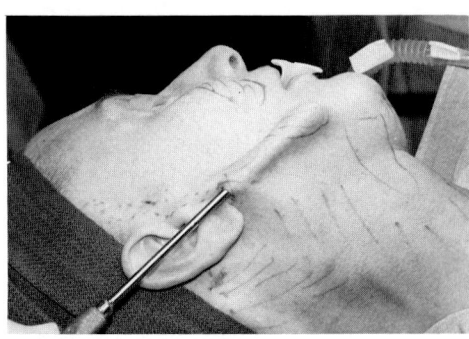

Fig. 14-50. Suction dissection of the jowl.

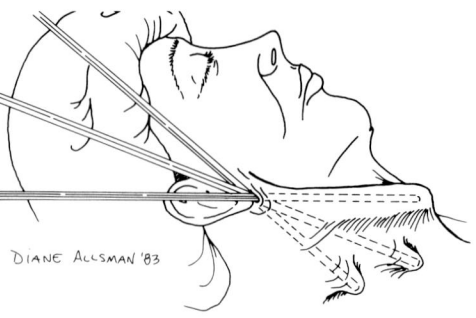

Fig. 14-51. Radial tunneling from infralobule incision.

Cervical-Facial Lipo-Suction

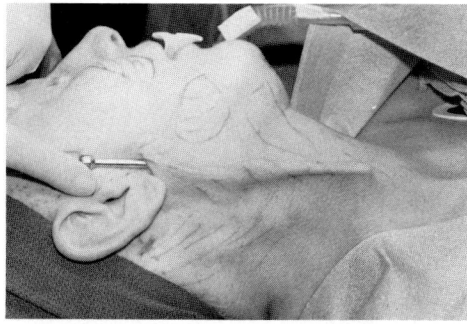

Fig. 14-52. The extractor is directed along the sternocleidomastoid muscle.

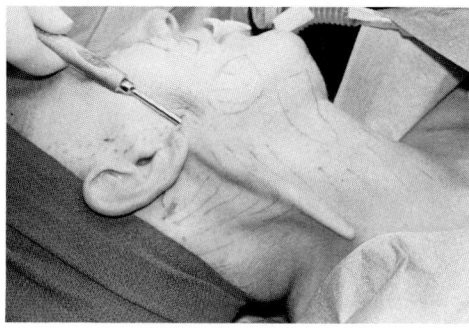

Fig. 14-53. Suction dissection in the area over the sternocleidomastoid muscle.

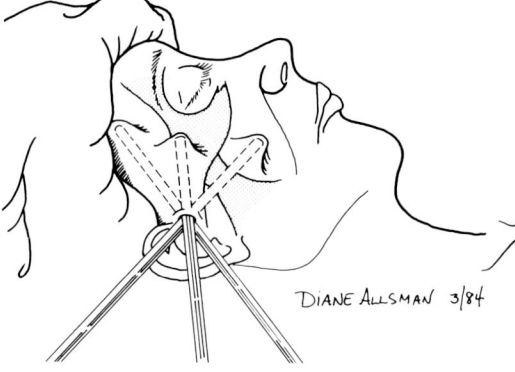

Fig. 14-54. Radial tunneling in the pretragal area.

vertical platysma bands in the neck. It is advanced superiorly and laterally to the rim of the mandible, reaching the anterior border of the sternocleidomastoid muscle (Figs. 14-48 and 14-49).

A 5 mm cannula is inserted from an infralobule incision and advanced toward the jowl for fat extraction and dissection (Fig. 14-50). The cannula is directed toward the lower neck in a radial fashion to create side-by-side tunnels in the lower facial flap (Figs. 14-51, 14-52, and 14-53).

Pretragal. A 4 mm cannula is introduced through a stab wound made in front of the tragus and advanced only 2 or 3 cm toward the temporal and malar areas (Figs. 14-54, 14-55, and 14-56). The suction machine is turned off. Too vigorous maneuvering of the cannula near the orbital rim may injure the zygomatic branch of the facial nerve.

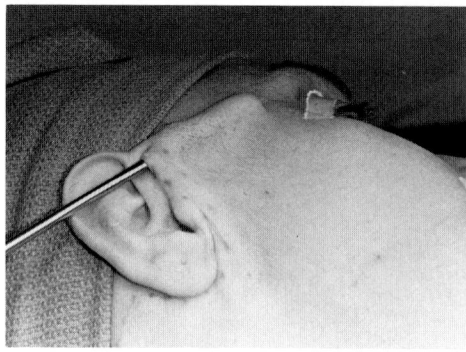 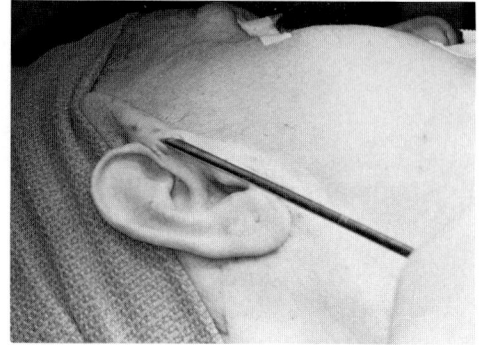

Figs. 14-55 and 14-56. The extractor is always kept in the subcutaneous tissue.

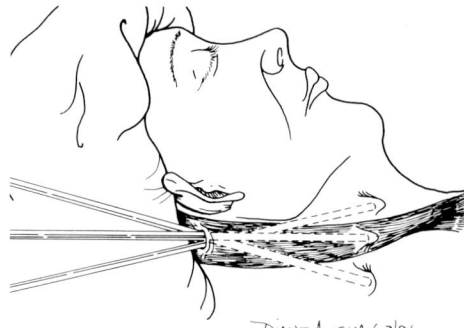

Fig. 14-57. Cannula dissection from a posterior cervical incision.

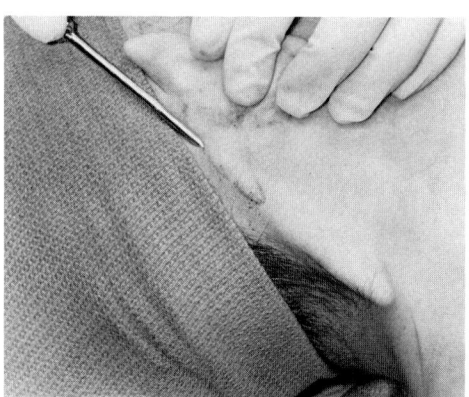 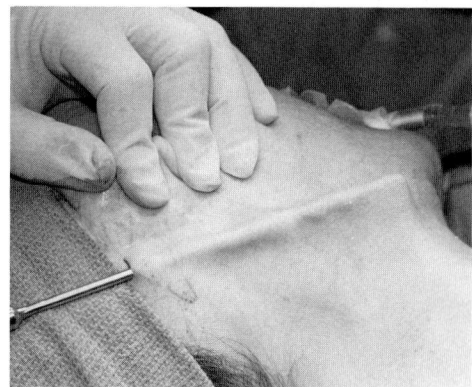

Figs. 14-58 and 14-59. The cannula is maneuvered in different directions in the posterior cervical area.

Posterior cervical. A stab wound is made on the outlined facelift incision near the hairline. A tunnel is created in the subcutaneous tissue. The suction machine is turned off. A 4 mm facial cannula is introduced and advanced toward the postauricular area and lateral neck in gradual, short, back-and-forth motions. The cannula is used for blunt dissection to separate the skin from the cervical fascia over the sternocleidomastoid muscle by creating a network of multiple cannula passages, one next to another (Figs. 14-57, 14-58, and 14-59).

Cervical-Facial Lipo-Suction

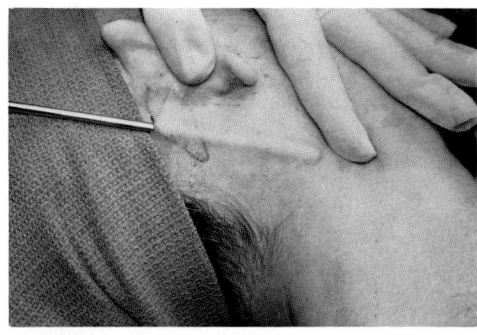

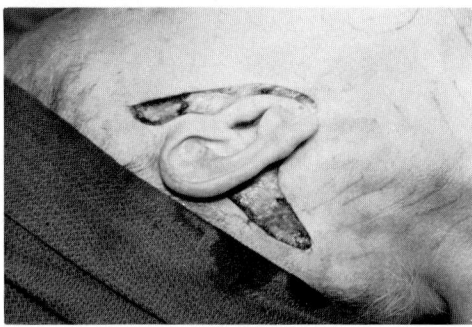

Fig. 14-60. The skin is kept under gentle traction between the thumb and index finger during cannula maneuvering.

Fig. 14-61. An island of redundant skin is excised.

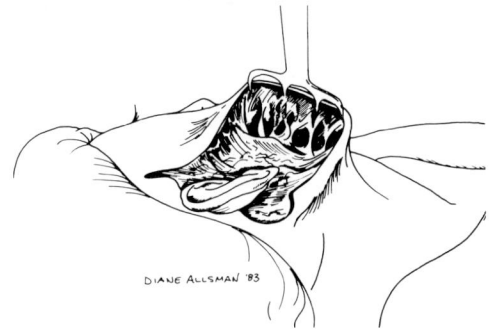
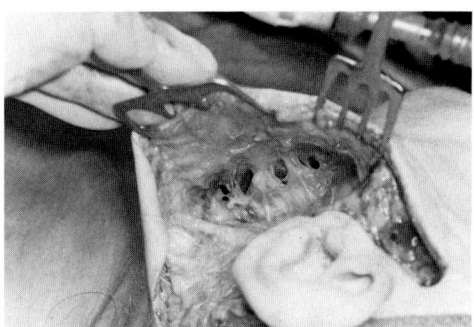

Figs. 14-62 and 14-63. Tunnels under the skin flap created by extractor passages.

The cannula tip must be aimed toward the skin and constantly be palpated. Injury to the great auricular nerve and the sternocleidomastoid is avoided.

When advancing the cannula through the dense subcutaneous tissue, the skin must be kept taut by gentle traction (Fig. 14-60). This prevents the skin from rolling under the cannula tip, which may result in skin perforation.

Completion of rhytidectomy. The standard rhytidectomy incision can now be performed. An island of redundant skin is excised (Fig. 14-61). Dissection under this area is not necessary.

The facial skin flap is raised, exposing entrance into criss-crossed tunnels and webs created by the cannula passages (Figs. 14-62 and 14-63). What the surgeon has to do next

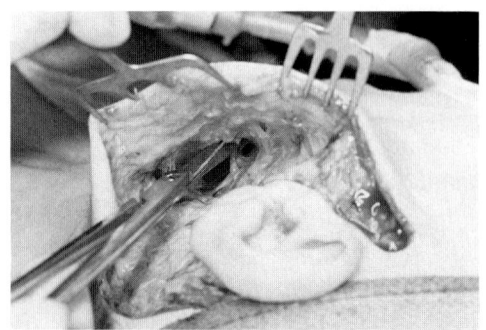

Fig. 14-64. The septa and webs between tunnels are transected.

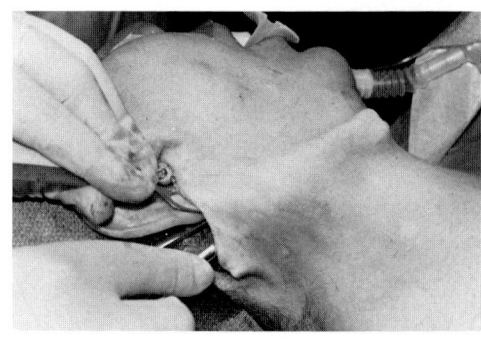

Fig. 14-65. The rhytidectomy scissor, with the tip slightly opened, follows and transects all tunnel webs, creating a facial skin flap.

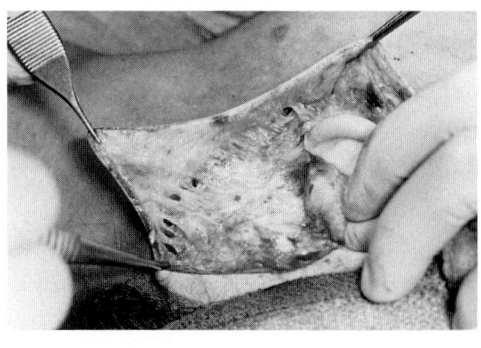

Fig. 14-66. Extractor tunnels in the lateral neck.

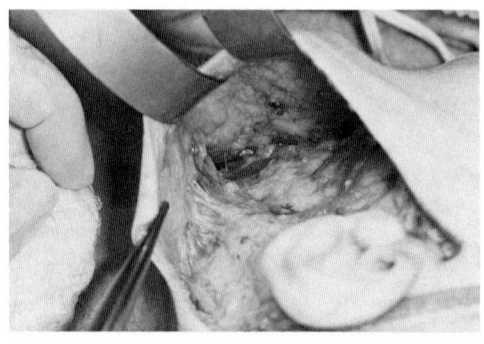

Fig. 14-67. Intact SMAS layer after cervico-facial suction followed by flap raising.

Cervical-Facial Lipo-Suction

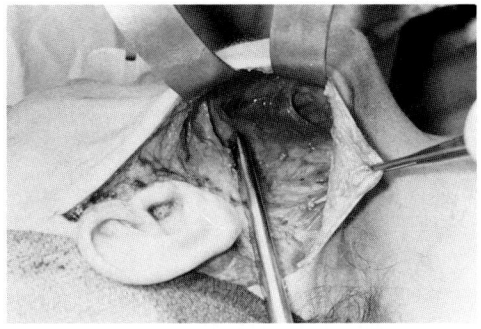

Fig. 14-68. Remaining fat lobules on the fascia are removed by open suction using 10 mm extractor.

is to follow and transect all the septa between the tunnels (Figs. 14-64 and 14-65) and consequently raise the entire flap to the neck without damage to the skin or underlying facial structures. Laterally, the flap over the postauricular region is raised without difficulty by dividing remaining septa over the sternomastoid muscle (Fig. 14-66). The great auricular nerve is usually seen underneath the thin cervical fascia undamaged.

The authors' experience shows that the suction cannula does almost half of the dissection work for the rhytidoplasty procedure. The SMAS and platysma layers are intact following appropriate lipo-suction techniques (Fig. 14-67).

Open lipo-suction. After the facelift flap has been raised, the suction extractor is again used to remove the excess of fat superficial to the playtysma muscle and the SMAS layer. This is named "open lipo-suction." This method uses the machine's capability of retaining high residual suction pressure in order to extract fat from an open wound. Open lipo-suction is done under direct visualization.

Residual fat lobules that were left from the closed lipo-suction are extracted using the 10 mm cannula. It has a large, flat surface that preserves significant residual pressure in an open system by its total sealing ability at the aperture. By firmly placing the aperture of the extractor directly on the fat lobules and using gentle back-and-forth motions, the loose fat tissue is ruptured and removed. The 10 mm cannula is applied on both the fascia (Fig. 14-68) and the skin flap (Fig. 14-69). Sometimes, a DeBakey forceps is used to break up encapsulated fat lobules and facilitate their extraction.

Residual fat in the cervico-facial area is extracted safely without any damage to the submandibular nerve or blood vessels. Direct observation has shown that there is practically no bleeding from any of the areas of lipo-suction extraction (Fig. 14-70).

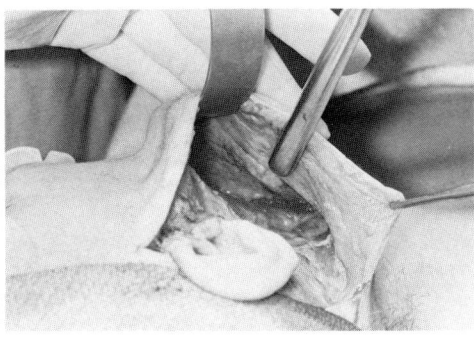

Fig. 14-69. Suction removal of fat lobules on the skin flap.

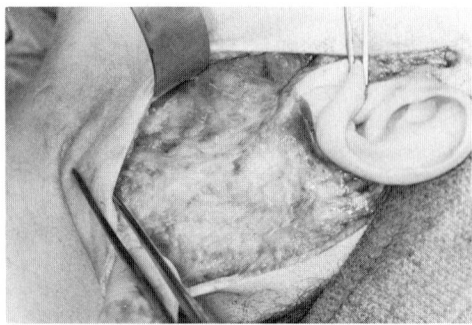

Fig. 14-70. Intact and dry field at the completion of dissection.

The completion of facelift using routine plication of the platysma and SMAS layer is carried out in a routine manner. Skin excision is tailored to achieve correction of the patient's poor skin tone and excessive sagging.

Dressings. The fluff dressing is placed on the postauricular, submandibular, and submental areas (Fig. 14-71). An elastic head garment is placed on the fluff dressing and is adjusted to provide appropriate compression (Fig. 14-72). An outer layer of 3-inch elastic bandage is gently wrapped around the entire head (Fig. 14-73). This layer of bandage is removed on the next day and the head garment is kept on for approximately 5 days. It is found that skin compression longer than 5 days is not necessary.

COMPLICATIONS OF CERVICAL-FACIAL LIPO-SUCTION

Skin Complications

Skin complications include skin dimpling and wrinkling from dermal injury, vertical wrinkling from taping, and skin reactions to molding tapes.

Early in the authors' experience,[11] when vigorous suction of the jowl and nasolabial folds was performed with the rounded-tip extractor, while aiming its aperture opening toward the skin, dermal injury was sustained. This caused excessive scarring and adhesions to underlying tissue, resulting in linear skin dimpling and wrinkling, especially in

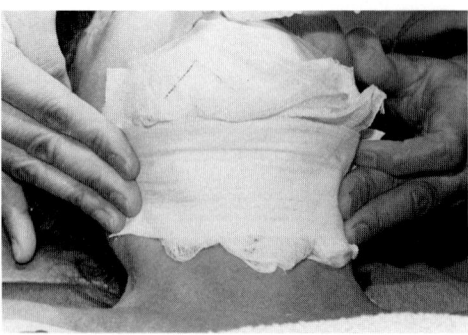

Fig. 14-71. Fluff dressing in place.

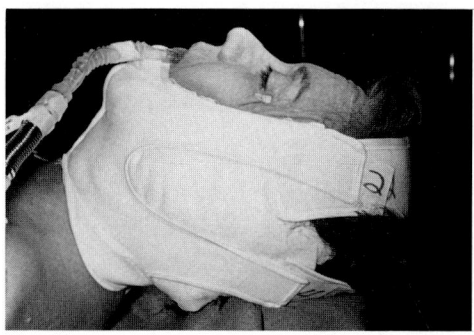

Fig. 14-72. Adjustable head garment in place.

the melolabial mound and in the submental area. This was noted approximately 3–4 weeks postoperatively after the edema had resolved. Successful treatment consisted of facial massage and intradermal injection of steroids. Triamcinolone Diacetate (Aristocort) intralesional solution at the concentration of 12.5 mg/ml was used. Using a 1 ml tuberculin syringe with a 26-gauge needle, the scarring area was injected with 0.1–0.2 ml of this steroid solution. The injections were usually repeated 1 or 2 times until the induration had softened.

Since the introduction of smaller extractors and the construction of a flat, spatula-shaped tip with the aperture turned down toward the fascia plane, and the creation of multiple side-by-side tunnels, dermal injury has not been seen in the authors' practice in recent years. It is important to leave adequate subdermal fat, because in this layer are found lymphatics and nerve endings which are necessary elements for the maintenance of normal cutaneous trophicity, tonicity, and sensation.

In the early days of facial lipo-suction, the molding tape was placed in one piece across the midline from one side of the mandible to the other. This caused vertical wrinkling of the submandibular area and the jowls. The wrinkling caused by taping usually disappeared with time and gentle massage.

The most common immediate postoperative complication was skin reaction to tape. It was manifested by severe itching, blister formation, and superficial excoriation when all brands of tape were used. Because of many adverse effects arising from taping, the authors are now replacing molding tape with the use of an elastic head garment placed over the fluff dressing. This provides adequate compression for skin molding and redraping after suction.

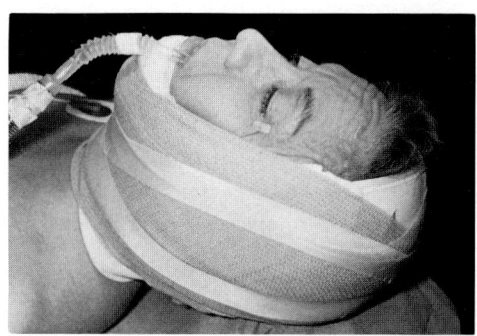

Fig. 14-73. Dressing is completed by elastic bandages, gently wrapped around the head.

Hematoma and Seroma Formation

The blood vessels are covered by a fibrous tissue adventitia which are rarely disrupted by the blunt cannula. There has been no incidence of hematoma formation of sufficient magnitude to require opening of the wound in the authors' series. There was a small incidence of seroma formation in the submental area which was removed by needle aspiration without any sequelae. By direct observation during open suction technique with rhytidectomy, the authors have confirmed an impression that a markedly dry field due to negligible amount of sharp dissection is usual.

Any penetration of the suction cannula into the platysma muscle and the cervical fascia will result in bleeding if the muscle fibers are injured by the extractor passages. If the platysma layer is violated, damage to major blood vessels in the neck could occur. Hemostasis appears to depend on the ability of the surgeon to keep the tip of the extractor within the fat layer and to extract the fat evenly and systematically.

Nerve Injury

Injury to the marginal mandibular branch of the facial nerve or to the greater auricular nerve is possible if the extractor penetrates the SMAS layer and enters the covering platysma muscle. It is found that the perineural tissue is not damaged by the blunt edges of the cannula aperture. During open lipo-suction combined with rhytidectomy, the authors have intentionally suctioned over the great auricular nerve using the facial extractors and vacuum force set at near 1 atm negative pressure. Postoperatively, no paraesthesia nor anesthesia was noted in the distribution area of this nerve.

Poor Patient Selection

Patient selection is of paramount importance in the avoidance of unfavorable skin wrinkling and folding in the submental region. In the younger age group with good skin tone and thick "bull" neck associated with significant subcutaneous fatty accumulation, good contouring can be predicted in most cases. The surgeon has to be more selective in the older age group with loose, redundant, poorly toned skin and hanging platysma bands. In these patients, it is necessary to do a combined cervico-facial lipo-suction and full face rhytidectomy. Age is not an absolute indication for the procedure chosen. A combination of age, skin tone and redundancy, and loose subcutaneous tissue is the basis for patient selection.

Other Complications

Infection and skin necrosis have not been observed in the authors' practice. Some patients lose sensation in the areas that have been treated, but sensation usually returns within 3–6 months.

Since cervico-facial fat is not voluminous, complications such as hypotension, pain, prolonged drainage, and thrombophlebitis are not seen. The amount of fat extracted rarely exceeds 100 cc at one time.

CONCLUSION

Cervico-facial fat extraction is an effective surgical method for aesthetic sculpturing of the submental, jowl, nasolabial and buccal areas. It can be done in both male and female, with no age limit. The operative procedure for suction of isolated facial fat accumulation varies from 10 to 20 minutes and requires only a small stab wound incision, which is placed below the mentum or earlobes, in the nasal vestibules, or in the mouth. If lipo-suction is done in conjunction with rhytidectomy, the cannula passages do most of the dissection work and markedly shorten the operative time. Minimal surgical trauma and stress allow for the patient's early return to activity.

Patient acceptance of lipo-suction has been exceptionally gratifying, with fewer complications, and quicker return to normality than with lipectomy by excisional methods. Proper use of the cannulas, basic understanding of the facial cutaneous-adipose complex, and careful patient selection are general guidelines for a pleasing aesthetic result.

REFERENCES

1. Maliniak JW: Is the surgical restoration of the aged face justified? Med J Rec 135:321, 1932
2. Newman J, Dolsky RL: Lipo-suction surgery: History and development. J Dermatol Surg Oncol 10:467–469, 1984
3. Fischer A, Fischer GM: Revised technique for cellulitis fat reduction in riding breeches deformity. Bull Int Acad Cosmet Surg 2:40, 1977
4. Schrudde J: Lipexeresis as a means of eliminating local adiposity. Aesthetic Plast Surg 4:215, 1980
5. Kesselring UK, Meyer R: A suction curette for removal of excessive local deposits of subcutaneous fat. Plast Reconstr Surg 62:305–306, 1978
6. Illouz YG: Body contouring by lipolysis: A 5-year experience with over 3,000 cases. Plast Reconstr Surg 72:591–597, 1983
7. Williams PL, Warwick R: Gray's Anatomy (ed. 36). Philadelphia: W.B. Saunders Company, p. 536, 1980
8. Jost G, Levet Y: Parotid fascia and face lifting: A critical evaluation of the SMAS concept. Plast Reconstr Surg 74:42–51, 1984
9. Ham AW: Histology (ed. 7). Philadelphia: Lippincott, p. 226, 1974.
10. Newman J, Dolsky RL: Innovations in platysma rhytidectomy. Arch Otolaryngol 109:637–641, 1983
11. Newman J, Dolsky RL: Complications and pitfalls of facial lipo-suction surgery. Am J Cosmet Surg 2:8–12, 1985.

Vijay K. Anand
Kenneth E. Lee

15
Voice Restoration

Voice restoration of the total laryngectomy patient has gained recent popularity due to the success of prosthetic phonatory devices. In the United States, there are about 10,000 new laryngeal cancer patients every year and the incidence in on the rise. Total laryngectomy is the treatment of choice in advanced laryngeal carcinomas and about 50 percent of these patients develop satisfactory esophageal speech with speech therapy. There are other methods of phonation and they are achieved with the use of the electrolarynx and the tracheoesophageal shunt procedures. This chapter will deal with the newer concepts of these procedures.

Billroth[1] in 1873 was the first surgeon to complete a successful total laryngectomy and his resident, Gussenbauer,[2] is credited as the first surgeon to attempt a tracheoesophageal shunt procedure. In recent years (1970), Staffieri and Serafini[3] have described refinements in the technique of creating a pseudo-glottis for phonation. Successful phonation without aspiration of food was described by Singer and Blom in 1979.[4]

The Singer-Blom procedure uses the principle of insertion of a one-way duckbill valve prosthesis at the site of the tracheoesophageal shunt. The indications for the procedure include patients who have no satisfactory speech or poor esophageal speech and who are motivated to improve the quality of their phonation. Age, sex, radiation therapy, and total laryngopharyngectomy do not appear to be contraindications for the procedure. This procedure can be carried out primarily at the time of the laryngectomy or as a secondary procedure following the ablative cancer surgery. Successful rehabilitation at the present time appears to be limited with the primary procedure, due to differences in the technique of the surgery, which varies with the individual surgeon performing it.

The patients for the procedure are carefully evaluated preoperatively in the office with the air-blowing test. The test is performed in the office by inserting a catheter (14 French) into the esophagus transnasally to the level of the tracheostoma. Air is then

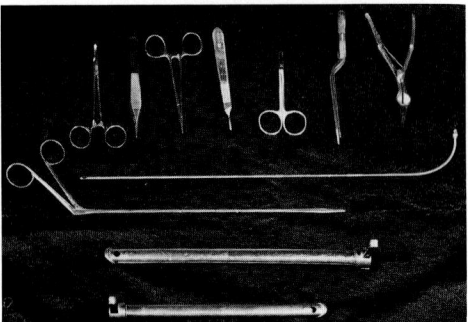

Fig. 15-1. Instrumentation for the procedure: special esophagoscopes with openings on the beveled ends, shown with other instruments used for the procedure.

blown into the catheter and the patient is instructed to phonate a sustained "ahhh."[5] If the patient is not able to phonate satisfactorily, there may be a spasm of the pharyngeal constrictors and a cricopharyngeal myotomy may be required at the time of the shunt procedure. This has not, however been found to be a contraindication in the authors' experience. Patients undergoing the shunt procedures are well counseled by both the surgeon performing the procedure and the speech therapist preoperatively.

The procedure is usually performed on an ambulatory basis when the cricopharyngeal myotomy is not indicated. General anesthesia is usually carried out with a carden tube and a venturi system.

METHOD I

A special esophagoscope with an opening on the beveled end is introduced and the spot of light from the endoscope is visualized at a point 5 mm below the junction of the skin and the tracheal mucous membrane (Fig. 15-1). A number 11 blade is used to make

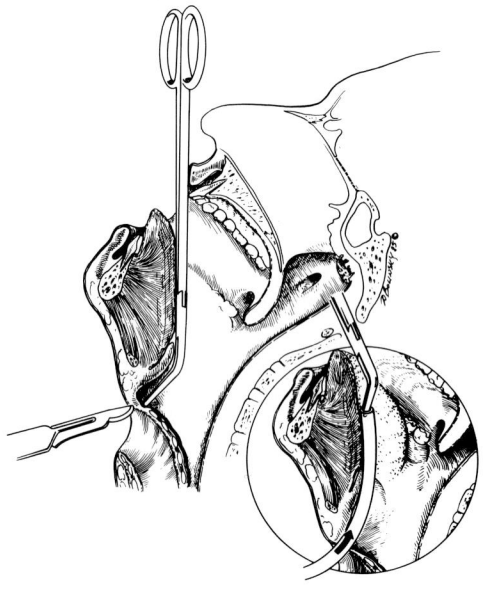

Fig. 15-2. The incision is made over the tracheal mucosa, at the proposed site of the tracheoesophageal fistula.

Voice Restoration

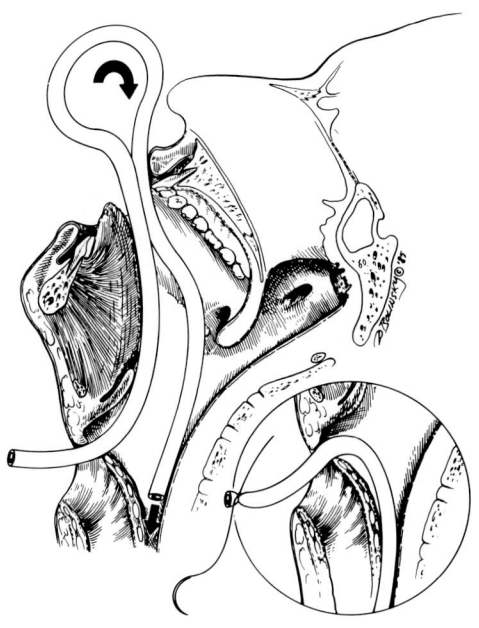

Fig. 15-3. The catheter is inserted through the site of the incision, retrieved through the mouth, and reinserted through the mouth into the esophagus.

the incision and the incision is dilated with a sharp hemostat. Under direct vision, a 14 French red rubber catheter is introduced and retrieved through the esophagoscope orally. A second catheter is introduced through the nasal cavity, and this is also retrieved through the oral cavity. The ends of the two catheters inside the oral cavity are now sutured, using silk sutures. The second catheter is then pulled out of the nasopharynx through the nose, bringing with it the first catheter, which is now tied to it. Once the second catheter is entirely out of the nasal cavity, the first catheter should extend from the trachea directly through the nasal cavity and out of the nose. Now, the second catheter can be disconnected from the first catheter and discarded. At the nasal end, the first catheter is secured over a dental roll, as in a posterior nasal packing, and, at the other end, the catheter is sutured to the neck, away from the tracheal stoma.

Patients treated by this method are discharged the same day and instructed to resume soft diet. A patient requiring an esophageal dilatation or cricopharyngeal myotomy is hospitalized for a few days and is maintained on nasogastric feeding or intravenous fluids before oral diet is resumed. A detailed description of the cricopharyngeal myotomy and its indications have been well reported by Singer and Blom in 1981.[6] The catheter is removed in 1 week in the office, and the prosthesis is inserted.

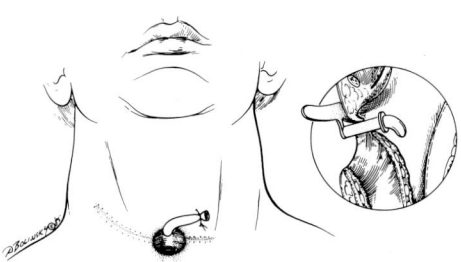

Fig. 15-4. The catheter is sutured to the neck away from the tracheal stoma. Placement of the Blaise-Raphael voice prosthesis is also shown.

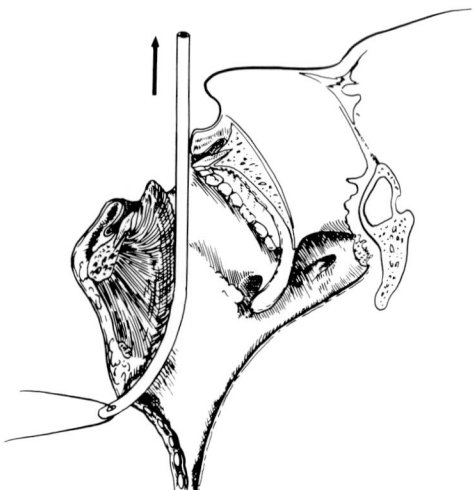

Fig. 15-5. The suction cannula can be used in place of the Mixter clamp to help make the incision and retrieve the catheter.

METHOD II

If the procedure is done at the time of laryngectomy, the Blaise-Raphael voice prosthesis is inserted immediately, and it is held in place by the tracheotomy tube.

If done weeks or months following laryngectomy, the procedure is done on an ambulatory basis under local or general anesthesia. A Mixter clamp is introduced intraorally to the level of the proposed site of the tracheoesophageal fistula. With the tips of the clamp slightly apart, an incision is made over the tracheal mucosa (Fig. 15-2). A rubber catheter is introduced at the site of the incision and is retrieved orally. The catheter is then reinserted through the mouth into the esophagus, so the catheter now extends from the site of incision directly to the stomach (Fig. 15-3). The catheter is sutured to the neck, away from the tracheal stoma. In 3–7 days, the catheter is removed, and the Blaise-Raphael voice prosthesis is inserted (Fig. 15-4).

For those patients in whom it is difficult to maneuver the Mixter clamp, an esophageal suction cannula with a side-suction can be used instead. The suction cannula is introduced to the level of the proposed site of the tracheoesophageal fistula, and the incision is made (Fig. 15-5). A string looped through the two suction ports is then tied to

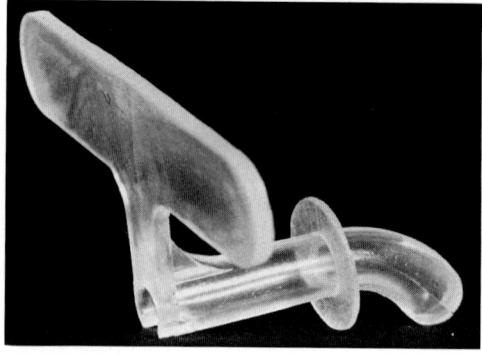

Fig. 15-6. The Blaise-Raphael voice prosthesis.

Voice Restoration

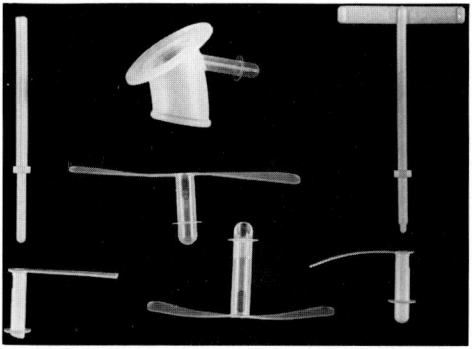

Fig. 15-7. The different varieties of voice prostheses available for ingestion, including the low-pressure varieties.

the rubber catheter. By withdrawing the suction cannula, the rubber catheter is pulled into the oral cavity, and the same procedure for management of the catheter illustrated in Figure 15-3 is followed.

The surgeon can also choose to implant the voice prosthesis as a secondary procedure without using a catheter. In this case, after the incision is made, the Mixter clamp or the esophageal suction cannula will be used instead of the nasogastric tube to retrieve and implant the Blaise-Raphael voice prosthesis. A tracheotomy tube is then used to push posteriorly the Blaise-Raphael voice prosthesis and hold it in place. In 3–7 days, the tracheotomy tube is removed, and the Blaise-Raphael voice prosthesis will stay in position by itself.

The Blaise-Raphael voice prosthesis has proven to be very convenient, as only minimum cleaning and minimum care are necessary (Fig. 15-6). At most, the patient has to clean the prosthesis with a Q-tip while the prosthesis is held in position. The downward curve of the Blaise-Raphael voice prosthesis discourages aspiration. Furthermore, patients have been able to use the device without any speech therapy. Most patients need to have the prosthesis changed once every 3–4 months. Four patients have had the

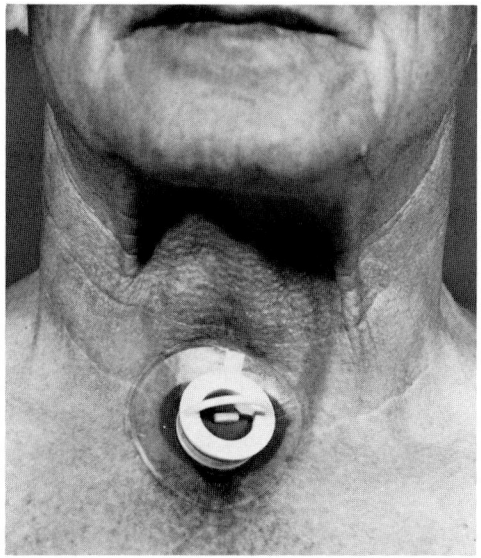

Fig. 15-8. Valve with housing over the stoma and the prosthesis which is useful for phonation.

prosthesis in position for over a year without ever having it removed. Other prostheses are shown in Figure 15-7. Once the patient achieves a certain level of fluency with regard to phonation, a valve with a housing is tried, and this valve eliminates the use of the finger for phonation (Fig. 15-8).

Complications from the procedure are minor. They include aspiration through or around the prosthesis, which is corrected by changing the prosthesis or cauterizing the tract with silver nitrate solution. Aspiration of a loose-fitting prosthesis into the trachea or the bronchus has been reported, and this is managed by removal with a bronchoscope and administration of antibiotics for infection. Patients who have undergone radiation prior to insertion of the prosthesis tend to develop stenosis of the tract or stenosis of the stoma. Tracheitis sicca has also been reported in the radiated patient. This is managed by revision of tracheostome prior to insertion of the prosthesis. Stenosis of the shunt area can be probed with a blunt probe, and the tract can be serially dilated in a select number of cases. If bleeding is encountered at the shunt area during dilatation, the probing should be abandoned and the procedure revised under general anesthesia.

Patients who have successfully developed good speech with the procedure should be seen periodically in the office, and instruction on the maintenance of the shunt hygiene should be explained to them. Some of the patients may require a change of prosthesis in 3 months or after that period, depending on their use of the device. Lastly, the physician performing the procedure should be cautioned that in the enthusiasm to help the patient, one should not underestimate the time and practice which must be expended by the patient to become proficient in the use of the prosthesis. Patients who undergo this procedure should also be carefully evaluated for any possible recurrence of the tumor or metastasis from it.

In conclusion, this procedure—the simplest and most reliable for surgical speech rehabilitation following laryngectomy—satisfies many important criteria in rehabilitation of the total laryngectomy patient: it is simple, can be done primarily or secondarily, does not compromise the original extirpative surgery, is well tolerated in conjunction with radiotherapy, and can be done in the office if the office has operating room facilities. Although the surgery itself is simple and reliable, the prosthesis is still being perfected, with refined models constantly being described.

REFERENCES

1. Miehlke A: Theodor Billroth, historical vignette. Arch Otolaryngol 84:354–358, 1966
2. Gussenbauer C: Uber die Erste Durch Th. Billroth an Menschen Ausgefuhrte Kehlkopf-Exstupation, und die Ambendung eines Kuntslichen Kehlkopfes. Verh Dtsch Ges Chir: 250, 1874
3. Staffieri M, Serafini I: La riabilitazione cherurgica della voce e della resperazione dopo laringectomia tatale. Bologna, Italy: Associazone Otologi Ospedalieri, Italiana, 1976
4. Singer MI, Blom ED: Tracheoesophageal puncture: A surgical prosthetic method for postlaryngectomy speech restoration. Third International Symposium Plastic Reconstructive Surgery of the Head and Neck, 1979
5. Johns ME, Cantrell RW: Voice restoration of the total laryngectomy patient: The Singer-Blom technique. Otolaryngol Head Neck Surg 89:82–86, 1981
6. Singer MI, Blom ED: Selective myotomy for voice restoration after total laryngectomy. Arch Otolaryngol 107:670–673, 1981

James H. Kelly
Marvin P. Fried

16

The Carbon Dioxide Laser in Outpatient Surgery

The carbon dioxide laser has been used extensively in the outpatient setting in gynecologic and otolaryngoltic procedures.

In order to safely perform these procedures in the ambulatory setting, meticulous attention to patient selection, safety precautions, in-service education, and instrument selection must be practiced. This is particularly true since carbon dioxide laser procedures in otolaryngology-head and neck surgery often have the potential to compromise the patient's airway. Careful patient selection, as discussed below, must therefore be practiced to determine which patients will be appropriate for the ambulatory setting.

Until the time that extensive experience is gained in the use of the carbon dioxide laser for ambulatory otolaryngology-head and neck surgery procedures, the burden of proof as to the appropriateness of these procedures will lie with the individual ambulatory units involved. The current need to diminish health care costs will allow this determination to proceed rapidly in the near future.

BASIC CONCEPTS OF THE CARBON DIOXIDE LASER

The laser is a scalpel that uses a light-emitting energy source. This light is an atomic-process-generated electromagnetic wave. When an atom makes a transition from an excited state of high energy level to a lower one, the light energy that is generated is a photon. This emitted light can be directed by a series of lenses to a specific focal point.

An atom at a low energy level may be struck by a photon and make the transition to a higher level. This absorption of light, such as is effected by objects in daylight, can impart a color to the object. If, however, an atom is at a high energy level (excited state) and is struck by a photon, 2 photons are released as the atom degrades to a lower energy level. If a population exists containing numerous excited atoms, and thereby emitting photons in increasing numbers, a chain reaction is produced. This process is light amplification by stimulated emission of radiation (LASER).

If this population of atoms (such as carbon dioxide molecules) is enclosed in a container with an electric current or similar energy source placed through this population, the atoms can be excited to a higher energy state, causing a "population inversion" with more atoms at the higher than the lower level. These carbon dioxide molecules will then produce photons in all directions. If 2 parallel mirrors are placed at each end of the laser container, some photons can be made to travel in a plane perpendicular to these mirrors. If one mirror is totally reflecting, while one allows partial photon escape, a beam of radiation is produced.[1]

The laser radiation beam emitted has certain specific properties. All of the waves in the light have the same wavelength, making it monochromatic. All of the wave forms are in phase with each other and parallel, making it coherent. These properties allow the laser light to be focused and concentrated by a lens imparting high energy to a very small cross-sectional area. The carbon dioxide laser has a wave length in the infrared range of 10.6μ. Tissue can absorb this radiation and dissipate the energy within a fraction of a millimeter. Since tissue is at least 80 percent water, the heat absorbed will cause evaporation or vaporization. The amount of tissue effect is determined by the power setting of the laser and the duration of exposure, regardless of the pigmentation of the tissue. Heat transferred to contiguous structures is minimal because of the low conductivity of the water and the vaporization to air that occurs.[3]

SELECTION OF A SUITABLE LASER UNIT

Carbon dioxide laser units are very expensive capital items ranging in cost from $40,000 to over $100,000. To this must be added the additional equipment necessary for their use, such as special instrumentation (bronchoscopes, laryngoscopes, anesthesia equipment, etc.) and the cost (in time) to train personnel and in maintenance.

Careful evaluation, therefore, must be made of the cost-effectiveness of any ambulatory center purchasing a laser. This should include the number of cases each year appropriate for the laser, space considerations, and whether or not third-party payers are willing to reimburse additional amounts for the use of the laser over conventional therapy.

After the decision is made to purchase a laser, considerable time and effort should be given to consideration of the particular type of laser to be purchased. Most manufacturers will provide a laser unit on a trial basis and several units should be compared. These should be the units that have features appropriate to the types of procedures that will be performed. A carbon dioxide laser with a high output (80–100 w) should be chosen, which will be adaptable. As important as (if not more important than) the laser unit itself is the service contract the manufacturer provides and the manufacturer's ability to live up to the contract. References should be obtained from the manufacturer for similar units, preferably in the same geographical area. These references should be thoroughly checked to determine the responsiveness to maintenance needs and the reliability of the equipment. This will prevent long periods in which the laser is unavailable for use.

The manufacturer should provide thorough in-service training for the personnel involved and should be available to update this as necessary. This availability can also be determined by a thorough questioning of the references provided.

The Carbon Dioxide Laser in Outpatient Surgery

ROOM ORGANIZATION

The use of the carbon dioxide laser requires that quite a few pieces of equipment be available: microscopes, endoscopic light sources, etc., as well as the laser itself. For this reason, a room large enough to hold all the equipment must be selected. It is preferable to have a single room designated for laser use in which all the equipment can be stored. This prevents unnecessary movement of equipment with loss of time and possible instrument damage to the equipment. Room layout is equally important. A diagram (or photograph) should be available to determine proper positioning of equipment to prevent clutter and to allow proper use of all necessary equipment. (See sample diagram, Fig. 16-1.)

PATIENT SELECTION FOR AMBULATORY SURGERY

It is obvious that patients must be selected who will be able to safely return home within several hours after surgery. Any patient, therefore, who has airway compromise prior to surgery is not a candidate for laser surgery in the ambulatory setting. This would include most patients with malignancies of the airway, and also patients with benign lesions such as laryngotracheal stenoses, in which the airway is reduced by 50 percent or more. Even more caution should be exercised in the pediatric age group, in which postoperative edema is of grave concern. Similarly, patients with lesions that are expected to bleed easily (e.g., cavernous hemangiomas) should not be considered for ambulatory laser removal. It should also be obvious that patients who would not be candidates for other ambulatory procedures, such as those with significant medical problems including cardiac and pulmonary disorders, should not be considered as candidates for ambulatory laser surgery.

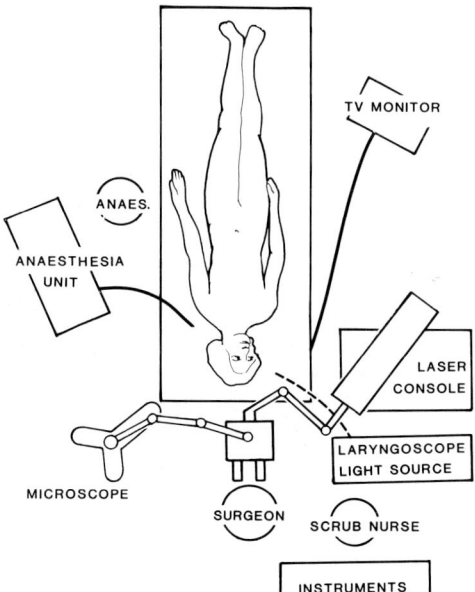

Fig. 16-1. Diagram of all necessary equipment in the suggested proper position.

An assessment should be made prior to scheduling regarding the feasibility of intubation of the patient. A patient with significant trismus, a short or inflexible neck, a large tongue, or other problems relating to ease of intubation should be carefully evaluated prior to the procedure.

Last, the general rule should be: if there is *any real question* of the safety of performing ambulatory laser procedures, the procedure *should not* be performed on an ambulatory basis.

ANESTHETIC CONSIDERATION AND TECHNIQUES

More than most other surgical procedures, head and neck/laser operations require good communication between the surgeon and the anesthetist. Competition for the airway and the possibility of laser hazards make these procedures more potentially hazardous than procedures in other areas of the body. The anesthetist, as well as the surgeon, should be thoroughly familiar with anesthetic techniques and safety precautions involving the laser.

When possible, Venturi ventilation should be utilized.[4] This reduces the risk of laser fire and allows the surgeon a much better view of the vocal cords. Venturi ventilation also eliminates the trauma of intubation and the endotracheal tube. Some patients, however, are not candidates for high-pressure Venturi ventilation. Patients with significant restrictive lung disease or lesions that compromise the airway (in the larynx, trachea, or bronchus), and patients with bullous emphysema are some examples of those who would not be suitable candidates.

Technique

A Venturi jet ventilator (Fig. 16-2A) is attached to the laryngoscope by means of a screw clamp. The patient is induced using mask ventilation and the laryngoscope is inserted to expose the airway. The anesthetist then ventilates the patient by way of a valve (Fig. 16-2B) attached to the anesthesia machine. The jet ventilation will cause some movement of the airway, so it may be necessary to use the laser in between the jets of ventilation or to ask the anesthetist to stop ventilating the patient for brief periods during laser use.

For those patients who require intubation, special precautions must be utilized with the endotracheal tube. The polyvinyl chloride (PVC) tube should be avoided, since in

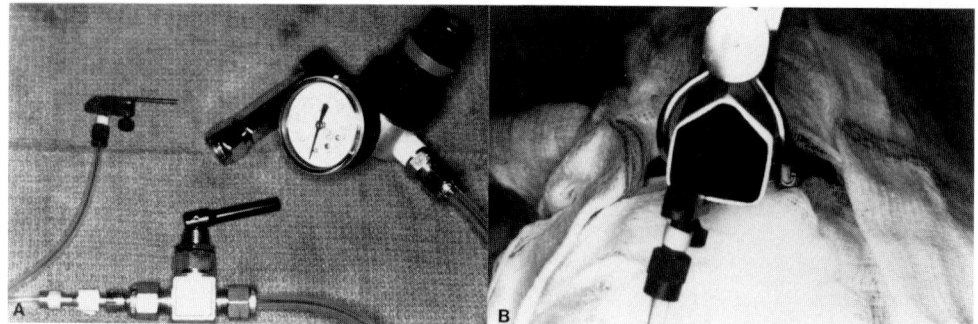

Fig. 16-2. (A) Venturi jet ventilator is attached to the laryngoscope by means of a screw clamp. (B) Ventilating the patient by way of a valve attached to the anesthesia machine.

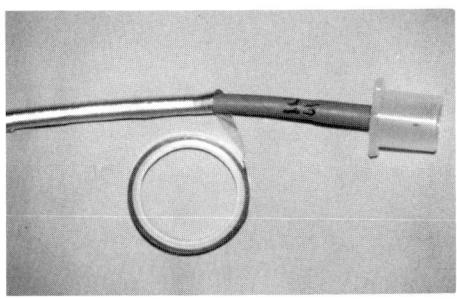

Fig. 16-3. A small red, rubber tube can be utilized and wrapped with metallic tape.

addition to its low kindling point, ignition of the tube produces toxic fumes that are further damaging to the patient. A small red rubber tube can be utilized and wrapped with metallic tape (Fig. 16-3). Care must be taken in wrapping the tube so that sharp edges are not produced and so that no area of the tube is left uncovered. The cuff cannot be wrapped; it should be filled with water (to extinguish a fire should the laser strike it). Some anesthetists prefer to use water colored with methylene blue, since it instantly alerts the laser surgeon when the cuff has been perforated. New tubes made of "noncombustible" material have been developed,[5,6] but are costly. Any new noncombustible tube should be tested prior to its general use.

A technique has been recently developed[7] using 5 percent nitrogen in the anesthetic gas mixture. Early reports indicate that this significantly reduces the danger of fire.

Even with new developments, the risk of combustion is present. Wet cotton patties should be packed around the cuff (and tube, when possible) and should be kept moist during the procedure (see below).

In all cases, the anesthetist, surgeon, and nursing staff should be constantly aware of laser safety and should be updated on recent developments.

INFORMED CONSENT

Informed consent is a significant cause for legal action against physicians. This is particularly pertinent in laser use, since, for the most part, alternative methods of treatment are available that do not share the hazards of the laser. Patients and/or family should be fully informed of these alternatives and risks both verbally and in writing and allowed to decide whether the anticipated benefits outweigh those risks. This information should be well documented, signed by both the patient (or guardian) and the surgeon, and witnessed. The anesthetist should also explain to the patient the specific complications related to anesthesia and should obtain similar documentation. Laser fires, burns, late scar formation, pneumomediastinum, pneumothorax, etc. (Table 16-1) should be specifically mentioned, as should complications of the procedure itself. If there is hesitancy on the patient's part in the use of the laser, alternate methods should be attempted.

INSTRUMENTATION IN LASER SURGERY

In addition to the laser itself, numerous instruments have been developed to extend the range of laser surgery and to provide more safety. Shields, retractors, mirrors, and

Table 16-1
Carbon Dioxide Laser Complications

Direct laser effects
  burn of tissue out of operative field (e.g., eye, facial)
  mucosal burn
  endotracheal tube ignition
  ignition of cottonoid
  pneumothorax
  subcutaneous emphysema
Secondary laser effects
  endotracheal tube obstruction by lasered tissue
  endotracheal tube ignition by flaming tissue
  burn from a reflecting surface
    outside of endoscope
    within endoscope
  mucosal charring with airway obstruction
  hemorrhage
  edema
  perichondritis
Delayed laser effects
  vocal cord web
  cicatrix and stenosis
  glottic incompetence due to excessive tissue removal

From Fried MP: A survey of the complications of laser laryngoscopy. Arch Otolaryngol 110:31–34, 1984. With permission.

smoke evacuation systems are among a few that are currently available.[8] Since these are expensive instruments, good judgment must be utilized in their purchase, use, and maintenance. Because of cost, instruments that are compatible with existing equipment should be selected when possible. When this is not possible and additional equipment is warranted, arrangements should be made with company representatives to "try" the equipment on loan to use in clinical situations prior to purchase. In all cases, instruments with nonreflecting surfaces are preferable. All personnel should become familiar with newly acquired equipment prior to the clinical application. Company representatives can be quite helpful in this regard.

As with most procedures, the surgeon should thoroughly check the available equipment to make sure the necessary instruments are available and in proper working order prior to beginning the case.

SAFETY PRECAUTIONS—COMPLICATIONS AND THEIR PREVENTION

As the laser gains more frequent utility, the incidence of actual as well as theoretical complications will increase. These potential, as well as real hazards, have been documented.[9] In a survey of one of the senior otolaryngology societies, 92 percent of the people questioned responded. Of these physicians, approximately one-half had used the laser without complications, 27 percent had not used the laser at all, and 23 percent reported a total of 81 complications. These included endotracheal explosion, laryngeal stenosis or web formation, facial burns, and hemorrhage. Five cases of pneumothorax and two of subcutaneous emphysema were also reported. Moreover, increased experience with the use of the laser did not necessarily guarantee fewer complications. It is difficult to assess the true incidence of complications, since not all have been reported or have come to litigation. It can be assumed, however, that up to this point, the general number of complications may reflect the number of cases performed each month.

The complications of laser endoscopy can be conceptualized into direct, secondary, and delayed effects (Table 16-1). One of the most serious of the direct effects is ignition of the endotracheal tube. This may occur with direct impact on the outside of an unprotected tube or due to a dehiscence in the wrapping. This also can occur as tissue embers are insufflated into the lumen of the tube, causing ignition internally. Other direct effects include burns of the eye, face, or mucosa, as well as ignition of substances in the operating field that have not been protected or moistened. Pneumothorax or subcutaneous emphysema is a consequence of air escape outside of the anatomic airway, either due to the disease process or the surgical procedure. The high-pressure Venturi system tends to propagate this air escape.

Secondary laser effects occur as a result of tissue alteration produced by the laser or the laser instrumentation. Delayed effects occur after healing has taken place.

Should a complication occur, the extent of injury must be assessed as soon as possible.[8] If this is an airway fire, the endotracheal tube should be removed and the source of oxygen disconnected. Ventilation can be resumed with a smaller endotracheal tube. Direct visualization of the airway should be performed by laryngoscopy and bronchoscopy and any debris removed. Antibiotics and steroids are needed for extensive mucosal injury. Reverse isolation, tracheal cultures, repeated endoscopy, and perhaps admission to an intensive care unit is needed for severe cases. Damage to pulmonary parenchyma may be assessed with polytomography, computed tomographic scanning, blood gas determinations, and ventilation-perfusion scans.

Prevention is best accomplished by adequate preparation. The entire surgical team must be familiar with the equipment used. All must be in readiness prior to having the patient enter the operating suite. Alternative surgical techniques should be considered. A plan must be available in case a complication should occur. All members of the operating team, as well as the patient, should have eye protection.

The anesthesiologist, in conjunction with the surgeon, should decide on a method of ventilation and make certain that the endotracheal tube is adequately protected.

All possible sources of combustion should be moistened. The patient's face should be covered with a moist gauze or cloth.

The surgeon should use binocular vision whenever possible in order to assess the depth of laser penetration. The laser should be kept in the center of the operative field so that reflection off of the side of the endoscope does not occur. It would be advisable to begin lasering at low power and with brief bursts so that the tissue interaction can be assessed and familiarity with a particular disease process can be obtained. If visualization is inadequate, then the laser and laryngoscope should be repositioned. Charred tissue must be removed to prevent excessive absorption of heat. Any areas of hemorrhage must be controlled, since this would obscure vision, as well as prevent adequate laser effect. Lasering 360° should be avoided in order to prevent cicatrix formation. Adequate aspiration of the laser plume must be available. Excessive tissue should not be removed since this may lead to an incompetent airway.

CONCLUSIONS

As was stated above, the carbon dioxide laser in otolaryngology-head and neck surgery has not been used widely as an ambulatory procedure. The authors feel that as the scope of ambulatory surgery is widened, the carbon dioxide laser will be increasingly utilized. It must be remembered, however, that in case of mishap, the burden of proof of the safety of ambulatory carbon dioxide laser treatments will rest with the surgeon, the anesthetist, and the ambulatory center. For this reason, extreme caution should be utilized until this procedure becomes routine and guidelines are set.

REFERENCES

1. Fuller TA: The physics of surgical lasers. Lasers Surg Med 1:5–14, 1980
2. Verschueren R: The CO_2 laser in tumor surgery. Amsterdam: Van Horcum and Co, pp. 1–11, 1976
3. Fried MP: Complications of CO_2 laser surgery of the larynx. Laryngoscope 93:275–278, 1983
4. Woo P, Strong MS: Venturi jet ventilation through the metal endotracheal tube: A nonflammable system. Ann Otol Rhinol Laryngol 92:405–407, 1983
5. Endelist G, Alberti PW: Anesthesia for CO_2 laser surgery of the larynx. J Otolaryngol 11:107–110, 1982
6. Norton ML, DeVos O: New endotracheal tube for laser surgery of the larynx. Ann Otol Rhinol Laryngol 87:554–557, 1978
7. Cassissi NJ: Personal communication, 1984
8. Ossoff, RH, Karlan MS: Instrumentation for microlaryngeal laser surgery. Otolaryngol Head Neck Surg 91:456–460, 1983
9. Fried MP: A survey of the complications of laser laryngoscopy. Arch Otolaryngol 110:31–34, 1984
10. Schramm VL Jr, Mattox DE, Stool SE: Acute management of laser-ignited intratracheal explosion. Laryngoscope 91:1417–1426, 1981

Richard L. Fabian

17
Cryosurgery in Outpatient Surgery

Cryosurgery is the branch of cryobiology in which extremely cold temperatures are used to treat a disease process. Historically, James Arnott (1797–1883) is credited with being the first physician to treat cancer with the application of cold. Since Arnott's initial use of iced saline, a variety of media have been utilized to deliver the cryoinjury. Today, the most effective medium is liquid nitrogen.

By definition, office or outpatient surgery is the performance of a surgical technique in the physician's office, surgical unit, or outpatient department of the hospital. In this setting, preoperative evaluation of the patient's medical status and proposed surgical technique indicates to the physician that there is no technical compromise or risk to the patient in the treatment of the disease process. Using either general or local anesthesia, the procedure is accomplished and the patient is allowed to return home the day of surgery. The decision to carry out such procedures must include the postoperative events expected after the procedure. The patient and family members should be provided with a written explanation of the procedure, what untoward complications and events are possible, and how they are to react to them. Dressing care, medication, and emergency back-up instructions are an essential part of good surgical practice. The arbitrary restraints of third-party payers or patient economics should not in any way influence good surgical judgment.

CRYOBIOLOGY

The purpose of the cryoinjury is to deliver a lethal blow to the tissue being treated. The size and degree of the injury can vary widely. This variation relates to the type of medium used, the time course of application, the number of applications, the sensitivity of the tissue being treated, and the vascularity of the tissue.

A wide variety of events occur in tissue in response to cryoinjury. Keeping in mind the variation of cellular response, the following events (biological and biochemical) in response to liquid nitrogen should be noted.

1. The formation of intracellular and extracellular crystals
2. Cellular dehydration and pH changes
3. Denaturation
4. Deactivation of cellular metabolism
5. Cell membrane lipoprotein disruption
6. Disruption of the nuclear and mitochondrial membranes
7. Secondary recrystalization injury

Permanent cell injury as shown above requires temperatures colder than $-20°C$. The rate of cooling should exceed $10°C/min$. The more rapid the freeze, the less chance there is for intracellular dehydration to occur, thus allowing intracellular crystallization to occur. Slow thawing allows small intracellular crystals to coalesce into larger crystals with a subsequent greater lethal effect. The repetition of rapid freezing and slow thawing increases the lethal effects exponentially.

In vitro, the cryoprobe or liquid nitrogen acts as a heat sink. During the thaw cycle, initial vasoconstriction is followed by vasodilation, stasis, and small-vessel (venule) damage. Platelet agglutination and stasis result in microvascular thrombosis. Direct cellular damage and vascular stasis are the summary events responsible for necrosis.

The variation of tissue resistance to cryoinjury is to be considered. Sperm, cartilage, and sensory nerves are extremely sensitive, in contrast to the high degree of resistance of bone.

CLINICAL APPLICATIONS

The following facts should be considered as advantages of cryotherapy.

1. Sensory nerve sensitivity decreases the need for general anesthesia.
2. The integrity of major blood vessels is not affected.
3. With closed probes, the size of the cryolesion is easily controlled.
4. The equipment and liquid nitrogen is inexpensive.
5. Cryotherapy may be repeated in more than one session.
6. Postoperative pain is minimal.
7. Tissue repair occurs as tissue necrosis dissipates.
8. There is minimal intraoperative and postoperative bleeding.

The following facts should be considered as disadvantages.

1. Tissue protection with open spray techniques is more difficult.
2. Tissue healing is by secondary intention and may be more deforming.
3. Both normal and abnormal tissue is affected.
4. Tissue type, temperature, and vascularity limit effectiveness.
5. Treatment of malignant disease is local and not regional.
6. Tissue margins are not available for pathologic analysis.

APPARATUS

A wide variety of apparatus and media are available for the cryosurgeon. The experience of this author has been exclusively with liquid nitrogen. The apparatus used is the Brymill unit (Brymill Company), which is used for major applications (Fig. 17-1) and the smaller, self-contained hand unit (Fig. 17-2). A frequently used instrument is the thermocouple (Fig. 17-3). The larger unit is complemented by a variety of closed probes to adapt to the variety of clinical problems possible (Fig. 17-4).

THERAPEUTIC APPLICATIONS

Nasal Pathology

Severe vasomotor rhinitis with turbinate hypertrophy is amenable to the application of cryotherapy utilizing a specially adapted closed probe. Because of the difficulty in protecting the adjacent normal tissue, its usefulness is quite limited. When possible, the nasal septum and floor of the nose are protected with strips of styrofoam. Vaselinated guaze is used to protect the alar rims. Using a thermocouple, 2 freeze-thaw cycles of 90 seconds after $-20°C$ has been reached are recommended. Care must be taken to check the apparatus for leaks before therapeutic application, since raw liquid nitrogen intranasally can result in severe injury to the septum, nasal floor, and underlying palate. The patient should be warned about crusting and obstruction during the necrosis stage. Frequent office follow-up during healing is recommended.

Familial hemorrhagic telangiectasia has been controlled with selective cryotherapy. Using a hand-held closed cryoprobe, telangiectatic areas are treated with one 2-minute cycle. The subsequent scarring results in vessel obliteration and strengthening of the overlying mucosa. For more severe cases, septal dermoplasty, vessel ligation, and septectomy is recommended. Troublesome areas of bleeding intranasally following more radical treatment can be controlled with selective cryotherapy as indicated above.

Local anesthesia with topical cocaine and 1 percent plain xylocaine for a greater palatine foramen nerve block allows the surgeon to accomplish the previously listed cryotreatments as an outpatient-office procedure.

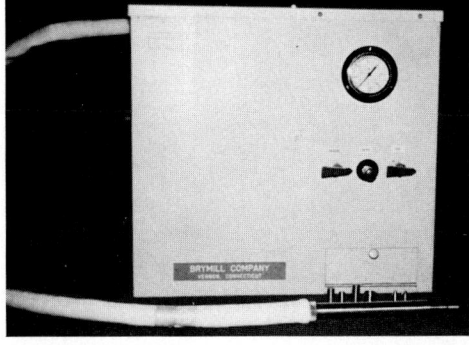

Fig. 17-1. Brymill unit used for the major application of cryosurgery in the head and neck area.

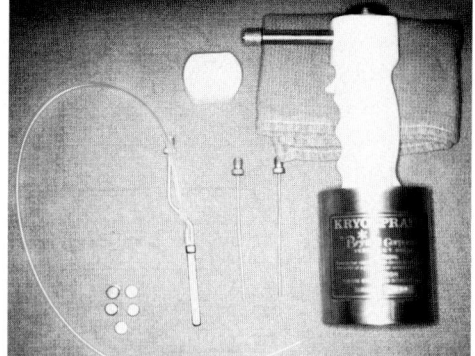

Fig. 17-2. Self-contained hand unit that is useful in both office and out-patient procedures. Also shown are the variety of tips and a nasal probe which can be used in the application of cryo to the nasal turbinates.

Laryngeal Pathology

Isolated lesions of in-situ carcinoma or papillomatosis of one vocal cord, false cord, or a solitary epiglottic focus can be successfully treated with cryotherapy. The advent of the laser has virtually eliminated the usefulness of cryotherapy in these situations, however. Under a general anesthetic, the entire endolarynx outside the lesion is protected with 8-ply vaselinated guaze. Using the hand-held laryngeal unit, an open spray is applied to the lesion for two 2-minute cycles. Steroids are given intraoperatively and for 24 hours postoperatively to prevent significant laryngeal edema. Under the clinical circumstances listed above, outpatient surgery can be safely accomplished.

Benign Oral Pathology

Painful herpes simplex eruptions can be effectively treated by an office procedure with the selective application of cryotherapy. A 30-second application time, using a closed probe or open spray (D opening), with the hand-held unit after the surrounding tissue is protected with 8-ply vaselinated gauze will facilitate rapid healing and pain control. The patient should be warned about transient edema of the tongue and cheek mucosa following treatment. The use of steroids if they are not contraindicated by the patient's medical condition is recommended. Areas of intraoral leukoplakia can be treated in a similar manner, providing a biopsy has confirmed the diagnosis. When done selectively, the resulting necrosis and healing process of the mucosa should obliterate the leukoplakia. This, coupled with good oral hygiene and avoidance of noxious stimuli such as smoking and alcohol, can provide effective control of this premalignant process.

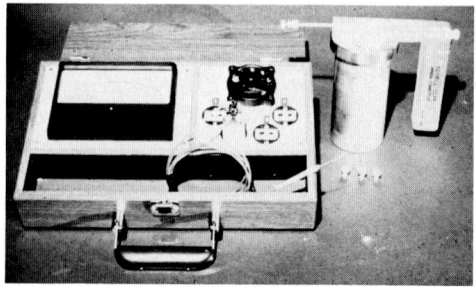

Fig. 17-3. Thermocouple unit and the Brymill hand held unit (older model).

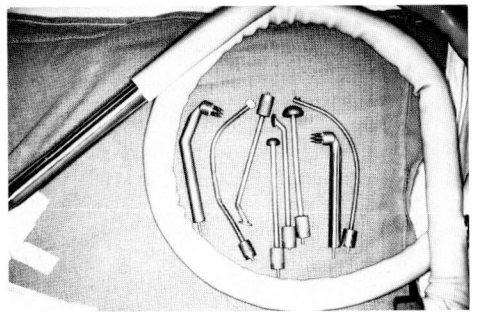

Fig. 17-4. Large unit closed probes which are encircled by the coiled insulated delivery arm.

Malignant Skin Lesions

Squamous cell carcinoma of skin of the head and neck can be effectively treated with cryosurgery. However, the potential for deep invasion and regional nodal spread, as well as the absolute necessity for pathologic margins, dictates against its use as initial therapy except in very select clinical circumstances. Patients with unresectable disease in which pain, ulceration, and bleeding have become a problem are candidates. In these circumstances, local anesthesia in an outpatient setting is feasible. Necrotic exophytic tumor is debulked by excision and open liquid nitrogen spray is applied to the base. At least 2 freeze-thaw cycles with thermocouple control are recommended. Daily home dressing care and weekly office debridement sessions are required. Repeat cryotherapy is used when clinically safe and efficacious.

Basal cell carcinoma is a locally malignant and invasive disease which, if not initially treated effectively, can result in massive tissue loss, deformity, and death. In keeping with good oncologic principles, biopsy confirmation should always precede treatment plans. Patients with basal cell carcinoma of the head and neck who are not candidates for cryosurgery are those with recurrent resectable disease, multicentric disease, basal cell carcinoma of the scirrhous type, and postradiation failures. In these circumstances, excisional surgery using Moh's fresh tissue technique with primary repair is the treatment of choice. Indications for cryosurgery in the treatment of basal cell carcinoma are as follows.

1. Recurrent unresectable postradiated disease for pain and bleeding
2. Superficial well-circumscribed disease
3. Treatment of a lesion in a cosmetically sensitive area
4. Patients medically unstable and poor candidates for long procedures
5. Alternate therapy to formal excision and repair

Prior to the use of cryotherapy in the head and neck area, the patient should be told that, because of the lack of pathologic control, the volume of tissue treated will be larger and deeper than that treated by formal surgery. Secondary healing may lead to deformity, although the cosmetic results are usually excellent. Depigmentation in the area of cryotherapy may sometimes occur. Treating any area of the face or scalp within 6 cm of the orbit will result in transient eyelid swelling. A prolonged healing time of up to 12 weeks may be experienced.

The surgeon should be aware that cartilage is extremely sensitive to the effects of cold. This is particularly true of the cartilages of the nose and pinnae. The use of a thermocouple is recommended. The protection of surrounding normal tissue is essential.

If the area to be treated is greater than 2 cm, adjacent tissue protection is best accomplished with 8-ply vaselinated gauze. Eye protection is accomplished with a scleral shield on the globe, styrofoam for the conjunctiva surface of the eyelid, and vaselinated gauze for the normal eyelid skin. In lesions less than 2 cm, a beveled cut of appropriate size is removed from the base of the styrofoam cup. By compressing the cup to the surrounding normal skin, the lesion to be treated is isolated in the opening at the base of the cup. Liquid nitrogen is applied to the lesion within the confines of the cup, with suction being used to remove excess liquid nitrogen. As in all areas, the application of liquid nitrogen results in the vaporization of excess accumulation of liquid nitrogen, which must be removed by suction. To avoid freezing of the suction apparatus, hot water must be constantly used to flush the suction during treatment. A rapid freeze followed by a slow thaw increases the effectiveness of treatment.

Steroids have little effect in diminishing the possible periorbital edema or transient fluid accumulation after cryotherapy in the facial region. Postoperative dressing changes and debridement sessions are as discussed earlier.

Head and Neck Malignancy

Malignancy of the oral cavity is amenable to cryotherapy in a variety of situations on an outpatient basis. Patients in this group are usually those who have undergone definitive therapy (surgery and radiation) and have evidence of recurrent disease. Bleeding, necrosis, secondary infection, and pain are but a few of the major problems with which the patient and oncologic surgeon must deal. These problems in a patient with recurrent carcinoma of the anterior tongue, anterior floor of mouth, retromolar trigone, buccal space, alveolar ridge, postmaxillary cavity, or exenterated orbit are amenable to cryotherapy, particularly for gross tumor reduction and pain control. Associated postoperative edema is usually not sufficient to cause an upper airway problem. Postoperative steroids are used to help minimize this edema. As a rule, a general anesthetic and the use of the large cryo unit is selected for patient comfort and effectiveness of treatment. Open liquid nitrogen spray or large, hand-held cryoprobes are selected, depending on the extent and site of the recurrence. Thermocouple documentation and control is used intraoperatively with an average freeze of 2 freeze-thaw cycles. Each freeze ranges from 2 to 4 minutes. Same day discharge is usually possible after adequate post anesthetic recovery. If a postoperative upper airway problem is suspected or if the patient's medical condition is unstable, then overnight hospital observation is required. Steroids for 1 or 2 days postoperatively in addition to weekly debridement sessions are recommended. Lesions posterior to the anatomical areas outlined previously (base of tongue, posterior tongue, etc.), if treated, will require a tracheostomy and in-hospital observation.

Miscellaneous

Small superficial skin hemangiomas, small areas of skin hyperpigmentation, and actinic changes on the lips and skin can be effectively handled with short duration (30–45 second) freeze-thaw cycles using the hand-held unit with the "C" or "D" size aperture. The treatment of multiple skin papillomas or coalescent seborrheic keratosis also falls in this treatment plan.

CONCLUSION

Cryotherapy is a valuable tool in the treatment of a variety of disorders in the head and neck. Many cryotherapeutic procedures can be safely performed on a patient in an outpatient or office setting provided that good surgical judgment is exercised. Familiarity with the equipment and the characteristics of the cryocoolant by the surgeon is mandatory.

BIBLIOGRAPHY

DeSanto LW: The curative, palliative and adjunctive uses of cryosurgery in the head and neck. Laryngoscope 82:1282, 1972
Holden HB: Cryosurgery in E.N.T. practice. J Laryngol Otol 76(8):821–827, 1972
Miller D, Meltzer D: Tissue penetration studies using liquid nitrogen. Trans Am Acad Opthal Otolaryngol, pp 300–309, 1969
Miller D: Cryosurgery for the treatment of neoplasms of the oral cavity. Otolaryngol Clin North Am 5:377–388, 1972
Neel BH III: Cryosurgery for the treatment of cancer. Laryngoscope 90(8:2) (Suppl. 23), pp 1–48, 1980
Sherman JK, Kim KS: Correlation of ultrastructure before freezing, while frozen and after thawing in assessing freeze-thaw induced injury. Cryobiology 4:16, 1967
Zacarian SA: Cryosurgery in dermatologic disorders and in the treatment of skin cancer. J Cryosurg 1:70–75, 1968

Denise Metz
June Bubier

18
Allergy Skin Testing

The importance of integrating allergy treatment and testing into the practice of otolaryngology is becoming more and more apparent as so many patients suffering from allergic diseases of the upper respiratory tract seek help. Skin testing by the serial dilution titration method was developed by Dr. Herbert J. Rinkel. It is based upon skin reaction to the injection of various dilutions of an antigen. The endpoint of reaction is considered the first wheal that is 2 mm larger than the preceding nonreacting wheal and followed by progressive 2 mm whealing.[1]

Serial dilution endpoint titration is an excellent method of determining a patient's sensitivity to an allergen. The starting dosage of immunotherapy based upon the endpoint of the reaction is safe and therapeutic.

Skin testing is easily introduced into the office practice. Nurses trained in this work can perform the tests, make the antigen dilutions, deliver the immunotherapy, and instruct and counsel the patient about dietary restrictions and environmental care.

EQUIPMENT

A quiet area in the office should be set aside for testing.

Equipment necessary for the successful completion of the skin test includes disposable 1 cc syringes, allergenic concentrates, sterile vials with saline diluent with phenol preservative, titration boards to hold the vials, a timer, a millimeter ruler, antiseptic wipes, refrigerator, titration charts, and an emergency kit.

PREPARATION OF TESTING AND TREATMENT TRAYS

The commonly used allergens include dust, housedust mites, mold spores, pollens, and animal danders. Allergenic concentrates can be obtained from a reliable commercial supplier, but it is important to buy amounts of each antigen sufficient to last an entire season, as the potency of the product may vary from one lot to another.

To prepare testing and treatment vials of these antigens, label each 10 cc vial with a given antigen in dilutions of 1–9. In each vial should be 8 cc of a saline diluent with phenol preservative. Draw up 2 cc of the allergenic concentrate and inject it into vial #1. Continue in this manner, using 2 cc of vial #1 to make the #2 dilution, etc., through the remaining vials. For example, there will be nine vials of ragweed, each one five times weaker than the preceding one. These vials are then placed in successive order on the treatment board (Figs. 18-1 and 18-2 A and B).

PATIENT SELECTION AND PREPARATION

Prior to skin testing, the patient is given a complete otorhinolaryngological examination, including an IgE and nasal smear for cytology. If these findings point to allergic disease, the patient is scheduled for skin testing. At this time, the patient is given an allergy questionnaire to complete. This includes questions about home environment, work habits, hobbies, symptoms, medications, past history, and any known allergies. The patient is also requested to keep a 2-week food diary. It is important when testing and treating an individual to continually question that patient about symptoms, medication, and food. Review the history sheets; talk about work, hobbies, home environment, etc. You will be surprised at what you may learn. Unquestionably, one of the most important diagnostic tools is a careful history.

The patient is instructed to refrain from antihistamines, decongestants, aspirin, and tranquilizers for 48 hours prior to testing. These medications may alter skin response.

SERIAL DILUTION TITRATION TECHNIQUE

The outer aspect of the upper arm is the site of testing. The skin is held tautly with one hand. The needle is inserted bevel down into the superficial layer of the skin and enough antigen to produce a well-demarcated 4–5 mm wheal is injected (Fig. 18-3). This is approximately 0.01–0.02 cc of the test dilution.

To judge skin reactivity, it is wise to use controls. These are applied to the skin in the same manner as are the antigens. Normal saline without preservative, normal saline with a 4 percent phenol preservative, and histamine are used. The histamine used is a #3 dilution made from 0.275 mg as the concentrate: this is the positive control. Failure to react to histamine may indicate the prior use of medications. The two salines are negative controls. Occasionally, a patient may be phenol-sensitive and will react to the

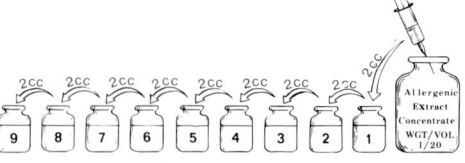

Fig. 18-1. Serial dilution titration solutions and how they are made.

Allergy Skin Testing

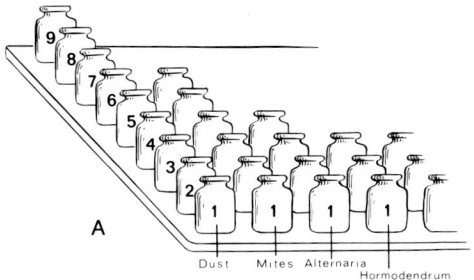

TITRATION SHEET

NAME

Date	Antigen	9	8	7	6	5	4	3	2	1
	Dust									
	Mites									
	Alternaria									
	Hormodendrum									
	Aspergillus									
	Penicillium									
	Helminthosporium									
	Trees									
	Grasses									

Fig. 18-2. (A) The titration board of antigens is set up in order, dilutions 1-9. (B) The titration sheet to record the skin test results is arranged in the same manner as the titration board of antigens, shown in Figure 18-2.

phenolated saline which is also used to dilute the testing antigens. If this should occur, testing should be done with nonphenolated antigens.

First testing is done in a vertical manner (Fig. 18-4). This is the application of several different antigens of the same dilution at the same time vertically on the arm. It is usually safe to start with a 6 dilution. The timer is set for 10 minutes and at this time the wheals are measured and recorded on the titration sheet. Testing continues in this manner

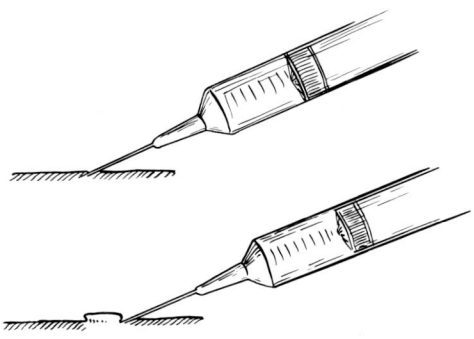

Fig. 18-3. Technique used to produce a well-demarcated wheal. The needle is inserted bevel down in the superficial layer of the skin, and enough antigen to produce a 5 mm wheal is injected.

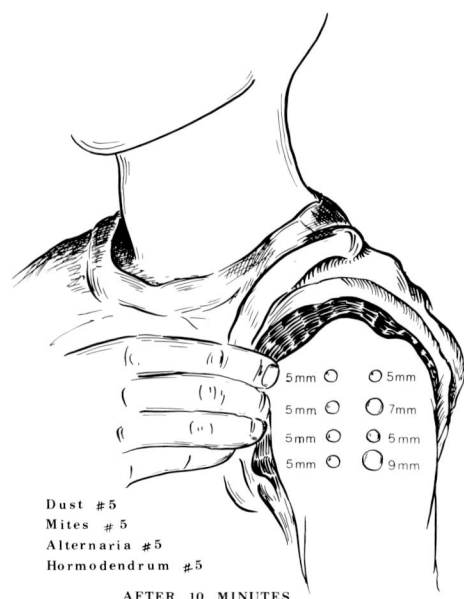

Fig. 18-4. The skin test is applied as a vertical test; i.e., the same dilution of several antigens at the same time in a vertical line.

using increasingly stronger dilutions, until a progressive 5, 7, 9, 11 mm whealing is established. The endpoint of a reaction is the dilution that gives a 7 mm wheal preceded by a 5 mm wheal and followed by successive 9 and 11 mm wheals (Fig. 18-5).

NORMAL RESPONSES

Serial dilution titration sounds easy and foolproof, and is in about 70 percent of the patients tested. However, all skin tests do not produce 5, 7, 9 mm progressions. There are normal and abnormal variations.

The normal responses include the 5, 7, 9, 11 mm whealing without erythema; 5, 7, 9, 11 mm whealing with erythema about each wheal; and progressive whealing with a variation in whealing size.

Erythema is not considered significant. Some skin reacts with redness, and the endpoint would still be the dilution that gives a 7 mm wheal preceded by a 5 mm wheal and followed by successive 9 and 11 mm wheals (Fig. 18-6).

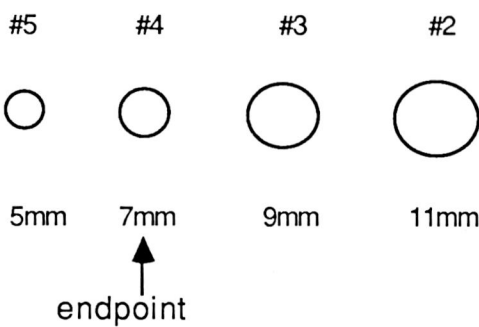

Fig. 18-5. Normal response with progressive 5, 7, 9, 11 mm whealing. The endpoint of reaction is the #4 dilution.

Allergy Skin Testing

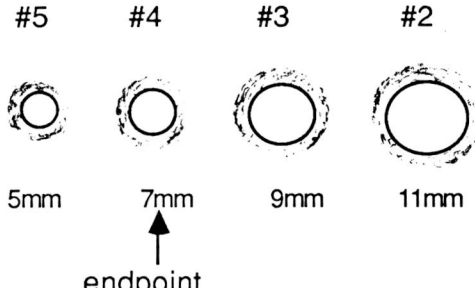

Fig. 18-6. Normal response with erythema about each wheal. The erythema is not significant. The endpoint of reaction is the #4 dilution.

With variations in whealing size, one can still obtain a progression in whealing. The first nonreacting wheal may only be 4 mm, which then may be followed by 6, 8, and 11 mm whealing. Here, the endpoint would be the dilution producing the 6 mm wheal (Fig. 18-7).

ABNORMAL RESPONSES

Abnormal whealing responses include the response with no endpoint, the flash response, the response with a short or long plateau, and hourglassing with a clear central zone and with erythema about the central zone.

The response with no endpoint means a 5 mm wheal has not been established. This patient probably has a phenol sensitivity and that is why it is important to test initially with saline with and without phenol preservative added. If the patient is phenol-sensitive, that patient should be rescheduled for testing with nonphenolated antigens.

The flash response can sometimes be quite dramatic and very often occurs when testing pollens or animal danders. This response will be either nonreacting wheals followed by a very large reaction or progressive whealing through 2–3 dilutions followed by a large reaction (Fig. 18-8). Often after such a response it is possible to do a linear test and obtain a normal 5, 7, 9, 11 mm whealing response. If flashing continues, that particular antigen can be checked by in vitro testing: either a radioallergosorbent test or an enzyme assay to obtain a safe starting dosage. Flashing often occurs when testing pollens in season.

With the plateau response, dilutions of different strengths produce wheals of identical size, called the plateau of the reaction. The plateau may by long or short, followed by

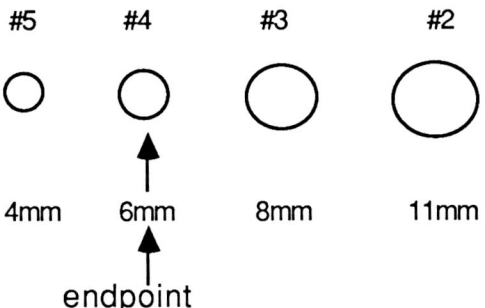

Fig. 18-7. Normal response with variation in whealing size. There is still progressive 2 mm whealing.

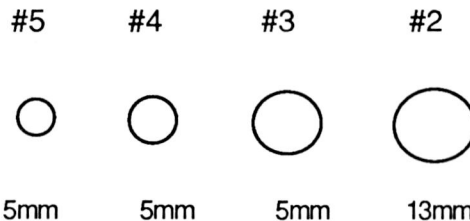

Fig. 18-8. The flash response. No endpoint is established.

progressive whealing. The endpoint would be the 7 mm wheal immediately preceding this progressive whealing (Fig. 18-9). This type of reaction suggests multiple sensitivities, especially foods.

An hourglass reaction with a clear central zone is a test that produces a large wheal with erythema on the weakest dilution applied. This is followed by smaller wheals on stronger dilutions to a clear central zone of nonreacting wheals after which the wheal size increases normally. The endpoint would be the first dilution below the nonreacting area that does react and is followed by normal increments (Fig. 18-10). The same is true of the hourglass linear erythema response, except that the central zone continues to produce erythema. The hourglass responses also suggest concomitant food allergy.

Repeat testing should always be linear. This is the immediate application of several different strengths of the same antigen, as opposed to the first testing, which is the application of several different antigens of the same strength. Often, repeating abnormal tests in a linear strip will establish a clearcut endpoint. If an endpoint is still not established, in vitro testing is advised.

There are several other problems that may be encountered during testing. They include patients with dermographic skin, active eczema, or other chronic skin disease. There are also some patients who are on medications for other problems, e.g., tranquilizers or steroids, and clearcut endpoints are difficult to obtain. Some patients will continue with bizarre whealing no matter how many times they are retitrated. Occasionally, an uncooperative patient will be encountered. If any of these problems arise, in vitro testing can establish a safe starting dosage.

Treatment

The initial dosage for immunotherapy is usually 0.05 cc of the endpoint dilution. Injections are given weekly while the dosage is being increased. The time between injections is lengthened as the symptoms decrease. Maintenance dose is the maximum

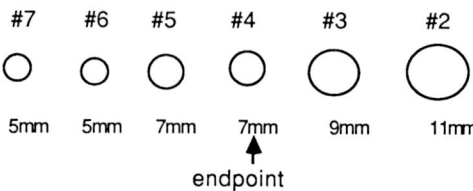

Fig. 18-9. Response with a short plateau. The endpoint of reaction is the first 7 mm wheal followed by progressive whealing.

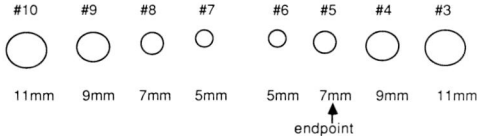

Fig. 18-10. Hourglass response. This response can be with or without erythema. The endpoint of reaction is the #4 dilution, which is followed by normal progressive whealing.

amount of extract needed to give the patient symptom relief without causing side effects. The interval between injections may be increased to 2–4 weeks, depending upon individual response.

Perennial therapy is recommended. This method allows for a larger cumulative dosage and seems to have a higher degree of successful immunotherapy than do either preseasonal or coseasonal therapy.

Many patients have no change in whealing response during treatment and can receive the same antigens on an escalated dosage schedule for 2–3 years with good response. At that time, if the patient remains symptom-free between injections, therapy is discontinued. There is, at present, no cure for allergy, but blocking antibodies produced by immunotherapy may alleviate symptoms for years.

Some patients show great variations in whealing response and symptom relief and require frequent retesting. Retitration is done when there is redness or swelling of the arm following an injection. This is usually caused by a shift to the left of one or more antigens. It is wise to separate antigens into several vials. Dust, mites, and animal danders may be mixed in one, molds in a second, and pollens in a third. An antigen to which a patient is extremely sensitive should be separated from all other antigens. This allows for the escalation of extracts at various levels. Each vial is given in a certain area in order to determine which vial is causing the problem. This allows for retesting using only the antigens in the troublesome vial.

If symptoms increase following an injection, each vial can be given at different times to see if it can be determined which vial is causing the problem. The patient can then be retitrated with the antigens from that vial. For example, a patient's pollen endpoints may shift to the left during pollen season and the dosage must be adjusted accordingly. On the other hand, a patient may not be experiencing relief after an injection and on retesting may show a shift to the right which would require a stronger dilution (Fig. 18-11).

The patient is continually instructed about the care to be taken with respect to the personal environment. It is helpful if printed material is available. This would include information on how to keep a dust-free room, reduce molds in and around the house, avoid pollen exposure, and reduce chemical irritant exposure. The offending allergens should be eliminated from or reduced in the patient's environment whenever possible.

After 12 weeks of treatment, the patient is examined by the physician. If there is no significant improvement at this time, food testing or retitration may be ordered.

There are also some patients who will have a positive skin reaction to a specific pollen only during that particular pollenating season. Therefore, if a patient is having symptoms during a certain season that patient should be retested for those pollens to which the response was originally negative.

The ingestion of foods may produce erratic responses if a patient has a concomitant food allergy. Each patient is an individual and this must always be considered when testing and treating.

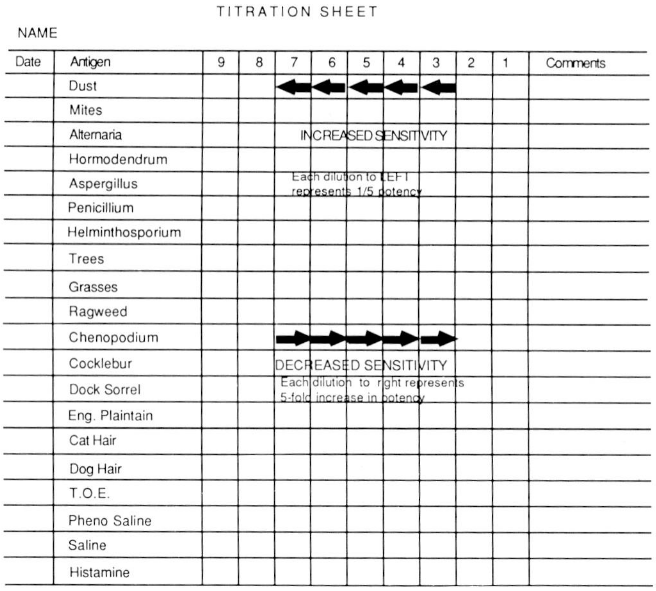

TITRATION SHEET

Date	Antigen	9	8	7	6	5	4	3	2	1	Comments
	Dust			←	←	←	←	←			
	Mites										
	Alternaria					INCREASED SENSITIVITY					
	Hormodendrum										
	Aspergillus					Each dilution to LEFT represents 1/5 potency					
	Penicillium										
	Helminthosporium										
	Trees										
	Grasses										
	Ragweed										
	Chenopodium					→	→	→	→	→	
	Cocklebur					DECREASED SENSITIVITY					
	Dock Sorrel					Each dilution to right represents 5-fold increase in potency					
	Eng. Plaintain										
	Cat Hair										
	Dog Hair										
	T.O.E.										
	Pheno Saline										
	Saline										
	Histamine										

Fig. 18-11. An endpoint shift to the left indicates increased sensitivity. An endpoint shift to the right indicates decreased sensitivity.

CONCLUSION

Serial dilution skin titration has been found to be an invaluable test for the otolaryngologist. It determines the antigens to which a patient is allergic and allows treatment to begin in a safe and therapeutic manner. However, the importance of continually questioning, searching, reviewing, and instructing cannot be stressed enough. Immunotherapy is only successful in conjunction with the education and cooperation of the patient.

BIBLIOGRAPHY

Rinkel HJ: The Management of Clinical Allergy, in Williams RI (ed) Archives of Otolaryngology 1963; 77 (January):42–75, Wyoming: Frontier Printing

Rinkel HJ: The Management of Clinical Allergys in Williams RI (ed) Archives of Otolaryngology 1963; 77 (February):205–225, Wyoming: Frontier Printing

Middleton E Jr, Reed CE, Ellis EF: Allergy, Principles and Practice. St. Louis: The C.V. Mosby Company, pp. 257–260; 877–898, 1978

Bickmore J: The integration of allergy into a surgical otolaryngologic practice. Otolaryngol Clin North Am 7:667–680, 1974

Williams RI: Skin titration and treatment. Otolaryngol Clin North Am 4:507–521, 1971

Willoughby JW: Serial dilution titration skin tests in inhalant allergy. Otolaryngol Clin North Am 7:579–614, 1974

Donald J. Nalebuff

19

The Modified RAST—An Aid in Diagnosis and Management of Allergic Patients

An increasing number of otorhinolaryngologists actively treat the allergic patients seen in their office practice. This is occurring because of a better understanding of the nature of the allergic response, coupled with the remarkable advances in technology available to the physician. The background events leading to this renewed interest will be reviewed in this presentation. Particular emphasis will be placed on the role of the modified RAST (radioallergosorbent test) procedure in the diagnosis and management of rhinitis patients.

BACKGROUND

Over 60 years ago, Prausnitz and Kustner demonstrated a transferable factor in the serum of allergic patients. The formerly nonreactive recipient of this factor was found to react with a positive wheal and flare response when suitably challenged with the appropriate allergen.[1] The search for the exact nature of this transferable protein continued until the mid-1960s, when the Ishizakas isolated a factor from the serum of an atopic individual which gave a P-K titer of 80,000—the reciprocal of the highest dilution of the serum capable of giving a definite positive transfer reaction. Since it appeared to mediate the erythema skin reaction and was different from the known immunoglobulins, they called it "gamma E globulin".[2] At about the same time, Johansson and Bennich isolated an atypical protein from the serum of a myeloma patient, minute amounts of which were found to be capable of blocking the P-K reaction.[3] The patient's initials (ND) were adopted by them as an interim label for this material. They observed that trace amounts of the material were present in the serum of patients with hay fever and allergic asthma. Subsequent study by both groups established that the "gamma E globulin" and the "N.D. myeloma protein" were the same substance. The research findings of the two teams were merged; a new class of immunoglobulins was formally established—officially designated "immunoglobulin E" (IgE) in 1968.

DIAGNOSIS

The complete evaluation of patients with allergic rhinitis demands a systematic approach. This starts with an understanding of the pathophysiology of the disease and includes a careful analysis of personal and family history data. A complete physical examination supplemented and confirmed by appropriate laboratory evaluation are also necessary for accurate diagnosis.

Pathophysiology

Allergic rhinitis is a disease of known pathogenesis. On exposure to inhaled allergens, predisposed atopic individuals mount high and prolonged IgE antibody responses within the lymphoid tissue of their respiratory tracts. This antibody becomes fixed to specific receptor sites on the surface of blood basophils and tissue mast cells. These latter cells are most numerous in the lining of the respiratory and gastrointestinal tracts, as well as under the skin—loci which, as might be expected, are the main sites of both the lymphoid cells that form IgE antibody and the major organs affected in IgE-mediated allergic reactions. Perturbation of the mast cell membrane receptor by IgE crosslinkage secondary to antigen binding is followed by a series of biochemical reactions, which leads to the degranulation of the cell with the release of potent chemical mediators such as histamine, the slow-reacting substance of anaphylaxis (SRS-A), eosinophilic chemotactic factor (ECF-A), and others. These pharmacologically active molecules released within the nose cause variable degrees of vasodilatation and edema (nasal congestion), an increase in mucous secretion (rhinorrhea), and increased capillary and mucosal permeability, permitting allergen contact with additional mast cells lying within the submucosa and thereby magnifying the reaction.[4]

While the IgE-mediated mechanism is the predominant trigger for disease, the degranulation of tissue mast cells may be initiated by several other factors, some immunologic (e.g., complement components such as the C3a and C5a anaphylatoxins) and several nonimmunologic (e.g., chemicals, physical factors, neurogenic stimulation, exercise, and infection). These factors then produce a disease state that is clinically indistinguishable from IgE-mediated allergy. Patients whose diseases are exclusively triggered by non-IgE-mediated factors are not atopic, usually do not have positive family histories, do not produce elevated levels of IgE, and do not demonstrate "positive" test results for specific IgE antibody. Most important, these patients do not respond to allergen immunotherapy.

Patient History

Rapid successions of paroxysms of morning sneezing—generally 10–50 sneezes each episode—associated with nasal blockage, rhinorrhea, and itching of the nose, eyes, palate, and pharynx are hallmarks of allergic rhinitis. Other manifestations of atopy, such as infantile eczema, wheezy bronchitis, or bronchospasm with exercise and cold, and serous otitis media, may precede the development of rhinitis. Important clues about what may be causing a patient's allergic rhinitis can be obtained through the timing, location, and exacerbating agents of symptoms. To a significant extent, clinical evaluation of patients is like detective work in that it involves gathering and sorting out clues from various bits of information.

Many physicians use patient history questionnaires to elicit pertinent information. This practice assures getting a comprehensive history and provides the basis for detailed questioning in selected areas. Use of such forms not only saves time for the practitioner and office staff, but also makes it possible to computerize the information to provide an immediate summary of relevant data for determining the most appropriate laboratory tests. Patients with year-round symptoms, however, present a greater diagnostic challenge than can be met by a questionnaire analysis. Such histories do not contribute as much to the etiologic diagnosis as do histories of patients with seasonal conditions.

Physical Examination

While there is no characteristic rhinoscopic finding in nasal allergy, pale, bluish, edematous nasal turbinates coated with a thin, clear secretion are often found in these patients. Children with year-round allergic rhinitis can sometimes be recognized by their "allergic salute," in which the palm of the hand rubs the nose in an upward and outward fashion, and by indication of nasal pruritus. This constant upward rubbing of the obstructed itchy nose may result in a permanent transverse crease across its lower part, just above the nasal tip. Other frequent findings include abnormalities of the oral cavity with overriding maxillary incisors, a high-arched palate, and hypertrophic lymphoid follicles on the posterior pharyngeal wall. Dark circles under the eyes—"allergic shiners"—due to chronic, nonspecific, vascular congestion are common. Transverse creases on the lower eyelid parallel to the lower lid margin (Dennie's lines) are another nonspecific sign of congestion. Tearing and conjunctival injection, lid edema, and periorbital swelling may also be present. Nevertheless, many persons with atopic disease do not have this finding and the diagnosis cannot be made without confirmatory laboratory findings.

THE ROLE OF THE LABORATORY IN ALLERGY DIAGNOSIS

For almost a century, in vivo skin test challenges have been employed to confirm sensitization to specific allergens. The basic principle of these tests is the demonstration that sensitized mast cells in the skin can be induced by a specific allergen to initiate a local allergic response characterized by a wheal and flare reaction. In the various skin testing methods, an allergen extract is placed into the skin by either scratching or pricking with a sharp device or by intradermal injection with syringe and needle. False-positive skin tests can result from improper preparation of the allergen material, the intradermal injection of solutions containing concentrations of glycerin (5 percent or greater), or the intradermal injection of too large a volume of allergen. A test using only diluent solution (4 percent phenolated saline) is usually included to assess skin reactivity resulting from the mechanical trauma. It is also advisable to use a 1:500 or 1:1000 w/v histamine base solution as a positive control. This helps identify any false-negative skin test result occurring from loss of potency of allergen solution or prior use of drugs that may suppress skin reactivity. Despite these precautions, the accuracy of all skin testing is limited by factors such as skin responsiveness related to the patient's age, the dampening effect of therapeutic agents, variables in technique, and interpretation.

In view of these problems, it was hoped that the measurement of total IgE levels would help in solving difficult diagnostic problems confronting the rhinologist. Unfortunately, elevation of IgE levels are not confined to allergic disease syndromes. As a result, such determinations have only limited clinical significance. The total IgE antibody level can only be correlated with clinical allergy in a general way; that is, patients with the higher concentrations of total serum IgE are usually positive to multiple allergens, and in these patients there is a greater incidence of extremely high levels of specific antibody detected, especially in patients with total IgE levels of 200 U/ml or more. However, in some patients with a total serum IgE level of over 400 U/ml, no positive specific antibody is ever found. On the other hand, 50 percent of patients with clinical evidence of allergy and detectable allergen-specific IgE have total IgE levels in ranges usually considered to be within normal limits and some patients with serum total IgE levels below 50 U/ml have significant specific antibody titers to a limited number of antigens. Patients with total serum IgE levels of 10 U/ml or less, however, rarely have detectable specific IgE levels. In contrast to the limited role played by total IgE determination, however, is the value of specific IgE antibody measurement.

The Radioallergosorbent Test (RAST)

The discovery of IgE as the antibody responsible for the classical immediate allergic reaction led to the development of the in vitro radioallergosorbent test for its detection in serum.[5] Wide et al. reported that this test had a clinical sensitivity, specificity, and overall efficiency of 96 percent. Since this initial report, the RAST has found worldwide acceptance for specific IgE antibody estimation; it is estimated that over 100 million tests have been performed. Investigators report a high correlation with the allergic history, the response to allergen challenge, and the results of skin endpoint titration and provocation.[6] Even the response to drug treatment and immunotherapy relates to the RAST score. The direct measurement of allergen-specific IgE has been applied in the diagnosis of allergy to such antigens as grass, weed and tree pollens, mold spores, animal danders, stinging insect venoms, and viral and bacterial components, as well as various food and chemical substances.[7-11]

Test Performance

Test principles are outlined in Table 19-1. In the first stage of the procedure, solid-phase allergens are reacted with a serum sample from suspected allergic individuals. IgE antibodies, as well as antibodies of other immunoglobulin classes, react with the allergens present on the solid-phase materials to form an antigen-antibody complex. Antibodies directed against allergens other than those on the solid-phase complex are washed away at the end of the first step of the reaction. In the second step of the procedure, the allergen-antibody complexes are reacted with radiolabeled rabbit or goat antibodies to human IgE. These purified antibodies react only with the IgE on the surface of the solid-phase complex and, after a second washing step to remove any unbound anti-IgE, the radioactivity associated with the complex is measured in a gamma counter. The quantity of residual bound radioactivity (count rate of the disc) is directly related to the quantity of specific IgE antibody present in the serum sample.

Table 19-1
Principles of the Radioallergosorbent Test

1. Soluble allergens are bound to solid-phase supports (e.g., a paper disc) to create a stable immunosorbent which then acquires the antigenicity of the allergen.
2. The passively created immunosorbent (insoluble allergen), on incubation with a test serum, will react with specific antibody to form a solid-phase complex.
3. Anti-human IgE serum raised in another species (e.g., rabbit) and radiolabeled will react with antigenic determinants on the Fc portion of the IgE antibody bound to the allergen-coated immunosorbent.
4. The greater the amount of radioactivity bound to the disc, the more specific IgE present in the serum sample tested.

The Modified RAST Scoring System

Since 1977, the author's group has utilized a modification of the commercially available RAST which has been described in detail elsewhere.[12] The Modified RAST (MRT) has an increased test sensitivity without a significant loss of specificity. This is accomplished by extending the initial incubation period from 3 to 18 hours and increasing the volume of serum used from 50 to 100 microliters. In the MRT, an additional step is routinely performed. After the second incubation period with the labeled-rabbit antibody against human IgE, and before counting the disc-bound radioactivity, the allergen-coated discs are removed from their original tubes and placed into fresh ones to ensure that only radioactivity immunologically bound to them is measured. Despite careful washing, a minute amount of radioactive residue adheres to the inner surface of the polystyrene carrier test tube and can take on significance in those sera with low levels of specific IgE antibodies. In the MRT system, the lower limit of detectable levels of allergen-specific IgE averages 1.5 times the binding of negative controls, consisting of either human cord serum, serum from nonatopic patients, or serum from highly atopic patients tested against an inappropriate allergen. Improved reproducibility of assay results has been accomplished by using a time or count control, i.e., the time used to count each disc matches that required by a known 25 unit/ml IgE sample to reach 25,000 counts when tested against an anti-IgE disc and run in parallel to the atopic sera under test. This step eliminates the day-to-day variation in results caused by isotope decay. With the availability in 1984 of improved reagents, the nonspecific binding in the system averages 300 counts. In the current MRT scoring system, 500 counts is at the 95 percent confidence level for the detection of specific IgE antibody. Counts greater than 500 and less than 750 are considered to be "equivocal". For convenience, scores above 750 counts have been divided into 5 distinct classes, each representing approximately a 5-fold increase in the amount of serum-specific IgE antibody present in the sample (Table 19-2). MRT Class One (750–1600 counts) is now considered to be a low-level positive score. While Class One levels are always associated with a positive skin test reaction, only 70 percent of affected patients will respond when suitably challenged. In contrast, MRT Class Two scores and above (1600–40,000 counts) represent positive scores with increasing levels of detectable specific-IgE antibody and degrees of clinical sensitivity.

Table 19-2
Modified RAST Scoring System

Class	Counts[a]	Interpretation
0	250–500	negative
1/0	501–750	equivocal
1	751–1,600	positive with increasing
2	1,601–3,600	levels of specific IgE
3	3,601–8,000	
4	8,001–18,000	
5	18,001–40,000	

[a] counts obtained when the time control of 25 units is run at 25,000 counts

Ninety-five percent of patients with these scores respond to a properly performed nasal or conjunctival provocation test.[13]

Advantages of In Vitro Tests

Although it has been shown that the various diagnostic procedures tend to give comparable results, they do have significant differences (Table 19-3). RAST has an advantage in patient convenience where one requires only a single blood sample which can be tested for multiple allergens. RAST is also the most reproducible procedure for identifying allergies, since the reagents can be kept for years without losing activity. Of the various procedures used for the quantification of the patient's sensitivity, measurement of IgE antibodies by the RAST seems to be the most practical. The RAST is less time-consuming for the patient than is the skin test and less expensive to perform than is histamine release procedure. The trauma (psychic and physical) and the hazards of direct skin testing are avoided. In the past, skin testing for allergy was considered to have a better sensitivity than the RAST, though such sensitivity without concomitant specificity can be a major disadvantage.

Table 19-3
Comparison of Skin Test and RAST Qualities in Diagnosis

Characteristic	Skin Test	RAST
Sensitivity	*	
Specificity		*
Reproducibility		*
Quantitation		*
Safety		*
Cost	*	
Speedy results	*	
Convenience		*

Both tests can be used in the diagnostic workup of allergic rhinitis patients. Each test has advantages as shown. The use of RAST allergen screens offsets the cost advantage of skin testing (see text).

Allergen Screening with RAST

Despite the many advantages of in vitro testing, some physicians question the use of such a potentially expensive approach to allergy diagnosis, particularly if a patient's serum is tested for 20 or 30 potentially clinically relevant allergens and is subsequently found to be negative to all allergens. King reports that 31 percent of his patients with head and neck or respiratory complaints have completely negative MRT responses to a battery of 16-20 allergens.[14] As a result, he described a screening method consisting of approximately one-third the number of tests ordinarily utilized in his full battery. In a retrospective analysis of 469 responders to a full RAST battery, King notes that the screening RAST would have missed 27 patients; only 4 of these, however, were definite "positives," with a MRT Class Two or greater score. Of the 23 "equivocal" cases, 12 had relatively low scores of less than 1000 counts. He speculated that a high level of total IgE may have contributed to the nonspecific background in these cases and caused an otherwise negative response to be read as a MRT Class One score. These observations led the author's group to incorporate RAST screening in the initial diagnostic work-up. To confirm the efficiency of a screening panel in diagnosis, a retrospective analysis was done on the diagnostic testing of 100 consecutive patients with rhinitis; total IgE levels were determined in all patients and their sera was subjected to 1784 individual MRT tests—an average of 18 suspected allergens examined in each patient. Ninety-two patients had detectable levels of specific IgE to at least 2 test allergens. Only 8 of the patients' sera were negative to all 152 allergen tests performed; these patients were then considered to be "nonatopic." Had an initial screen been done to demonstrate the presence of specific IgE antibody on those patients with the MRT atopy screen (one representative allergen from each of the major antigen groups, as shown in Table 19-4), 90 of the 92 patients with demonstrable levels of allergen-specific IgE would have been detected—an overall sensitivity level of 98 percent. Smaller mini-screens comprised of 3 or 4 individual allergens would have been only 85 and 90 percent effective, respectively.

Screening with Multiple-allergen Discs

In an attempt to further lower the cost of using RAST as a diagnostic tool, the regular battery allergen have been linked to a single paper disc to create a microscreen allergen disc. Initial analysis of the preliminary MRT data obtained from 85 patients in whom a complete battery of tests was also done with the individual allergens revealed that the single microscreen disc worked as effectively as the routine battery in identifying both negative and positive responders. By using either of these screening procedures in the initial diagnostic evaluation and limiting additional RAST testing to those patients symptomatic enough to warrant immunotherapy, the expense of allergy care is significantly reduced.

If the initial screen is positive, additional tests should be performed only on those patients deemed suitable for allergen immunotherapy. As a general rule, a total of 25-35 determinations will include the significant clinically relevant allergens (Table 19-4). In addition, those patients with perennial symptoms, high levels of total IgE, and high MRT scores often benefit from having additional testing done for common foods in the diet. Unusual exposure to animal danders may have to be evaluated by RAST to insure that pertinent allergens are not omitted from treatment.

Table 19-4
20 Common Clinically Relevant Allergens: A Typical RAST Battery

Grasses	Weeds
Bermuda	*Short ragweed*
Timothy	Lamb's quarter
June	Plantain
Molds	Trees
Penicillium	Maple
Mucor	*Oak*
Aspergillus	Birch
Cladosporium	Sycamore
Alternaria	Ash
Animal Danders[a]	Dust Components
Cat epithelium or	*Housedust mite*
Dog epitheliumd	Cockroach

A mini-allergen screen, composed of the representative example (as italicized) in each of the major allergen groups can be used to confirm whether or not a patient negative to these allergens will be positive to others when tested by RAST.
[a]as indicated by history

Inappropriate and Appropriate Uses of RAST

There are situations in which RAST data may be informative and yet not significantly contribute to improved patient care. The author sees no reason for using these tests when the diagnosis is apparent from the clinical history (e.g., symptoms on exposure to cat or on ingestion of a particular food) or when nonspecific therapy is found to be effective in alleviating symptoms. Furthermore, patients in whom properly performed skin tests have given negative results are not likely to have measurable levels of allergen-specific IgE antibody. On the other hand, the RAST is extremely helpful in many situations. It is of great benefit in apprehensive children, in patients with dermatologic problems for whom skin testing is contraindicated, and in those patients unable to stop medication that can potentially influence the test result. It has been found to be particularly valuable in evaluating individual sensitivity when initiating specific immunotherapy and in evaluating transfer patients already on immunotherapy and not doing well; more than one-third of these patients have undetectable levels of specific IgE antibody and immunotherapy is discontinued.

ALLERGEN IMMUNOTHERAPY

The symptoms of allergic rhinitis can be relieved in most patients by using a combination of antihistamines, decongestants, inhaled cromolyn, or synthetic steroids, along with the elimination or reduction of environmental factors such as animal danders, dust, and mold. When these measures do not provide satisfactory relief, allergen immunotherapy may still be effective. Specific clinical situations in which the use of allergen immunotherapy is appropriate include those involving patients with symptoms extending over

2 or more seasons who experience unpleasant side effects from pharmacotherapy. If such a patient consistently observes an increase in symptoms during certain seasons and has a positive skin test or RAST to aeroallergens present at that time, one may assume that the flare-ups are due to an allergic response and that immunotherapy will be useful.

The Effectiveness of Immunotherapy

The efficacy of allergen immunotherapy in the management of allergic rhinitis is well documented. Proven clinical benefits have been reported in treatment-resistant patients with known sensitivity due to ragweed, grass, and mountain cedar pollens, and house-dust mite and cat dander allergens.[15-20]

In the traditional method, an arbitrary safe starting dose of allergens is administered in high dilutions (1:100,000–1:10,000,000 w/v). Dosage increments are increased once or twice a week over several months until a maintenance dose is reached. During the first 2 or 3 months of such treatment, the titer of specific IgE antibody rises, usually twofold or more. As therapy is continued, the titer returns to or below its original level. Because therapeutically effective doses are not reached until 6–12 months, some physicians accelerate the dose schedule by administering injections several times a day—a variation called "rush therapy," with gradually increasing doses and concentrations, until a maximum tolerated dose is reached. An inherent disadvantage of these methods is that all patients are treated the same way.

For years, rhinologists have used an approach popularized by Rinkel in which each patient's sensitivity is measured by the graded response of the skin to allergen challenge. Doses of each allergen in a treatment set mixture are determined by this bioassay in an inverse relationship inversely related to patient sensitivity.[21] In the currently accepted method, treatment doses are increased incrementally until the maintenance level is reached—which may be several thousand times the amount of allergen found to cause the original endpoint response. A recognized weakness in this approach, however, is the selection of allergens for immunotherapy based on endpoints at low dilution and of questionable clinical significance.

RAST-based Immunotherapy

In 1975, Bernstein found that patients with high RAST scores could tolerate only the smallest amount of allergen extract; he advises that such patients be routinely started with extremely dilute material and that doses in such patients be raised cautiously.[22] These observations suggested to the author's group that individual sensitivity to clinically relevant allergens as determined by the in vitro RAST procedure could be used as a guide in selecting safe initial dose levels.[23-25] In the RAST-based method, the starting immunotherapy dose is based on the patient's serum level of allergen-specific IgE antibody (Table 19-5). When more than one allergen is mixed in a treatment vial, the various strengths are adjusted to be in inverse proportion to each individual serum antibody concentration. With this approach, the initial dose of allergen is usually higher than that of the other methods—often making it possible to reach therapeutically effective levels within a month. It has been found that by employing this technique, untoward reactions are avoidable. The author's patients are regularly started at allergen concentrations of 1:500 w/v for those allergens with low serum-specific IgE levels (MRT Class One scores). As the serum antibody concentration rises, the suggested initial dose is propor-

Table 19-5
Initial Immunotherapy Doses Based on the MRT Score

Class	Allergen Concentration	
	regular	aggressive
	w/v	
0		
0/1	1:100	—
1	1:500	1:100
2	1:2,500	1:500
3	1:12,500	1:2,500
4	1:62,500	1:12,500
5	1:312,500	1:62,500

The regular concentration schedule (one dilution weaker than possible to use) is the recommended initial dose in RAST-based immunotherapy (see text).

tionally decreased in 5-fold increments. For those allergens in which the specific antibody score is extremely high (MRT Class Five scores), the recommended initial doses is significantly lower, at an allergen concentration of 1:312,000 w/v. After the initial doses have been administered and tolerated, injections are usually doubled at subsequent visits (unless the clinical response suggests it would not be safe) until the dose reaches maximum levels. Before starting such immunotherapy, however, it is mandatory that a small amount of the incriminated allergen be placed intradermally as a skin-test challenge (enough of the allergen must be injected to produce a 4 mm skin wheal). The patient is then observed, and if in 10 minutes this in vivo challenge produces a wheal of 15 mm or less, the suggested dose is given subcutaneously. While this challenge is performed in all patients, it is especially important for Class One through Class Three allergens, where the suggested RAST-based doses are high (1:500–12,500 w/v). With Class Four and Five allergens, the in vivo challenges are less important because the suggested allergen doses (1:62,500–1:312,000 w/v) are consistent with levels considered safe even for extremely sensitive patients.[21] Nevertheless, even in these situations, the in vivo challenge serves the useful purpose of confirming the biological potency of the highly diluted allergen extract. Only rarely, in the author's experience, have the skin test challenge responses suggested that the RAST-based dose would be excessive. A technique of preparing stock and individualized treatment sets is described below.

Preparation of Serially-diluted Stock Solutions

The author's group uses 50 percent glycerinated allergen extracts because these maintain potency well; these are obtained at a 1:20 w/v concentration in the 30 ml vial size. To ensure a constant rotation of fresh solutions, the group works with small amounts of solution in both the stock and treatment vials (2.5 ml and 5.0 ml). The stock solutions are prepared as follows: 5.0 ml of the 1:20 w/v concentrated extracts is withdrawn from the large vials (30.0 ml) and placed into an empty sterile 5.0 ml vial for subsequent use. Five-fold dilutions of this material are then prepared as follows. Preparation of Stock Dilution #1 (1:100 w/v) is made from the concentrates as follows: 1.0 ml of the 1:20 w/v concentrate plus 4.0 ml phenolated saline diluent will make a total volume of 5.0 ml. of Stock Dilution #1. Stock Dilution #2 (1:500 w/v) is made from the #1 Stock Dilutions as follows: 1.0 ml of the 1:100 w/v concentration plus 4.0 ml phenolated saline diluent will make a total volume of 5.0 ml of Stock Dilution #2. Stock Dilution #3 (1:2,500 w/v) is made from the Stock Dilution #2 as follows: 1.0 ml of the 1:500 w/v concentration plus 4.0 ml phenolated saline diluent will make a total volume of 5.0 ml of Stock Dilution #3. Finally, Stock Dilution #4 (1:12,500 w/v) is made from the Stock Dilution #3 in a similar fashion: 1.0 ml of the 1:2,500 w/v concentration plus 4.0 ml phenolated saline diluent will make a total volume of 5.0 ml of Stock Dilution #4. These stock solutions are then used to create individualized treatment sets for atopic patients.

Preparation of Individual Patient Treatment Set Vials

The Modified RAST scores of a typical patient with perennial allergic rhinitis are listed in Table 19-6. An appropriate treatment set for this patient is made by taking 0.1 ml of one dilution stronger than the suggested initial concentration for each clinically relevant allergen to be included, and adding enough phenolated saline diluent to total a volume of 2.5 ml to dilute each allergen 25-fold; thus, a maximum of 25 allergens can be included in a single treatment vial. Low-sensitivity allergens (Classes One, Two, and Three) are placed in vial A, and highly sensitive allergens (Classes Four and Five) are kept together in vial B. Once the treatment set is made up according to this technique, initial treatment dosages are escalated until the maximum tolerated dose is reached.

Results of RAST-based Immunotherapy

A review of the MRT records of patients treated in the author's clinic between 1980 and 1985 revealed that, on an average, they were sensitive to 10 allergens. Eighty-five percent of the positive scores were at the lower levels (Classes One–Three). Since these allergens were unlikely to cause a constitutional reaction in therapy, initial treatment doses were administered at the regular suggested doses (Table 19-5). All patients toler-

Table 19-6
Typical RAST Results in a Patient with Allergic Rhinitis

Allergen	Score	Class	Allergen	Score	Class
Bermuda	1,250	1	Penicillium	225	0
Timothy	1,270	1	Mucor	250	0
June	2,750	2	Cladosporium	185	0
			Aspergillus	385	0
Maple	875	1	Alternaria	1,240	1
Oak	13,750	4			
Sycamore	2,300	2	Short ragweed	14,750	4
Birch	1,250	1	Mugwort	3,400	2
Elm	875	1	Lamb's quarter	1,750	2
			Dandelion	245	0
Cat epith.	18,650	5	Engl. plantain	400	0
H-D mite	21,500	5			

Note the high RAST scores for housedust mite, ragweed, oak, and cat epithelium. These are the allergens for which the patient is at risk in advancing doses. The patient should remove the cat from the home environment.

ated their initial high doses of these allergens and were readily advanced to doses of 0.1–0.25 ml of a 1:100 w/v concentration of the allergen material (equivalent to doses of 1000–2500 noon units) without untoward reaction. In these same patients, the remaining 15 percent of incriminated allergens were associated with high levels of specific IgE antibody (Class Four and Class Five MRT scores) and the patients were started in therapy at the regular lower dose levels. These allergens were advanced on a more deliberate schedule. The author's group was not able to routinely raise these allergens to the high levels achievable with the others in these same patients. They commonly caused large local and even mild constitutional reactions when high dosage levels were attempted—even after a year's course of allergen immunotherapy. During the past 7 years, the only constitutional reactions requiring medical intervention in the author's practice have occurred with those allergens associated with high Modified RAST scores (Classes Four and Five) in whom an attempt was made to raise the dose above the 1:500 w/v concentration.

Length of Treatment and Prognosis

The extent to which patients respond remains unpredictable in any given patient. Usually therapy is continued through 2 or 3 years of reduced or symptom-free seasons. It is also evident that few patients receive enough benefit from this modality to enable them to discontinue all medication. While for some patients there is a permanent relief, permanent "cure" is rare; it has frequently been observed that relapses occur once therapy has discontinued and relapsed patients may require a repeat course of immunotherapy. Immunotherapy should be discontinued, however, if after 2 years of uninterrupted maintenance dosage the patient shows no clinical improvement. A patient who has not responded by then is unlikely to do so should immunotherapy be continued. The measurement of specific IgG antibody should be helpful in deciding the course to be followed in such patients. One must be sure, in those not responding, that other forms of rhinitis are not coexisting and that any physical factors contributing to symptoms, such as septal deviations and turbinate enlargements, are corrected.

CONCLUSION

Gleich and Yunginger, writing about the role of the RAST in the practice of allergy, state that " . . . the introduction of RAST has been a milestone in the transition of allergy from a practice based on subjective judgments related to history and skin tests to one based on definitive biochemical information derived from the clinical chemistry laboratory.[8] With the availability of these reagents in kit form, many rhinologists have elected to carry out this procedure in their offices. It should be stressed, however, that the diagnosis of atopic allergy and the selection of patients to be started on immunotherapy must be made in conjunction with the physician's clinical judgment; detection of allergen-specific IgE levels by the RAST is not in itself sufficient evidence for making such assumptions. Nevertheless, reaginic activity and the development of sensitive and specific tests for its measurement have resulted in improved diagnosis and cost-effective care for allergic patients.

REFERENCES

1. Prausnitz K, Kustner H: Studien uber die Uberempfindlichkeit. Zentralbl Bakteriol Parasitenk Infektionskr 86:160, 1921
2. Ishizaka K, Ishizaka T, Hornbrook MH: Physicochemical properties of reaginic antibody. V. Correlation of reaginic activity with the E-globulin antibody. J Immunol 97:840, 1966
3. Johansson SGO, Bennich H: Studies on a new class of human immunoglobulins. 1. Immunological properties. In Killander J (Ed.): Gamma Globulins. Structure and Control of Biosynthesis, Nobel Symposium 3. Stockholm: Almqvist & Wiksell, p. 193, 1967
4. Wasserman SI: Mediators of immediate hypersensitivity. J Allergy Clin Immunol 72:101, 1983
5. Wide L, Bennich H, Johansson SGO: Diagnosis of allergy by an in-vitro test for allergen antibodies. Lancet 2:1105, 1967
6. Johansson SGO, Bennich HH: The clinical impact of the discovery of IgE. Ann Allergy 48:325, 1982
7. Aas K: The diagnosis of hypersensitivity to ingested foods. Reliability of skin prick testing and radioallergosorbent test with different materials. Clin Allergy 8:39-50, 1978
8. Gleich GJ, Yunginger JW: The radioallergosorbent test: Its present place and likely future in the practice of allergy. Adv Asthma Allergy 2:1, 1975
9. Eriksson NE: Diagnosis of reaginic allergy with house dust, animal dander and allergens in adult patients. III. Case histories and combinations of case histories, skin tests, and RAST compared with provocation tests. Int Arch Allergy Appl Immunol 53:441, 1977
10. Berg TLO, Johansson SGO: Allergy diagnosis with the radioallergosorbent test. J Allergy Clin Immunol 54:209, 1974
11. Welsh PW, et al: Preseasonal IgE ragweed antibody level as a predictor of response to therapy of ragweed hay fever with intranasal cromolyn sodium solution. J Allergy Clin Immunol 60:104, 1977
12. Nalebuff DJ: An enthusiastic view of the use of RAST in clinical allergy. Immunol Allergy Pract 3:18, 1981
13. Hoffman DR: Comparison of methods of performing the radioallergosorbent test: Phadebas, Fadal/Nalebuff and Hoffman Protocols. Ann Allergy 45:343, 1980
14. King WP: Efficacy of screening radioallergosorbent test. Arch Otolaryngol 108:81, 1982
15. Frankland AW, Augustin R: Prophylaxis of summer hay fever and asthma: A controlled trial comparing crude grass-pollen extracts with the isolated main protein component. Lancet 1:1055, 1954
16. Johnstone DE: Study of the role of antigen dose in the treatment of pollenosis and pollen asthma. J Dis Child 94:1, 1957
17. D'Souza MF, et al: Hyposensitization with Dermatophagoides pteronyssinus in house dust allergy: A controlled study of clinical and immunological effects. Clin Allergy 3:177, 1973
18. Taylor WW, Ohman JL, Lowell FC: Immunotherapy in cat induced asthma. A double-blind trial with evaluation of bronchial responses to cat allergen and histamine. J Allergy Clin Immunol 61:283, 1978
19. Levy DA, et al: Immunologic and cellular changes accompanying the therapy of a pollen allergy. J Clin Invest 50:360, 1971
20. Van Metre TE, Adkinson NF, Lichtenstein LM, et al: A controlled study of the effectiveness of the Rinkel method of immunotherapy for ragweed pollen hay fever. J Allergy Clin Immunol 65:288, 1980
21. Rinkel HJ: The management of clinical allergy. Arch Otolaryngol 76:289, 1962
22. Bernstein IL: Experience with RAST in the diagnosis and management of inhalant allergy. In Evans R III (Ed.): Advances in Diagnosis of Allergy: RAST. Miami: Symposia Specialists, p. 17, 1975
23. Nalebuff DJ, Fadal RG, Ali M: Determination of initial immunotherapy dose for ragweed

hypersensitivity with the modified radioallergosorbent test. Otolaryngol Head Neck Surg 89:271, 1981
24. Fadal RG, Nalebuff DJ: A study of optimum dose immunotherapy in pharmacological treatment failures. Arch Otolaryngol 106:38, 1981
25. Nalebuff DJ, Fadal RG: RAST-based immunotherapy. Rhinology 22:11, 1984

Lori Wills

20
The Clinical and Practical Aspects of Auditory Brainstem Response

The auditory brainstem response (ABR) is an evoked potential occurring within the first 10 msec following auditory stimulation. It is the sum of synchronous discharges in nuclear groups that ascend the auditory brainstem pathway. ABR is embedded within ongoing electroencephalographic (EEG) activity, but can be magnified and recorded through computer averaging techniques. As synchronous neural activity occurs, the evoked potential is seen as a series of generated waves. Through analysis of these waves, the integrity of the eighth nerve and auditory brainstem can be assessed.

TERMINOLOGY

Auditory brainstem response is widely used as the accepted terminology for the auditory evoked potentials, but other acronyms abound in the literature. These include auditory evoked potentials (AEP), brainstem evoked response (BSER), brainstem electric response audiometry (BERA), brainstem auditory evoked potentials (BAEP), brainstem auditory evoked response (BAER), and similar variations. Auditory brainstem response is a relatively new test procedure and nomenclature is not standardized to date.

HISTORY

ABR became known clinically in the U.S. in the 1970s. Its history stems back to the 1800s when Caton first described electrical potentials in the brains of rabbits.[1] For decades, investigators were restricted in their discoveries because of limited instrumentation. It was Berger who, in 1929, recorded the EEG from the human scalp using the galvanometer.[2] Not until the discovery of amplifiers and digital averagers was it possible to extract the comparatively minute auditory potentials from background EEG activity. In 1954, Dawson reported findings on auditory potentials using an electronic averager.[3] This discovery was revolutionary, for it allowed auditory responses to be separated from spontaneous EEG and other physiological noise. Sohmer and Feinmesser wrote the first article, appearing in 1967, on a noninvasive electrode placement that recorded auditory responses to click stimuli.[4] It was Jewett and Williston in 1971 who described the auditory evoked responses as "farfield potentials" and labeled them as a series of seven positive vertex waves corresponding to brainstem generators.[5] (See Figure 20-1.)

WHY INVEST IN CLINICAL ABR EQUIPMENT?

ABR has established a foothold as an important and versatile tool within the audiological test battery. It is reliable and sensitive, providing specific information in a relatively short amount of time. ABR is an objective test, unaffected by attention, sleep, or sedation, and resistant to many drugs.[6] This makes it applicable to not only the cooperative adult, but also to malingerers, neonates, small children, the mentally retarded, and multihandicapped populations.[8]

Unlike its forerunner, electrocochleography (ECochG), ABR is a noninvasive procedure that can be completed safely and efficiently in the office. It is widely used for detecting and localizing lesions along the retrocochlear pathway and for predicting auditory sensitivity within the upper speech frequency range. Recently, it has been applied to hearing aid selection in difficult-to-test patients. Clinical ABR equipment is compact and mobile and can be transported to the hospital bedside or the intensive care unit (ICU) or operating room for monitoring effects of accidental head trauma and surgical and pharmacological intervention on auditory and brainstem function.[7,8]

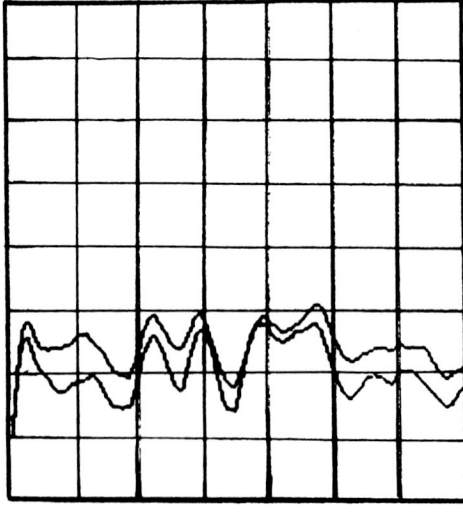

Fig. 20-1. The results above typify the morphology of a normal ABR. In this example, Wave I is present at 1 msec (each vertical line on the graph represents 1 msec in time), Wave II appears at approximately 2 msec, Wave III at 3 msec, and Waves IV and V approach 4 and 5 msec, respectively.

INTERPRETATION

Waveform Origins

Jewett and Williston reported that "farfields at least 10 cm from the brainstem generators can be recorded"[5] The oscilloscope displays the ABR as 7 positive vertex waves occurring within the first 10 msec of stimulus presentation. The Roman numeral nomenclature of Jewett and Williston, labeling positive Waves I-VII has become the convention in the United States.[5]

The anatomical origins of these waveform generators are still being studied. Recent work in this area has been done by Møller and his colleagues. Through studying ABR in patients undergoing neurosurgical operations, Møller has proposed that Wave I originates from the cochlear hair cells and the distal region of the auditory nerve. Wave II represents the more proximal portion of the VIII nerve.[9,10] Previous studies had attributed Wave II to the cochlear nucleus.[11] Møller presents evidence that it is Wave III that corresponds to the neurons of the cochlear nucleus. Wave IV is attributed to the superior olivary complex as well as neurons from the cochlear nucleus, and possibly the lateral lemniscus. Wave V is believed to be generated by the lateral lemniscus.[9,10] Origin of Waves VI and VII is thought to be the inferior colliculus and medial geniculate bodies.[9,11] Møller cautions against regarding the above as more than a working hypothesis, because evoked potentials represent compound action potentials of the auditory nerve that have not been precisely pinpointed.[9]

ABR represents normalcy or alterations in function related to these generating sites. Interpretation depends upon the ABR technique applied. Through studies such as Møller's, it is possible to attribute a lesion to a general site by analyzing specific parameters of the ABR. The following characteristics of the waveforms are studied in determining conductive, cochlear, and retrocochlear pathology.

Waveform Morphology

Morphology refers to the overall appearance of the 7 waves. The configuration is predictable and affected by age, gender, pathology, and test parameters.[12] Waves IV and V are often fused in normals. Wave V is the most important, prominent, and stable of the waves. Normative data is typically obtained on Waves I, III, and V, as they are the most reliable. Waves VI and VII are assessed for general morphology, but their latencies are not reviewed as often in routine clinical ABR.

Absolute Latency

Each wave occurs within a certain amount of time following stimulus onset. The time period needed for a wave peak to emerge is referred to as its absolute latency. These latencies are very stable and reliable among normal subjects. Wave I occurs within a range of 1.5-1.7 msec, and each successive wave follows approximately 1 msec later.[13]

Test technique and parameters will affect latencies. Each clinic should have its own normative data for the equipment and test protocol it uses.

Interwave Latency

The time difference between primary peak components Waves I–V, I–III, and III–V are assessed. On the average, 2.0 msec is the difference between Waves I–III and III–V, with I–III having a slightly longer conduction time. The I–V interwave latency is approximately 4 msec.[14] Each clinic should refer to its own norms.

Interwave latency is also referred to as interwave interval (IWI) or interpeak latency (IPL).[13]

Amplitude

Amplitude of wavepeaks shows great variability, and, for this reason, amplitude is not used as a strong determining factor in clinical assessment at the present time. Waves III and V are generally the most prominent waves. Wave V is approximately twice the amplitude of Wave I. This is referred to as the I–V amplitude ratio. Wave amplitude is dependent upon intensity and electrode montage as well as age and gender.[12,13]

Interaural Latency

Comparing latencies between ears should show latencies within approximately 0.2–0.3 msec of agreement. If the loss is greater than 65 dB HL, 0.4 msec may be considered acceptable. Asymmetrical hearing loss has to be considered when making comparisons.[15]

Replicability

Waveforms should be replicable. The ABR test is always repeated at least twice at a given intensity level and parameter arrangement. If waves show poor replicability, this could indicate the presence of artifact, equipment problems, or physiological abnormality. The interpreter must rule out artifact and equipment problems before calling an ABR abnormal.

All patient responses are compared to the clinic's normative data. Normal limits for absolute and interwave latencies are usually considered to be plus or minus 2 standard deviations from the mean values of normal subjects tested.

Test Results

ABR's strongest application is in detecting the presence of retrocochlear disorder. The test is presented at a moderately loud to loud intensity level and the wave features are compared to clinic norms.

Another application of ABR is estimating hearing sensitivity. Although this is somewhat less accurate than is the use of ABR to detect lesions, it can provide a good estimation of hearing within the mid to high frequencies. To establish threshold estimation, the stimulus intensity is presented at an assumed suprathreshold level and an ABR is obtained. If there is clear morphology and wave latencies are within normal limits, the intensity level is dropped in gradations of 5 or 10 dB until Wave V, the most robust of the waves, can no longer be clearly seen. As intensity decreases, Wave V latency increases. In normal hearers, Wave V is within 5–6 msec at 80 dB HL and increases to 8–8.5 msec at 10 dB HL.[16] The lowest intensity producing Wave V is predicted to be within 5–15 dB HL of the patient's threshold for the 1000–4000 Hz region of hearing.[17]

The Latency-intensity Function

If the Wave V latency obtained at each intensity level is plotted on a latency versus intensity graph, a function emerges that can typify the existing type of hearing loss. By using the latency-intensity (L-I) function, only a low, mid, and high intensity presentation may be used, and the complete function extrapolated as a time-saving method.

The L-I function can give threshold estimation information, as well as display patterns for predicting site of lesion. Typical patterns of waveform characteristics and L-I functions for conductive, cochlear, and retrocochlear ABRs are discussed below.

Conductive Hearing Loss

Due to the presence of the conductive loss, the sound intensity presented to the ear is reduced, causing a longer conduction time for the waveforms. Sound is transmitted to the ear at a softer level, resulting in the displacement of the L-I function the same degree as the conductive hearing loss. As a latency shift of all the ABR waves occurs, the function parallels the normal shape but is shifted out in time.[18] (See Figure 20-2.)

Although the latency-intensity function can be useful in predicting type of hearing loss, other tests must be used in conjunction with ABR to verify the nature of the loss. Because the ABR click presentation is within the 1000–4000 Hz region, a low frequency conductive loss may not be discovered through ABR testing. A mild sensorineural loss with a flat audiometric configuration could be mistaken for a conductive loss if viewed only on the L-I function. Whenever possible, tympanometry and bone conduction testing should be administered to differentiate conductive losses. If this is not possible, as is often the case with a very young child or multihandicapped individual, an ABR using bone conduction stimulation provides a reasonable alternative to demonstrate an air-bone gap.[19]

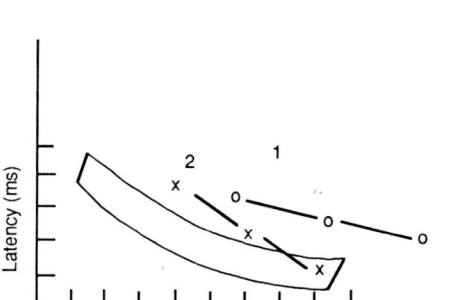

Fig. 20-2. An L-I function, showing the latency of Wave V plotted at various intensity levels, is shown below. The boxed-in region represents the range of normal.

Numeral 1 exemplifies a conductive hearing loss. The L-I function for a conductive loss has the same configuration as a normal ABR, but latencies are prolonged. They are shifted out in time on the L-I function. Conductive hearing loss causes a reduction in the presentation level of the ABR test stimuli to the ear. Sound is transmitted to the ear at a softer level, causing the longer conduction time.

Numeral 2 shows an example of a sensorineural hearing loss plotted on the L-I function. Wave V latencies shorten more than the normal ear at higher intensity levels, attributed to the recruitment phenomenon. This abnormal decrease in latencies, once above threshold, results in a steeper L-I function for sensorineural losses.

Cochlear Hearing Loss

In cochlear hearing loss, the L-I function is extremely steep. Wave V latency shortens abnormally rapidly once above threshold, and joins the normal curve. This is attributed to the phenomenon of recruitment, an abnormal loudness growth occurring in damaged cochlear hair cells.[18] A shallow function with an abrupt, steep rise can be indicative of a predominantly high frequency cochlear loss.[2]

Latencies of earlier waves are generally prolonged in cochlear losses greater than 40 dB Hl. Depending upon the degree of loss, morphology of Waves I and III may be poor.[15] It is theorized that click stimuli excite lower frequency components in high frequency losses due to cochlear hair cell damage. As a result, the components travel longer on the basilar membrane and latencies are increased.[20]

Although absolute latencies may be delayed, the I–V interwave interval is within normal limits for cochlear losses.[15]

Evaluating cochlear loss takes expertise. The audiometric contour, etiology of hearing loss, and special techniques applicable to testing cochlear site of lesion are reviewed. In cochlear losses over 50 dB HL established correction factors may be added to normative data to allow for degree of hearing loss.

Retrocochlear Disorder

Eighth nerve and low brainstem abnormalities, such as the acoustic neuroma, intra- and extra-axial tumors, and vascular lesions, can greatly alter ABR results.[14] Interwave latency delay, especially I–V, is a strong indication of retrocochlear disorder. A delayed Wave V is another salient retrocochlear sign. Inter-ear latencies for Wave V are often significantly prolonged, and wave morphology and replicability may be poor, with reduced wave amplitude present. Total absence of waves can occur in retrocochlear lesions.[14,21] (See Figure 20-3.)

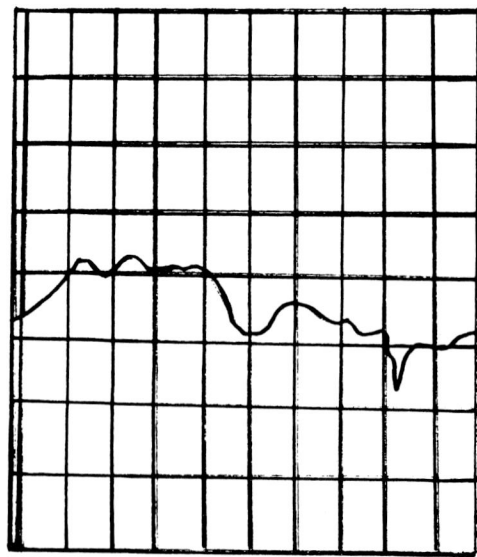

Fig. 20-3. Waveforms are delayed and poorly defined.

msec

Speculation exists concerning why these ABR abnormalities occur. Nerve fibers may be stretched or compressed due to the presence of a tumor, slowing nerve impulse conduction time. The tumor may interfere with high or low frequency fibers and alter traveling wave patterns, resulting in increased latencies. Vascular compression may result in decreased oxygen supply.[15]

The retrocochlear L-I function is often shifted out in time in the absence of a conductive loss.

Low versus high brainstem lesions can be predicted from the ABR. Low brainstem lesions may show an absence of earlier waves, or all waves could be absent. The I–III interwave latency is typically prolonged on the ipsilateral side. High brainstem lesions may show earlier waves, but later waves may be absent. Waves III–VI may be prolonged.[15]

As mentioned, it is essential to obtain an audiogram whenever possible. A profound hearing loss, as well as retrocochlear disorders, can cause absence of waves.

Infant ABR

ABR interpretation in neonates is unique to this population only. The ABR reflects an immature auditory system that responds differently than does an adult's. A reliable ABR can be recorded by 27–28 weeks gestation.[2,22] Waves I, III, and V are seen, with differing morphology and longer latencies than observed in an adult ABR.[22] Amplitude of Wave I is twice the size of a typical adult Wave I, while Wave V is smaller.[2] Jacobson speculates that an abnormally large Wave I amplitude may be due to small infant head size, resulting from electrodes closer to the auditory nerve in infants than in adults.[23] ABR maturity changes are attributed to improved transmission from absorbed mesenchyme, greater myelination, and greater synaptic synchrony arriving at wave generators.[24] Wave I approximates adult latency and amplitude by 2 months of age. Wave V is comparable to an adult Wave V by 12 months. (See Figure 20-4).

INSTRUMENTATION

Quality equipment will aid in ABR sensitivity. The following explanation of instrumentation will introduce the reader to computer averaging techniques. Suggestions for purchasing clinical ABR equipment are included.

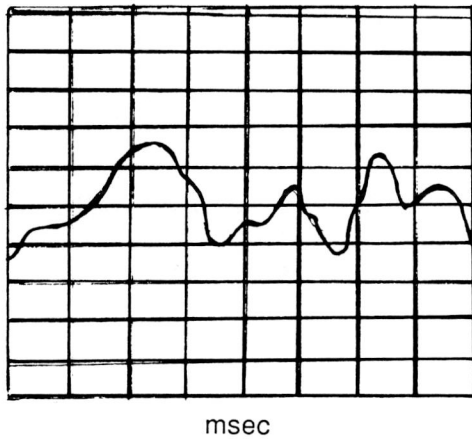

Fig. 20-4. The recording to the left typifies a normal ABR for a neonate.

In this example Wave I is the largest waveform, present at 2.5 msec (each vertical line on the graph represents 1 msec in time), Wave III present at almost 5 msec, and Wave V at 6.5 msec.

ABR is called a far-field recording because electrodes are removed from their generator sites.[5] Other electrical activity contaminates and obscures the ABR, intervening in this distance between the surface electrode and the response origin. The EEG is approximately 10 microvolts in amplitude, compared to the ABR at only 0.01–0.05 microvolts.[25,26] Through computer techniques, the ABR emerges from these larger potentials. The ability of the computer to do this is based upon its ability to increase the ABR while effectively decreasing the EEG and other unwanted artifact.

In 1964, Borsanyi and Blanchard described computer averaging in biological data processing.[27] Until the introduction of computers, ABR could not be extracted from other physiological responses. Today, small computers are commonplace, and commercial ABR equipment that utilizes computer averaging for clinical use is easily accessible. Important components of the ABR instrumentation include the amplifier and filter system, the stimulation system, and the signal averager. The amplifier, common-mode rejection, bandpass filter, and time-locked averager can all serve to enhance the ABR.[28]

Preamplifier and Amplifier

The preamplifier increases the signal by utilizing the principles of common mode rejection. At least 3 surface electrodes are needed for this technique. The electrodes are placed on the head, where the ABR differs but where other potentials and unwanted artifact remain constant. Two electrodes are connected to the preamplifier and one serves as ground.[29] The first electrode, the positive, noninverting electrode, should be positioned as close to the generating source as possible. Although electrode montage has not been standardized to date, best results have been reported with the positive electrode on the scalp vertex (Cz).[30] Another acceptable placement is the high forehead at midline (Fz). The inverting electrode should be placed on assumed inert, inactive tissue. This placement is usually on the earlobe (A_1 or A_2) or mastoid (M_1 or M_2) of the ear being stimulated.[29,31] This is a bipolar arrangement. The differential preamplifier subtracts the electrode voltages from the noninverting and inverting electrodes. The difference between these electrical potentials is measured. Irrelevant electrical noise is greatly reduced because this random activity tends to average to zero, with the desired potential remaining. Repeated sampling allows the random activity to be eliminated and the ABR emerges through this common mode rejection.[25,27,29]

Filters also play an important role in rejecting unwanted electrical activity. The filter serves as a bandpass. It allows certain frequencies to be averaged while rejecting others. Incoming activity outside a preset frequency band range is attenuated in an attempt to reduce the amount of noise being averaged with the ABR.[13]

Stimulation System

The stimulus onset is time-locked to the computer onset. The sound stimulus is presented to the patient via earphones while, simultaneously, the timer is activated and the digital averager records for a predetermined amount of time (usually 10 msec for ABR). It is the onset of the stimulus that evokes the electrical potential. Electrical potentials are evoked best when the onset of the stimulus is rapid. The broadband click is used most commonly in ABR testing. Its rapid onset activates both high and low threshold fibers at once.[16]

Signal Averager

Signal averaging operates under the assumption that the ABR remains constant each time an auditory stimulus is presented, while unwanted noise is random and does not produce a pattern. When an acoustical signal evokes a potential, a small direct current potential is triggered and a waveform occurs. In order for this waveform to be seen, the averager begins sampling as soon as the stimulus click begins, and stops at a set interval (10 msec) after stimulation. This time-locked sequence is repeated over and over for a predetermined number of times. Each sequence is called a sweep, or repetition. Often, 2000 repetitions or more are used. Time-locked responses build up while random noise is cancelled out.[16,27,31] During this process, the analog, or waveform, signal is converted to a digital signal. The computer averages all responses in digital form, superimposes and averages them, then converts the signals back to an analog form, where their averages appear on the oscilloscope.[26,28] Through utilization of the above methods, extraneous electrical activity shrinks to a minimum. Unfortunately, there is always some residual noise that hasn't been cancelled out. Figure 20-5 shows a schematic of ABR Instrumentation.

Selecting ABR Equipment

When choosing an ABR clinical system, several factors should be taken into account. The system should be designed as an evoked potential instrument foremost and a computer second. Computers can be slow and programming may not keep up with the test procedures if the computer hasn't been specifically designed for that purpose.

Look for high-speed digitizers, digital filters, and amplifiers with optimum filter rolloff. Analog filters, found in older ABR equipment have inferior filter rolloff and can cause phase distortion; notch filters can be the source of even greater distortion. While a notch filter may be a desired feature in certain noisy test situations, it should be used only as a last resort technique for decreasing artifact.[32]

The screen (oscilloscope) will ideally permit observation of input as well as output. The number of repetitions averaged and rejected should be displayed. Cursors, one to pinpoint latency, and two for interwave and amplitude measurements, should be available.[32]

Systems that allow inspection of emerging waveforms, and manipulation of cursors

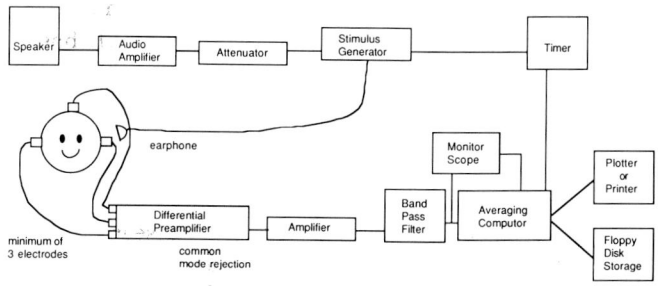

Fig. 20-5. A schematic illustration of ABR instrumentation.[1,26,28] Basic equipment components are shown.

and plotters at the same time averaging occurs, save time. Automatic plotters and floppy disc storage of data are recommended.[13,32]

Choose earphones with a flat frequency response. Spectral contents of earphones will affect waveform morphology, latency, and amplitude.[13]

The instrument should have capabilities for monophasic and alternating polarity. Look at stimulus rates and intensity level ranges. The system should have the capacity to process 1–80 or more clicks each second, at levels from 0 to 100 or greater dB HL.

If hearing estimation will be done routinely, an installation jack for a bone vibrator, and masking and bandbass noise, as well as broadband clicks, are features to include.

Current systems on the market include several types of evoked potential capabilities, so that auditory, visual, and somatosensory potentials can be completed using the same piece of equipment.

FACTORS INFLUENCING ABR OUTCOME

Once a good clinical system has been chosen, ABR appearance is further dependent on stimulus parameters, recording techniques, and subject characteristics. ABR is a relatively new field and no standardizations of parameters are in existence to date. It is important to be aware of the effect of changing parameters on ABR.

Stimulus Parameters

Intensity

Intensity and waveform latency have an inverse relationship. As intensity of the stimulus decreases, the latency increases. At lowest intensities, only Wave V, the most stable of the waves, may be seen. For every 10 dB HL drop in intensity, Wave V latency increases by approximately 0.4 msec.[13] It is theorized that latency increases at lower presentation levels because neural firing is less rapid.[13]

To obtain optimum latencies, suprathreshold intensity levels are routinely used in ABR testing. As with routine audiometry, masking in the nontest ear must be used when there is the possibility that the intensity of the stimulus in the test ear could be at a sufficient level to cross over, via bone conduction, to the nontest ear and affect test response. A conservative interaural attenuation level for the click stimuli has been established as 50 dB HL. Masking noise in the nontest ear can affect the response of the test ear. A short duration click in the test ear and long duration broadband noise in the nontest ear are recommended. They will not interact; research has shown that they follow different afferent pathways of the auditory system.[33]

Polarity

Stimulus click polarity has been found to alter wave amplitude and morphology. Stockard et al. reported that rarefaction clicks caused shortened latency of Wave I with increased amplitude and waveform appearance.[34] Other researchers showed no advantage to using one polarity over another.[2,13] Wave I is clearer in some subjects for positive than for negative clicks; in other patients, negative clicks produce a clearer Wave I. More research is needed in this area.

Repetition Rate

The number of clicks presented each second will affect the appearance of the waveforms. A slow click presentation rate (below 12 clicks/second) enhances clarity and amplitude of waveforms. Rates above 20 clicks/second (c/s) decrease the amplitude of Waves I–III. Latencies have been noted to increase by 0.4 msec as click presentation is increased from 10 to 80 c/s.[13,35] Rates greater than 50 c/s are considered high click rates. It is believed that rapid click presentation stresses the auditory system. In normal hearers, Wave V latency shifts at rates above 50 c/s, but morphology remains intact. A Wave V that shifts dramatically or shows morphology degradation could be exemplifying a system breaking down under stress. Musiek speculates that this may be due to a longer than normal absolute refractory period in a malfunctioning nerve cell.[15] The high click rate has been found to be a good test for neurological involvement. Abnormal functioning may include a reduced refractory period and inefficiency of neural synchrony.[15]

Type of Stimulus

The broadband click, with its rapid onset and short duration, is effective in acquiring the ABR. Longer rise times can desynchronize neural activity, decreasing amplitude and increasing latencies.[36] The click is not frequency specific, as its rapid onset activates both high and low neural fibers.[16]

Stimuli that can improve frequency specificity include notched noise, high-pass noise, bandpass noise, pure tones, and masking. Unlike tone pips, tone bursts, and filtered clicks that potentially cause wide spread of energy (spectral splatter), these stimuli appear to restrict noise to particular frequency regions, at least among normal hearers.[2]

Two problems have existed with ABR stimulation other than clicks. Many averaging systems don't have the capabilities to use other forms of stimulation, and frequency specificity does not necessarily have a direct correlation with place specificity within the inner ear. In the normal cochlea, a frequency-specific stimulus may also be place-specific. In ears with damaged high frequency hair cells, the traveling wave may allow high frequencies to be received by stimuli in areas of the cochlea that usually receive low frequency information.

Subject Characteristics

Age

Separate data pools should be obtained for infants, young children, young to middle aged adults, and the geriatric population. Infant ABR responses reflect an immature auditory system and have a different appearance than does an adult ABR. Effects of aging on the auditory system may demonstrate an increase in latencies among geriatrics.

Gender

One should control for sex differences in adults. On the average, males have a 0.14 msec increase in Wave V latency over females. This is believed to be due to a woman's smaller head circumference and foreshortening of the brainstem pathway between the auditory nerve and midbrain.[13] An equal number of female and male adults should be tested when pooling norms.

Recording Techniques

ABR is an objective measure, but clinical application introduces subjective variables. Obtaining an accurate and informative ABR depends upon the clinician's expertise; the clinician's knowledge of the many factors that can affect the response and of how to use these to best advantage; on the upkeep of equipment; and on norms that are established for the equipment. Administration of ABR is ideally performed by an audiologist, an individual with firm knowledge regarding hearing loss and its effect on the auditory system. Calibration of the ABR equipment is essential to its upkeep. All components and parameters, including stimulus, intensity, rate, polarity, etc., should be calibrated by a trained professional.

Norms

ABR is interpreted by comparing results to normative data. This is an established clinical procedure. As far back as 1968, Yoshie stressed the importance of classifying an ABR as abnormal by comparing it to normal responses.[37] The limited variability of latencies within and between patients makes ABR a valuable diagnostic tool.

Each clinic needs to establish its own norms, which become the standard for the population; recording parameters; and methods it uses. This includes consistency in electrode placement and earphone use. A pool of at least 10 subjects is used. The behavioral threshold to the click stimulus is obtained for each subject. The mean threshold becomes the intensity reference: n dB HL. This value can be more closely referenced to audiometric HL by testing the same subjects on a calibrated audiometer. The mean of the ABR click threshold is referenced to HL on the audiometer dial.[38]

A set suprathreshold intensity level (generally 70–80 dB HL) enhances the ABR components and is used to measure absolute, interwave, and interaural latencies.

Normal limits for these measures are generally considered to be plus or minus 2 standard deviations from the mean. No standards are available on ABR at this point in time, but the above has become an accepted procedure.

If a latency-intensity function is desired, means are obtained at 5–10 dB intensity level increments until the slope of the function and its range is normed.

New procedures in ABR are constantly emerging. Norms must be kept updated.

Amplitudes of waves and the I–V amplitude ratio are used in research clinics; as more data are collected, they will be routinely used in clinical application. Other techniques that are comparatively new include norming the troughs following Waves I and V (I_N and V_N). If Waves IV and V are fused, or if I is difficult to find, comparing trough latencies can clear confusion.[39]

Test Preparation

Prior to ABR testing, an audiogram should be obtained to establish the existence and degree of hearing loss.

ABR testing requires proper electrical grounding. Equipment should be kept away from copy machines, x-ray equipment, 60 Hz line noise from house current, radio waves, and other possible sources of electrical interference. Overhead lights are turned off during testing.

A quiet test room with a low ambient noise level should be selected. The patient is instructed to lie down and remain as relaxed and still as possible, with eyes closed. Swallowing, blinking, and chewing can cause artifact. Infants can be tested when sleeping, but very young children may require sedation such as chloral hydrate.

Quality electrodes are applied with care. Impedances at electrode and skin interface must be low and similar, or an imbalance can occur, disturbing the common mode rejection process and increasing the input noise level.[1,13] Low impedance is most easily obtained by preparing the skin with a liquid abrasive and using an electrolyte between the scalp and electrode, using tape or collodion to secure it in place. Once electrodes are applied, placement should be checked on the electrode impedance meter. The most accepted electrode arrangement is a vertex, earlobe placement. Vertex placement of the positive electrode may increase the amplitude of Waves V, VI, and VII.[13] A bilateral recording which simultaneously records responses ipsilaterally and contralaterally will separate a IV/V complex on the contralateral recording.[26] This can be a useful technique when Wave V appears to be delayed, but (due to a fused IV/V) the Wave V peak is difficult to determine. An example of an ipsilateral versus contralateral ABR recording is shown in Figure 20-6. Wave I may be enhanced by a horizontal montage, achieved by placing the positive electrode on the nontest ear and the negative electrode on the test ear.[26] Wave I is the reference point for all other waves. An obscured Wave I makes detecting other waves much more difficult.

Filters suppress frequency components containing high amounts of noise energy, but they also alter the signal. (See Figure 20-7.) Some signal frequency components can be filtered, altering phase of these components and resulting in phase distortion. The bandpass filter setting should be based upon the evoked potential being recorded and upon the nature of the unwanted noise. Low pass filters smooth out high frequency components, serving to diminish unwanted noise artifact. High pass filters can reduce 60 Hz artifact, but should be used cautiously, as they decrease wave amplitude and shift latency.[13] ABR equipment often has a notch filter designed to suppress 60 Hz line power. Notch filters can cause phase distortion and should be used only after all methods of reducing the noise source have failed.[13] Appropriate click rates and bandpass settings are usually sufficient to squelch 60 Hz artifact. ABR filters are set above 60 Hz. The low

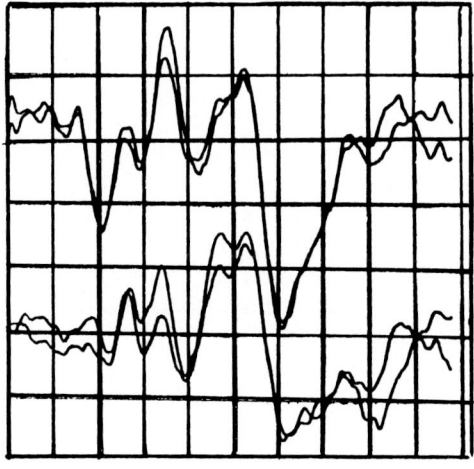

msec

Fig. 20-6. The ipsilateral recording (top recording), measured from the same ear, results in a Wave IV/V complex in this example.

The contralateral recording below it, measured from the same ear and the opposite ear, serves to separate Waves IV and V into individual waveforms.

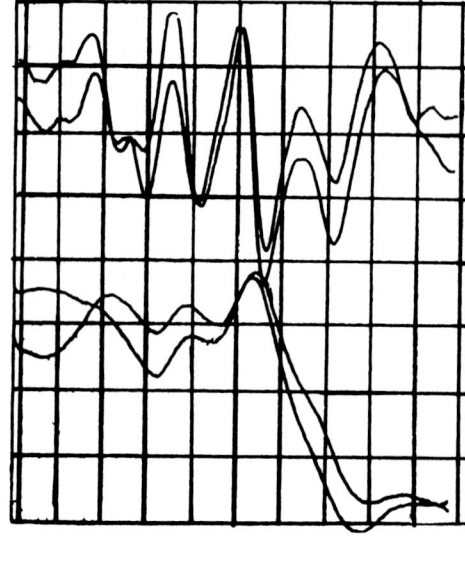

Fig. 20-7. The top recording shows the affects of a low filter at 150 Hz and a high filter at 1500 Hz. The ABR morphology is distorted. The recording below it, with a low filter setting at 30 Hz and a high setting at only 250 Hz further distorts the ABR.

band filter will filter out 60 Hz noise. Using an odd-integer click repetition rate, not easily divisible into 60 Hz, helps eliminate 60 Hz and its harmonics.

Test Administration

Test parameters chosen depend upon the purpose of the ABR. If the purpose is to test for retrocochlear disorder, high intensity levels are used with a relatively low stimulus rate. If threshold assessment is desired, higher stimulus rate is used and latencies are recorded in increments of intensity until Wave V, the most robust of all the waves, can no longer be detected. Wave V can be seen almost to threshold level.

Once the ABR is obtained, it is immediately repeated under the same exact conditions. This retest will ensure an actual response and reveal a random occurrence. The oscilloscope should be closely monitored during test administration. A true ABR builds slowly during the averaging process, while artifact often occurs abruptly.[40] If the patient is extremely tense or active, it may be difficult to discern the ABR from the overlaying artifact. A control run without sound displays the waves that are due to artifact. To obtain optimum waveform morphology and amplitude, 2 runs of 2000 repetitions are often used. Noisy environments or restless patients may require additional repetitions.

A binaural ABR presentation is useful when testing young children. The binaural threshold is obtained to click stimuli. Each ear is then tested separately at 20 dB HL above the binaural threshold. If the monaural thresholds are equal, testing can be terminated. If there is a discrepancy between ears, a threshold search is done only on the poorer ear. This approach saves time, an important consideration when a child is only under mild sedation, the effects of which may wear off quickly.[41]

Bone conduction ABR is applicable when earphone use is impossible, as in a patient with atresia or microtia. Bone conduction can be compared to air conduction ABR results to detect a conductive hearing loss. Special precaution should be used in comparing bone conduction versus air conduction stimuli: bone conduction latencies are longer and spectral content of the two is not the same.[2,19] Norms are needed for bone conduction latencies, type of bone vibrator used, and its routine placement (mastoid or forehead).

In asymmetrical losses, the same intensity levels are obtained in both ears, so that latencies can be compared. If one ear has a profound loss and cannot be tested using ABR, the good ear still should be tested. A large tumor can prolong Waves IV and V in the opposite ear.[15,42]

Acquiring effective test techniques is a skill. When interpreting results, a technical or procedural problem is always ruled out before attributing the abnormality to the patient. Poor waveform morphology may be resolved by reinstructing the patient to relax. Checking electrode contacts and inspecting earphone fit, increasing the number of repetitions, decreasing the stimulus rate, changing stimulus polarity, or adjusting the electrode montage may improve resolution.

Combining ABR results with pure tone audiometry and acoustic reflexes helps further in preventing ambiguity.[43]

In hostile ABR environments such as the operating room or intensive care unit, the clinician must be aware of additional variables such as anesthetic agents used, and the effects of reduced body temperature and oxygen supply. Different filter settings, polarity changes, insert earphones, and electrical isolation equipment may be needed.[7,44,45]

CLINICAL APPLICATIONS

Test Sensitivity

ABR sensitivity has surpassed the traditional special audiometric tests, having a higher hit rate in detecting retrocochlear disorder than do all classical tests, including acoustic reflex decay testing. Barrs et al. reported the ABR was 98 percent effective in revealing abnormalities among 305 patients with acoustic neuromas. Acoustic reflex decay testing in these same patients yielded an 80 percent success rate.[46] This study agrees with an earlier report by Glasscock et al., conveying a 98 percent hit rate for ABR.[42] Similarly, Musiek reported the accuracy of ABR as being 92 percent or higher in several recent studies of retrocochlear pathology.[15]

Although it is sensitive, the ABR needs to be interpreted in conjunction with other audiological tests. As mentioned, it is essential to obtain an audiogram to account for the effects of hearing loss. In addition, speech testing and acoustic immittance are important tests in the test battery approach used in ruling out auditory nerve and brainstem tumors.[43]

Newborn hearing screenings utilizing ABR are routine in many hospitals. Advantages include the fact that ABR is objective and can test 2 ears separately at conversational loudness or below. Disadvantages include a high false-positive rate due to late maturation or resolving middle ear disease.[23]

The ABR is used for auditory assessment only after conventional audiometry fails to provide sufficient information. This may be the case with the very young child or the multihandicapped. Smith et al. used ABR to predict hearing in young children. They used the presence of Wave V on the latency-intensity function to estimate the pure tone average that would be expected from the audiogram. The same children were retested years later with conventional audiometry. The pure tone average had been predicted accurately with ABR in 76 percent of the children.[47] Pure tone audiometry gives threshold information with more accuracy over discrete frequencies and in a broader frequency range than does any current ABR technique.

The ABR threshold for click stimuli measures the upper speech frequency range. It does not reflect sensitivity below 1000 Hz. Other stimuli, such as tone pips, etc., can provide some degree of lower frequency information and greater frequency specificity. Hayes and Jerger reported a low frequency tone pip overestimated degree of hearing loss at 500 Hz in 28 percent of 32 hearing-impaired children tested with ABR. Without accurate information regarding hearing loss at 500 Hz, hearing aid fittings could result in overamplification.[48]

Hearing Aids and ABR

To combat the problems of overestimating hearing loss and possibly damaging residual hearing, a comparatively new application of ABR is in use in some clinics. Instead of predicting hearing loss from the ABR and attempting to select a hearing aid that may or may not be appropriate, a child or multihandicapped individual who cannot undergo a standard hearing aid evaluation is tested with ABR while wearing a hearing aid. Speakers or earphones are used to administer an aided ABR. Click stimuli are presented to the hearing aid aid worn on the patient's ear while the patient is in a sound-treated room. By making proper adjustments to the output, gain, and compression settings of an appropriate aid, the ABR approaches normality. Using a latency-intensity function to estimate normal dynamic loudness function, the aided ABR can be correlated to speech intelligibility by its latencies and closeness to a normal L-I function. More research is being developed in establishing positive correlations between ABR results and successful use of hearing aids.[49]

Monitoring Techniques

Monitoring the lower auditory pathway during operations that put the inner ear, eighth nerve, or auditory areas in the brainstem at risk gives important information of the condition of these areas due to anesthesia and surgery. Similarly, ABR is independent of level of consciousness and can be used to monitor the neurological status of patients comatose due to brain injury, no matter the degree of coma.[7,44,45] ABR is also being used to monitor patients on special diets. Hecox notes that dietary therapy can improve ABR results in children with metabolic diseases.[50]

CONCLUSION

Although ABR has appeared in the literature for almost 20 years, it is still in its infancy in many respects. Standardization is just beginning. ABR should never be viewed in isolation, but it is the best single test procedure available for retrocochlear testing and for testing those of all ages who will not or cannot cooperate with conventional audiometry. New monitoring techniques attest to the amazing versatility of ABR. No otolaryngology practice should be without access to ABR.

REFERENCES

1. Glasscock ME, Jackson CG, Josey AF: An introduction to brainstem electric response audiometry. In Glasscock ME, Jackson CG, Josey AF (Eds.): Brainstem Electric Response Audiometry. New York: Thieme-Stratton, pp. 3–7, 1981
2. Hecox K, Jacobson JT: Auditory evoked potentials. In Northern J (Ed.): Hearing Disorders (2nd ed.) Boston: Little, Brown and Co., pp. 57–73, 1983
3. Dawson GD: A summation technique for the detection of small evoked potentials. Electroencephalogr Clin Neurophysiol 6:65–84, 1954
4. Sohmer H, Feinmesser M: Cochlear action potentials recorded from the external ear in man. Ann Otolaryngol 76:427–435, 1967
5. Jewett D, Williston JS: The auditory evoked far fields averaged from the scalp of humans. Brain 94:681–696, 1971
6. Koizumi S: Consistency of auditory brainstem responses in young children during sleep. J Otolaryngol 78:9, 1975
7. Hall JW, Huangfu M, Gennarelli TA: Auditory function in acute severe head injury. Laryngoscope 92:883–890, 1982
8. Gibson WPR: The (acoustic) brainstem electrical responses—BER. In Gibson WPR (Ed.): Essentials of Clinical Electric Response Audiometry. New York: Churchill Livingstone, pp. 107–132, 1978
9. Møller AR, Jannetta PJ, Møller MB: Intracranially recorded auditory nerve response in man: Interpretations of BSER. Arch Otolaryngol 108:77–82, 1982
10. Møller AR, Jannetta PJ: Neural generators of the auditory brainstem response In Jacobson JT (Ed.): The Auditory Brainstem Response. San Diego: College-Hill, Inc., pp. 13–31, 1985
11. Stockard JJ, Stockard JE, Sharbrough FW: Detection and localization of occult lesions with brainstem auditory responses. Mayo Clin Proc 52:761–769, 1977
12. Jerger J, Hall J: Effects of age and sex on auditory brainstem response. Arch Otolaryngol 106:387–391, 1980
13. Schwartz DM, Berry GA: Normative aspects of the ABR. In Jacobson JT (Ed.): The Auditory Brainstem Response. San Diego: College-Hill, Inc., pp. 65–97, 1985
14. Musiek FE, Gollegly KM: ABR in eighth nerve and low brainstem lesions. In Jacobson JT (Ed.): The Auditory Brainstem Response. San Diego: College-Hill, Inc., pp. 181–202, 1985
15. Musiek F, Sachs E, Geurkink N, et al: Auditory brainstem response and eighth nerve lesions: A review and presentation of cases. Ear Hear 1:279–301, 1980
16. Stapells DR, Picton TW, Pérez-Abalo M, et al: Frequency specificity in evoked potential audiometry. In Jacobson JT (Ed.): The Auditory Brainstem Response. San Diego: College-Hill, Inc., pp. 147–177, 1985
17. Jerger J, Mauldin L: Prediction of sensorineural hearing level from the brainstem evoked response. Arch Otolaryngol 104:456–461, 1978
18. Galambos R, Hecox K: Clinical applications of the auditory brainstem response. Otolaryngol Clin North Am 11:709–722, 1978
19. Mauldin L, Jerger J: Auditory brain stem evoked responses to bone-conduction signals. Arch Otolaryngol 104:656–661, 1979
20. Gorga MP, Worthington DW: Some issues relevant to the measurement of frequency-specific auditory brainstem responses. Semin Hear 4:353–362, 1983
21. Jerger J, Neely JG, Jerger S: Speech impedance, and auditory brainstem response audiometry in brainstem tumors. Arch Otolaryngol 106:218–223, 1980
22. Galambos R, Hicks GE, Wilson MG: The auditory brainstem response reliably predicts hearing loss in graduates of a tertiary intensive care nursery. Ear Hear 5:254–260, 1984
23. Jacobson JT, Seitz MR, Mencher GT, et al: Auditory brainstem response: A contribution to infant assessment and management. In Mencher G, Gerber S (Eds.): Early Management of Hearing Loss. New York City: Grune & Stratton, pp. 151–181, 1981

24. Kaga K, Tanaka Y: Auditory brainstem response and behavioral audiometry. Arch Otolaryngol 106:564–566, 1980
25. Coats AC: Instrumentation. In Moore EJ (Ed.): Bases of Auditory Brain-stem Evoked Responses. New York City: Grune & Stratton, pp. 197–220, 1983
26. Jolly M: Personal communication, 1984
27. Borsanyi SJ, Blanchard CL: Auditory evoked brain responses in man. Arch Otolaryngol 80:149–154, 1964
28. Sanders JW: Personal communication, 1982
29. Berlin CI, Dobie RA: Electrophysiologic measures of auditory function via electrocochleography and brainstem-evoked responses. In Rintelmann WF (Ed.): Hearing Assessment. Baltimore: University Park Press, pp. 425–458, 1979
30. Terkilden K, Osterhammel P: The influence of reference electrode position on recordings of the auditory brainstem response. Ear Hear 2:9–14, 1981
31. Parker DJ: Dependence of the auditory brainstem response on electrode location. Arch Otolaryngol 107:367–371, 1981
32. DeCristoforo DA: Personal communication, 1985
33. Humes LE, Ochs MG: Use of contralateral masking in the measurement of the auditory brainstem response. J Speech Hear Res 25:528–535, 1982
34. Stockard JE, Stockard JJ, Westmoreland BF, et al: Brainstem auditory evoked responses: Normal variation as a function of stimulus and subject characteristics. Arch Neurol 36:823–831, 1979
35. Hyde ML, Blair RL: The auditory brainstem response in neuro-otology: Perspectives and problems. J Otolaryngol 10:117–125, 1981
36. Don M, Eggermont JJ, Brackman DE: Reconstruction of the audiogram using brainstem responses and high pass noise masking. Ann Otol Rhinol Laryngol 56:1, 1979
37. Yoshie N: Auditory nerve action potential responses to clicks in man. Laryngoscope 78:198–215, 1968
38. Dalzell LE: Personal communication, 1984
39. Gardi J: Personal communication, 1985
40. Weber BA: Interpretation: Problems and pitfalls. In Jacobson JT (Ed.): The Auditory Brainstem Response. San Diego: College-Hill, Inc., pp. 99–112, 1985
41. Hayes D: Personal communication, 1983
42. Glasscock M, Jackson C, Josey A, et al: Brainstem evoked response in clinical practice. Laryngoscope 89:1021–1034, 1979
43. Jerger J, Neeley JG, Jerger S: Speech, impedance, and auditory brainstem response audiometry in brainstem tumors. Arch Otolaryngol 106:218–223, 1980
44. Grundy BL, Lina A, Procopia PT, et al: Reversible evoked potential changes with retraction of the eighth cranial nerve. Anesth Analg 60:835–838, 1981
45. Grundy BL, Procopia PT, Jannetta PJ, et al: Evoked potential changes produced by positioning for retromastoid cranectomy. Neurosurgery 10:766–770, 1982
46. Barrs DM, Brackmann DE, Olson JE, et al: Changing concepts of acoustic neuroma diagnosis. Arch Otolaryngol 111:17–21, 1985
47. Smith LE, Simmons FB: Accuracy of auditory brainstem evoked response with hearing level unknown. Ann Otol Rhinol Laryngol 91:266–267, 1982
48. Hayes D, Jerger J: Auditory brainstem response (ABR) to tone-pips: Results in normal and hearing-impaired subjects. Scand Audiol 11:133–142, 1982
49. Mahoney TM: Auditory brainstem response hearing aid applications. In Jacobson JT (Ed.): The Auditory Brainstem Response. San Diego, College-Hill, Inc., pp. 349–370, 1985
50. Hecox KE, Cone B, Blaw ME: Brainstem auditory evoked response in the diagnosis of pediatric neurologic diseases. Neurology 31:832–839, 1981

Kenneth H. Brookler

21

The Clinical and Practical Aspects of Electronystagmography

A room should be set aside solely for the performance of vestibular testing utilizing electronystagmography. The room need not take up too much space, but should accommodate all of the equipment conveniently located for the testing staff. On the average, a space of 8 feet by 10 feet should be sufficient. The room must be adequately ventilated, with a comfortable temperature year-round. It is important to control the temperature at about 70°F to allow patients who sweat easily with caloric stimulation to feel comfortable and for the water baths to easily maintain 30°C.

There should be an adequate electrical supply to the room. It should be conveniently located for the equipment. Depending upon the source of the electricity, conditioning may be required to prevent voltage surges and to keep power, even if brownouts are a common occurrence.

The room lighting should be easily controllable. The lighting should not be too bright and the switches should be near the technician should the need arise to test in total darkness.

The control switches should be clustered in the vicinity of the equipment and be convenient to the technician. This arrangement should allow the technician to monitor the equipment and the patient simultaneously.

Last, the plumbing should be located, if possible, near the water baths. This is especially necessary if an open irrigation system is utilized. Closed-loop systems do not need frequent filling and air systems do not need water at all.

EQUIPMENT

The first piece of equipment to consider is a table on which to perform the test. Some will recommend that the patient be seated in an examining chair, but this may introduce the influence of the neck upon the spontaneous and induced nystagmus. A table with an electric motor to elevate the head to the 30° supine position for caloric testing is preferable. The motor reduces the strain on the back of the technicians attempting to raise the heads of patients. It may be necessary to place an on-off switch near the motor, since the electrical field of the motor may interfere with the recording. In addition, it is helpful to have brackets on the table to house the elements of the equipment attached to the patient, such as the electrode cables and the outputs of the caloric stimulator.

The recorder is the most important piece of equipment. The quality of the recordings and the consistency of that quality are mainly related to the recorder and almost equally to the technician. Recorders are basically either AC (alternating current) or DC (direct current) coupled. The AC coupled machines were initially recommended because of the ease of use in the clinical setting. However, it is important to seek a long time-constant, since the decay of the signal which is part of an alternating current can produce tracings which suggest eye movements not actually present. The time-constant should be at least 5 seconds and preferably 10 seconds. The DC recorders initially used in electronystagmography needed special shielding and tended to have major baseline drift which was a problem in the clinical setting. In addition, it was necessary to allow the electrodes to "set," which was not necessary with the AC electrodes. Currently available DC recorders do not need the special shielding and do not have major drift problems. The newer DC electrodes require less time to set than do AC electrodes and are therefore clinically more attractive. The DC recordings reveal actual eye movements and will record eye position as well. In general, the differences between the two systems are small, involving a tradeoff between the ease of application of the electrodes (without waiting for electrodes to set) versus the minimal constant error related to the time-constant and the inability to record eye position.

Recorders also have channels. The most basic is the single-channel recorder. This, by definition, records eye movement in one plane, i.e., horizontal or vertical. There are some recorders claiming to be 2-channel, but they contain the raw channel and the derived (discussed further) channel of that raw recording. A true 2-channel recorder should record 2 channels of raw nystagmus, allowing for simultaneously horizontal and vertical tracings. The main advantage of this sort of recording is that the clinician may look at both channels for spontaneous and positional testing. In addition, this sort of recording may aid in identifying eye blinks with caloric induced nystagmus (when the test first begins). The 2 channels also allow for basic recognition of disconjugate eye movements in a given plane, i.e., disconjugate horizontal or disconjugate vertical eye movements. To look at both vertical and horizontal disconjugate eye movements simultaneously would require a 4-channel system. A derived channel allows for the calculation of the nystagmus by measuring the slope of the slow phase and providing a calculation for each nystagmus beat. An alternative today is the computer analysis on-line of the nystagmus. Currently produced programs promise to obviate the need for mechanical calculations.

At this time, caloric stimulation remains the standard stimulus for evaluating the vestibular system. By common usage, the bithermal stimulus of Fitzgerald and Hallpike[1] is utilized. This provides a water thermal stimulus of 30° and 44°C. Water caloric stimulators come as open or closed loop irrigators; the open systems are in more general usage. The ideal system should have thermostatically controlled water baths with the water recirculated to the irrigation tip. If the water is not recirculated, it may be necessary to purge the system before each use. When the baths are initially installed, the temperature should be checked with standard mercury thermometers and from time to time thereafter, to satisfy the accuracy of the control system. With the open system, a satisfactory collection method should be employed. Either kidney basins or funnels efficiently collect the discarded water. The closed system has all of the advantages of a water thermal stimulus without the mess of water collection and the need to refill the baths.[2] This allows for caloric testing with safety in draining ears and ears with perforations or cavities.

Air caloric systems are now a reality as a result of modern technology. In practice, however, the air stimulus does not enjoy the reliability and reproducibility of water.

It is advisable to permanently install calibrating lights to allow for accurate calibration. Some laboratories utilize dots on the wall, which do not compel the patient to be as conscientious as in following the lights. The distance between the calibrating lights should be calculated to subtend an angle of 20° where the gain on the recorder can be adjusted so that each degree of eye movement produces 1 mm of excursion of the tracing.

Some prefer to obtain information about the optokinetic system. As such, there are very few of the stimulators that provide more than a very coarse stimulus. Many investigators cannot agree on the best stimulus. Generally, the stimulus should surround the subject. However, the stripe size, i.e., the width, and the speeds to be tested are very variable from investigator to investigator. Last, the degree of subject cooperation, as with other eyes-open testing, can produce variable results.

TECHNICAL STAFF

For many years it was felt that a high school education was adequate for the performance of the standard electronystagmography. Experience has taught that audiologists produce a more reliable product. They are more diligent with respect to detail and take pride in the quality of the study. However, the physician should have a full understanding of the testing procedure and direct the daily function of the laboratory.

The specific training should come under the purview of the physician. The technique to be utilized, as well as the concepts to be adhered to, should be set up by the physician in conjunction with the needs of the practice. If the laboratory is to provide service to more than one physician, then the technician should be fully aware of the many physicians' preferences. If the physician is not adequately grounded in the fundamentals of electronystagmography, then attendance at a course, preferably with the technician or subsequently by the technician, will allow for the smooth set-up of the laboratory and its procedures.

TESTING ROUTINE

The testing routine here described is the one that has evolved in the authors' practice. It is not suggested as *the* routine, but as one of many possible. Where there appears to be a definite deviation from others, an attempt will be made to explain the reasoning in arriving at the difference.

The patient is ushered into the electronystagmography (ENG) room and seated on the ENG table and the ears are examined. A search is made for occluding cerumen or other pathology to be taken into consideration in testing the patient or interpreting the results (Fig. 21-1).

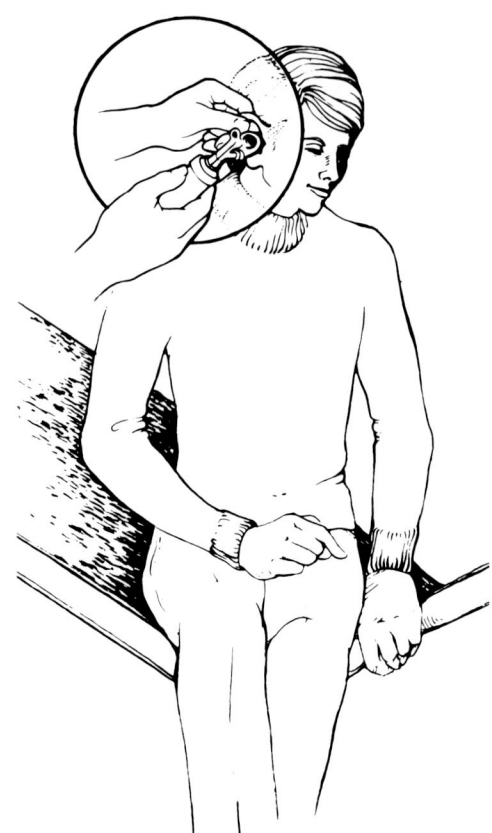

Fig. 21-1. The patient is ushered into the ENG room, seated on the ENG table, and the ears examined for cerumen or pathology.

Next, the skin is carefully cleansed of any make-up or skin oils which may interfere with good skin-to-electrode contact (Fig. 21-2). This is not as important with AC electrodes as with DC. In addition, the DC electrodes need to "set" for a while after application (Fig. 21-3).

Once the electrodes have been applied, the calibration must be undertaken (Fig. 21-4). At the very least, the horizontal eye movement should be calibrated, and the

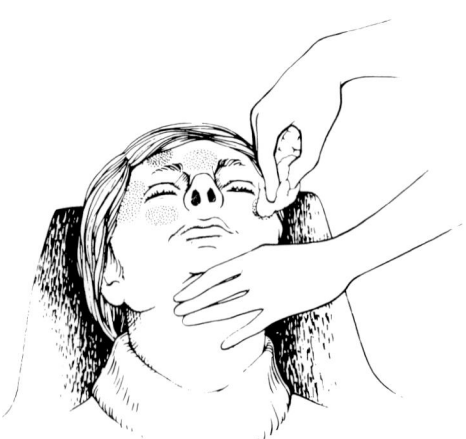

Fig. 21-2. The skin is cleansed where the electrodes will be placed.

The Clinical and Practical Aspects of Electronystagmography

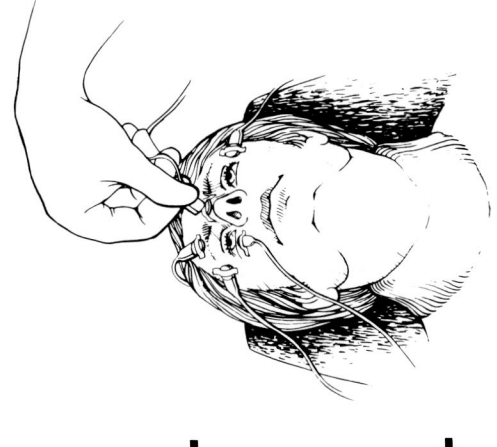

Fig. 21-3. The electrodes are attached to record 2 raw channels of nystagmus: horizontal and vertical.

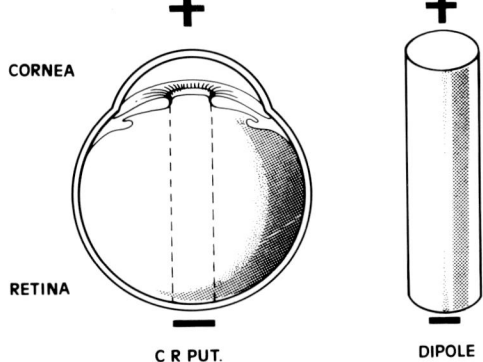

Fig. 21-4. The electrical potential between the retina and the cornea allows surface electrodes to record the movement of this dipole in the field and thus the eye movements.

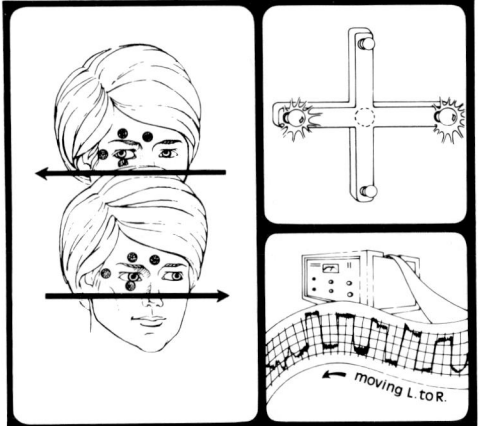

Fig. 21-5. The eye movements are calibrated with flashing lights. The paper moves from right to left and the gain is set so that 1° of eye movement equals 1 mm of pen deflection. Both horizontal and vertical eye movements are calibrated.

vertical when it is being utilized (Fig. 21-5). Calibration overshoots suggestive of a central lesion should be sought only in the horizontal channel, since other channels may indicate the same morphology of eye movements and not represent an abnormality.

By convention, the nystagmus is labeled by its fast phase. The paper moves from right to left and a fast phase moving up on the horizontal channel is right beating (Fig. 21-6). With the fast phase moving down on the horizontal channel, a left beating

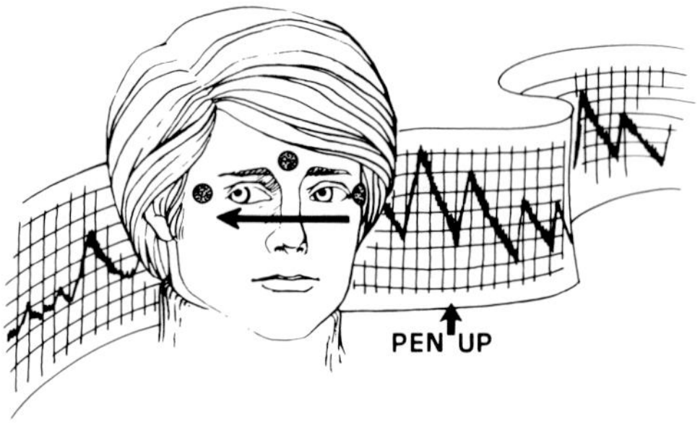

Fig. 21-6. By convention, nystagmus is indicated by the quick component. When the pen is deflected upward, this signifies a right beating nystagmus in the horizontal channel.

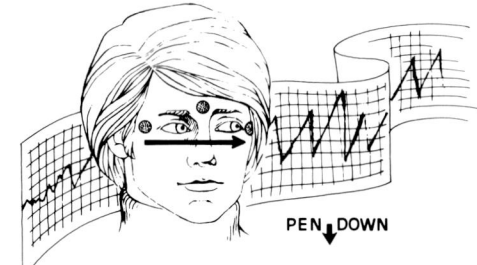

Fig. 21-7. A left beating nystagmus is seen when the pen is deflected downward in the fast phase in the horizontal channel.

Fig. 21-8. When the pen is deflected upward in the fast phase in the vertical channel, an upbeating nystagmus is recorded.

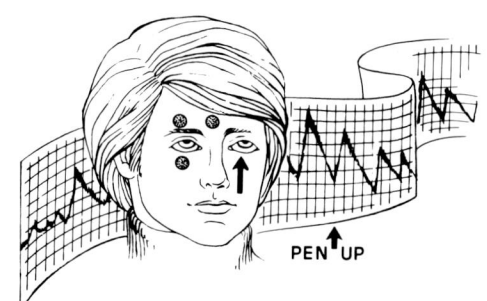

Fig. 21-9. Downbeating nystagmus in the vertical channel occurs when the quick component deflects the pen downward.

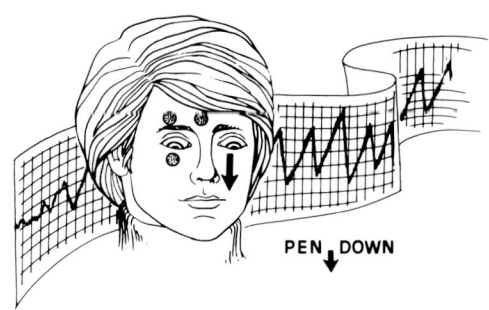

nystagmus is recognized (Fig. 21-7). The vertical channel recognizes an upward fast phase as upbeating (Fig. 21-8) and a downward fast phase as downbeating (Fig. 21-9).

Next, a search is made for nystagmus while the patient is in various positions. The positions are both 0° (Fig. 21-10) and 30° supine, right and left lateral (Fig. 21-11), with neck torsion to the left or right in those positions (Fig. 21-12). From these findings, a definition of spontaneous nystagmus becomes clear. Rather than nystagmus in a particular spontaneous position, the presence of nystagmus in all positions, of the same direc-

The Clinical and Practical Aspects of Electronystagmography

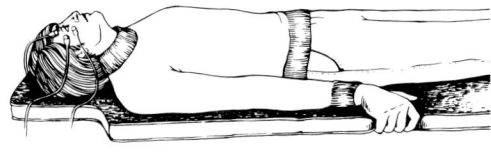

Fig. 21-10. A patient in the 0° supine position with the eyes open. A search is also made for nystagmus with the eyes closed. The portion used in the report is the eyes-closed tracing.

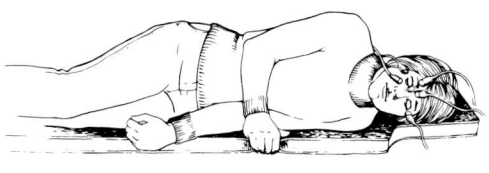

Fig. 21-11. A search is made for nystagmus while the patient is on each side, with eyes both opened and closed. The tracing is of the eyes-closed recording.

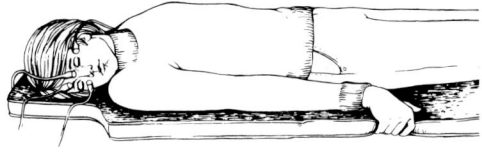

Fig. 21-12. The effect of the neck torsion is also recorded, eyes opened and closed, with the eyes-closed on the report form.

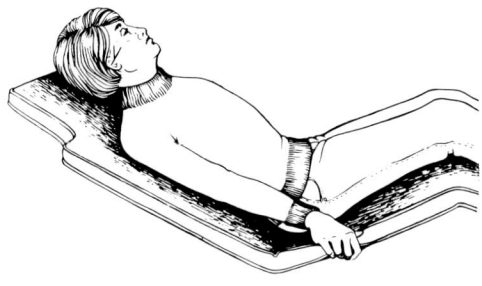

Fig. 21-13. A patient in the 30° supine position revealing the vertical orientation of the lateral semicircular canal: *The Caloric Position.*

tion and of similar velocity, defines spontaneous. That is, nystagmus unaffected by head position.

Neck torsion nystagmus is defined by means of the maneuver above and is nystagmus occurring only in that position or with changes in direction or significantly in velocity from the equivalent lateral position. Often, this neck torsion nystagmus does not represent a primary neck lesion but a modulation of the nystagmus by the input of the cervical nerves.

The 30° supine position is only important with relation to the caloric stimuli. This places the lateral semicircular canal in the vertical position, providing a maximal caloric stimulus (Fig. 21-13). This can also be performed with the patient in the seated position, but neck extension may influence the caloric responses (Fig. 21-14). A search is made for a pre-existing nystagmus in this caloric position, from which to add or subtract the induced response (Fig. 21-15).

The caloric irrigation can be performed with differing techniques. With the open system, a Y-connector comes off the line from the irrigator and some intravenous tubing brought to each ear (Fig. 21-16). The tubing is pinched off to the nontest ear in the alternate stimuli and the water goes to both ears in the simultaneous binaural bithermal stimulation. The funnels are used to collect the discarded water. The closed-loop irrigator needs no water collection system, since the water is constantly recirculating.

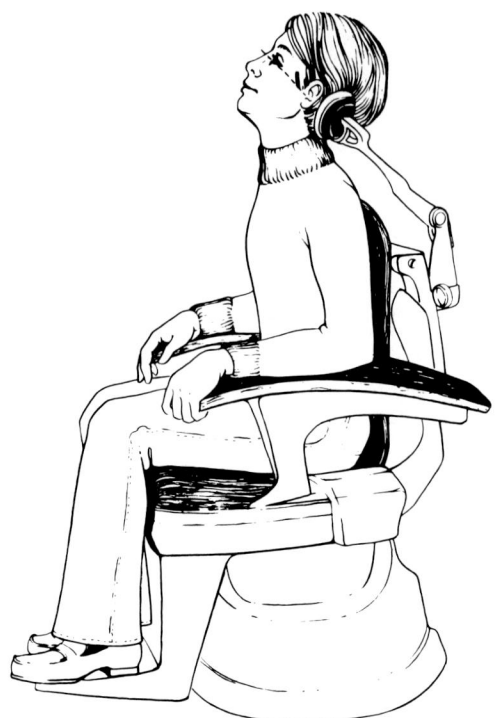

Fig. 21-14. A patient seated in an examining chair with the head tilted back 60° to bring the lateral semicircular canal vertical. The effect of neck extension could modify the induced caloric response.

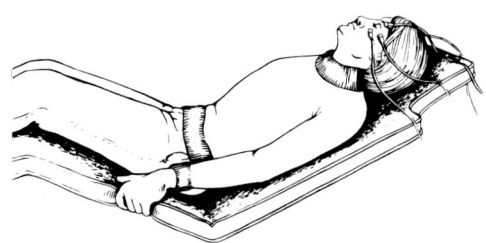

Fig. 21-15. Prior to caloric irrigation, a search is made for a pre-existing nystagmus with the patient in the 30° supine position.

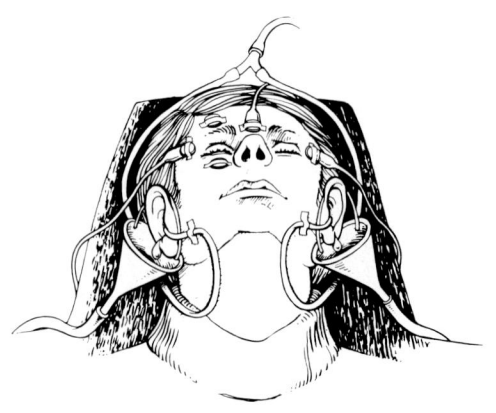

Fig. 21-16. The open caloric irrigator and its funnels for collection of discarded water are attached. The electrodes for measuring vertical eye movements may be disconnected.

The Clinical and Practical Aspects of Electronystagmography

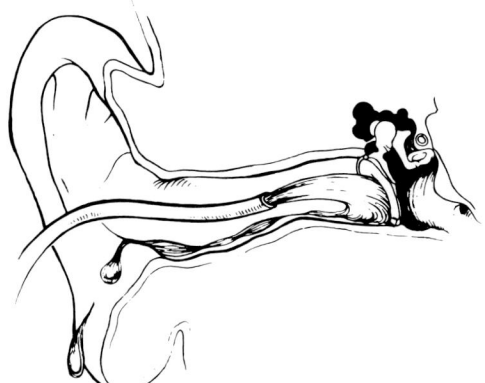

Fig. 21-17. An artist's rendering of an open caloric irrigation in an ear with a normal tympanic membrane.

This technique looks at the alternate binaural bithermal (ABB) in 3 major areas. The first is the velocities of the individual responses. A retrospective computer analysis revealed the individual responses to range between 5° and 25°/sec.[3]

Those below 5°/sec were considered hypoactive responses and those above 25°/sec, hyperactive. These responses were considered normal if the tympanic membrane was intact (Fig. 21-17). However, if a perforation was present, then the caloric stimulus was directly applied to the inner ear and should have produced a hyperactive response (Fig. 21-18). If not, then the response might indicate the source of the symptoms.

Cool stimuli, i.e., below body temperature, produce an utriculofugal flow with the lateral canal vertical yielding nystagmus with its fast phase away from the ear stimulated (Fig. 21-19). The opposite occurs with warm stimuli, which produce an utriculopetal flow and nystagmus with its fast phase toward the stimulated ear (Fig. 21-20).

The responses were then placed in Jongkees' formula and assessed for a reduced vestibular response (RVR) and for directional preponderance (DP). In addition, the individual nystagmus was examined for central dysrhythmia, i.e., nystagmus in which each successive beat bears no relationship to the other beats either in velocity or amplitude.

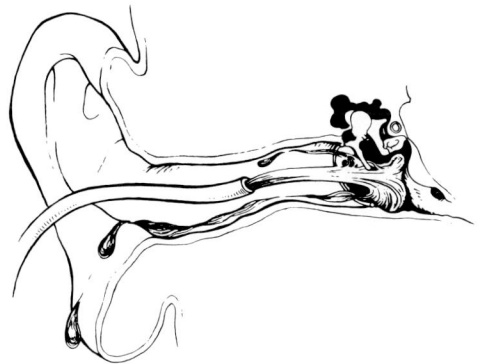

Fig. 21-18. With a tympanic membrane perforation, the caloric stimulus is directly applied on the inner ear. A normally functioning vestibular labyrinth will produce a hyperactive response in that ear.

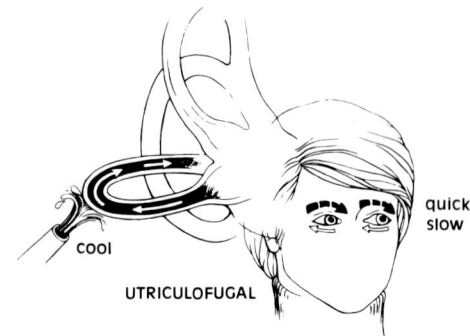

Fig. 21-19. Surrealistic rendering of a movement of endolymph in the lateral semicircular canal and the direction of nystagmus produced when a cold stimulus is applied in the caloric position.

With the head in the 30° supine position, the simultaneous binuaral bithermal is also performed.[4] The temperatures utilized are the same as are utilized for the alternate binural bithermal. The difference is the manner of stimulation. The same stimulus i.e., 30°C water, is irrigated in both ears at the same time with the same flow rate. The duration of the stimulus is 30 seconds and the clinician searches for nystagmus in the next 60 seconds. After a suitable rest (5 minutes), the other temperature of water, in this instance 44°C water, is irrigated in both ears simultaneously and the nystagmus recorded for the 60 seconds after the stimulation is stopped.

When the response to the cool stimulus is below the 5°/sec expected as the norm, an ice water stimulus is utilized to see if there is any further response to possibly indicate recruitment or a markedly reduced response.[3] The stimulus used is 30 dl of ice water over 20–30 seconds.

NONROUTINE TESTING

The necessity of eyes-open testing utilizing electronystagmography can be questioned, since these observations can be made without it. Also, in the test situation in which subject cooperation is essential, the eyes-open tests are subject to wide variability. In some instances, these test results have shown indications of dire central lesions—only to have them disappear with extraordinary alerting. For this reason, gaze nystagmus, optokinetic nystagmus, and eye tracking are not considered in the routine examination.

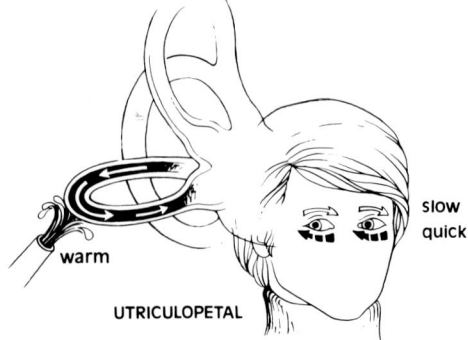

Fig. 21-20. Similar to Fig 19. Showing endolymph flow with a warm water stimulus in the caloric position and the direction of nystagmus produced.

A search for the fistula sign with electronystagmography can be helpful, when positive, in identifying a perilymph fistula. The test can be performed 2 ways. The first utilizes a pneumatic otoscope with the patient in the 30° supine position. The ear canal is sealed with the speculum and a negative and later a positive pressure applied to the otoscope. During the pressure changes, the tracing is observed for nystagmus related to the pressure. The other method utilizes the impedance bridge. This allows for a more controlled stimulus, in that the seal can be assessed and the pressure limited and measured by the bridge, whereas the pneumatic otoscope may produce stimuli in excess of those necessary or desirable in performing the test.

When a patient presents with disabling vestibular symptoms and there is no response to warm (44°C), cool (30°C), or ice water, it is helpful to find out if there is any residual vestibular function. This is assessed by the massive caloric stimulation. This stimulus uses 2 temperatures of water, but to a more intense degree. The cool water is 300 dl of ice water and the warm is 300 dl of hot water, i.e., between 46° and 48°C. Each stimulus is applied immediately after the other while the recorder is recording for the entire stimulation. The subject is in the 30° supine position for stimulation and recording. If there is a pre-existing nystagmus, then the first temperature employed is the stimulus that will further drive the nystagmus in the pre-existing direction when that ear is stimulated. This is then rapidly followed by the other temperature of water to determine if a response is indicated by the nullification or reversal of the pre-existing nystagmus.

The Hallpike maneuver can be performed with electronystagmography as well. The main need is to measure both horizontal and vertical nystagmus simultaneously, since there may be a rotary nystagmus which can be partly measured by a dual array of electrodes. In addition, it is helpful to have extra-long cable lines to allow for the movement necessary to perform the test adequately.

There may be some patients with symptoms occurring in head or body positions not ordinarily used in the test procedure. In addition, the remainder of the test results may not reveal a vestibular abnormality. The specific positions should then be replicated in the electronystagmography laboratory. This will frequently expose an abnormality not previously seen.

PREPARATION OF THE TRACING

The ideal manner in which to communicate the results of the testing is a standard report form. The standard to be used should reflect the orientation of the testing laboratory. A preprinted form allows for the insertion of the data as the evaluation is routinely performed. Where there are nonroutine tests, blank spaces should be available to insert these results. It is best to attach the actual tracings to the form. The presence of the tracings allows an experienced observer to interpret many of the findings and get a feel for the functioning of the vestibular system. The inexperienced observer looking at these tracings repeatedly and studying them could then learn more about the vestibular evaluation. By pregumming the portions of the report form where the tracings are to be affixed, their insertion is facilitated and the messiness of gluing avoided.

In order to provide neat tracings for mounting in the report form a cutting board should be used. Some prefer not to "chop up" the entire tracing. For those, a method of stacking the rolls and filing them should be considered. In practice, the rolls are rarely looked at again and present a storage problem. Once confidence is gained in saving the important part of the tracing on the report form, the unmounted remainder of the tracing can be discarded. Others may record the results on magnetic tape as a form of storage. These are rarely looked at again. The advantage of the magnetic tape is that they enable the clinician to play back the tracings as they were produced and to compare them to current tracings in the same patient. One has to decide how important this is in the overall management of the patient. Also to be considered is the confidence of extracting the important data and inserting this in a mounted report form to which future repeat tests in the same patient can be compared.

INTERPRETATION

The interpretation of the vestibular evaluation has several levels. The first level revolves around the selection of the nystagmus and the calculation of the intensity of the nystagmus. This can be taught to the person performing the test routine. In fact, computer programs are able to assess these parameters in most studies. There are instances in which the raw nystagmus needs to be studied in order to gain an understanding of the vestibular system under study. The identification of nystagmus requires looking at many wave forms where clearcut nystagmus is present and where there is no nystagmus present. From this perspective, the questionable nystagmus can be studied. There are those who teach: "if there is any question, it is not likely nystagmus."

Once the presence of nystagmus is identified, the calculation of the intensity should be undertaken. This helps in understanding the vestibular system, and in cases in which the caloric responses are concerned, the calculations allow for the determination of the percentage response. There are several methods of determining the intensity; these usually involve some measure of the intensity of the response. The maximum intensity is frequently represented as the maximum slow phase velocity. This is calculated by measuring the slope of the fastest slow phases of the nystagmus under question. This can be represented by a single beat, but is more accurately characterized by an average of the fastest slow phases. The methodology chosen for its convenience in working with raw nystagmus looks at 10 seconds of the most intense nystagmus. The total amplitude as measured by the cumulative length of the fast phases is measured. This gives the distance the eyes have moved in 10 seconds. Then, if the calibration shows that 1° equals 1 mm deflection, the maximum velocity in degrees per second is one-tenth the total amplitude in millimeters. The advantage of averaging this out over a time period is that it gets around a single fast beat which does not characterize the intensity of the response. Computer programs are increasingly available to perform these calculations with less error than when manually performed. These programs must be thoroughly understood with respect to their mechanics, since artifact rejection, particularly unrelated saccades, may introduce a degree of inaccuracy. For this reason, there should be an indication of the nystagmus beats examined in reaching the calculated intensity.

Other parameters of nystagmus less frequently examined are the number of beats each second at the maximum intensity. The other parameters look at the entire response from the beginning of the stimulus to the end of the response. The problem is in estimating when the response has ended if there is a pre-existing nystagmus in the same direction as the induced response.

The physician's responsibility in interpreting the vestibular evaluation goes beyond the mechanics outlined above. In some instances, the tracings and their calculations take on a different importance when the patient history, neuro-otologic examination, and results of laboratory evaluations are collated.

Is the Evaluation Abnormal?

If there is nystagmus in any of the positions, a significantly abnormal alternate caloric response, or an abnormal simultaneous caloric response, then the evaluation is abnormal. It is with this information that one can assure the patient that there is an organic vestibular disorder. Many times, the patients have lost selfconfidence or have been led to believe that their symptoms are psychiatric, and they need to be reassured as to the genuine nature of their vestibular problem.

Is the Abnormality Central or Peripheral?

The absence of strong central signs generally will lead to diagnosis of a peripheral site for the disorder. It must be pointed out that the biphasic nature of the hair cells in the peripheral vestibular apparatus, and the marked influence of the efferent vestibular nerve fibers, together are the central regulatory influence on both the recording of nystagmus and the vestibular symptoms produced. Since eye movements are the mode of measuring vestibular response, the central processes are always at work to some degree. The failure of optic fixation to suppress caloric or other induced nystagmus is a strong central sign. Along similar lines, the appearance of nystagmus with eyes open and not evident with the eyes closed, is a similar sign of a central abnormality. The exact location cannot be discerned by the character of the sign. The presence of a direction-changing positional nystagmus suggests, although not strongly, a central etiology. This must be closely examined, since endolymphatic hydrops can mimic several central signs. With clearcut peripheral signs, a direction-changing positional nystagmus is a less important central sign. However, if the direction-changing positional nystagmus is the only finding, a search for a central etiology is indicated.

Consistent hyperactive caloric response to all 4 alternate bithermal stimuli suggests a lack of central inhibition and may lead one to search in that direction for an etiology.

Last, one needs to closely examine the character of the nystagmus. Alerting dysrhythmia, in which well formed nystagmus is interrupted by intervals of no nystagmus, defines a lack of alerting during the testing. However, central dysrhythmia is characterized by each successive beat showing no repeatable morphology in amplitude, wave form, or velocity. This finding needs to be further qualified. Children whose vestibular system has not fully matured will show this. Therefore, this finding is considered normal for children up to 9 years of age. Thereafter, this may be a sign of delayed maturity and have a bearing in the understanding of the symptoms. Not infrequently, where the induced nystagmus is weak, the waveform may undertake this form and should be overlooked or repeated until clarified. At times, patients will present themselves for testing under extremes of fatigue which can produce central dysrhythmia. Once fatigue has been ruled out, this dysrhythmia can be considered a central sign.

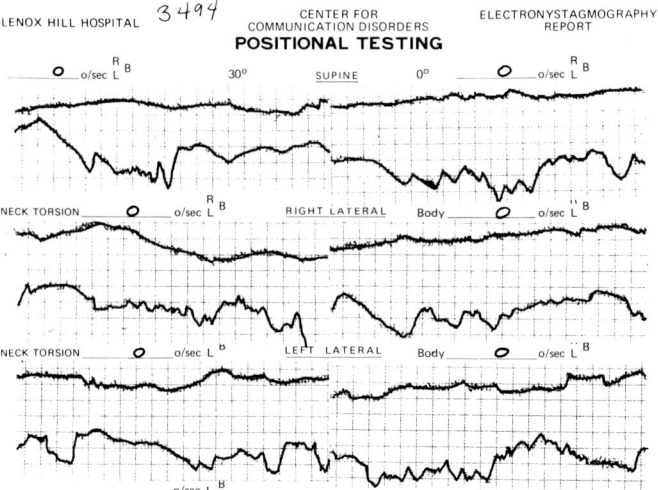

Fig. 21-21. Actual tracings from a patient without evidence of spontaneous, positional, or neck torsion nystagmus. Note that the upper tracing in each position records horizontal eye movement while the lower records simultaneous vertical eye movement.

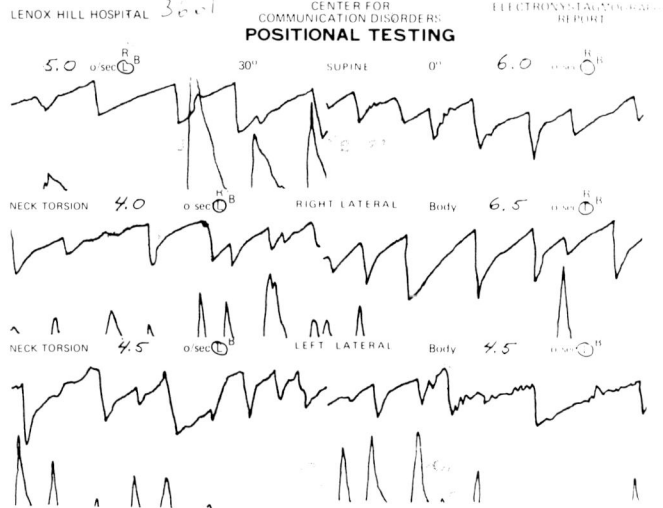

Fig. 21-22. The tracing of a patient demonstrating spontaneous nystagmus, i.e., nystagmus in the same direction without significant changes in velocity no matter what the head position. The occasional vertical channel tracing demonstrates simultaneous eye blinks.

The Clinical and Practical Aspects of Electronystagmography 261

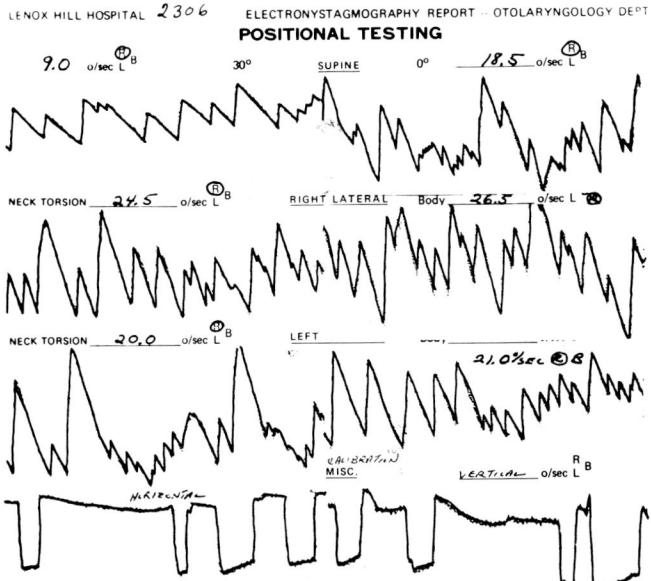

Fig. 21-23. The tracing of a patient with a direction-fixed positional nystagmus. Note each of the lateral and supine positions reveals significantly differing velocities. Also note the difference in the calculated caloric induced response which could be expected if the 0° supine nystagmus were the only supine nystagmus recorded.

Is This a Peripheral Lesion?

If there are no central signs, a peripheral lesion should be considered. If there is a direction-fixed nystagmus, this may lead you to a peripheral lesion, though not consistently often enough to be considered a strong sign. A reduced caloric response on one side with the alternate binaural bithermal is a strong peripheral sign. The presence of directional preponderance in response to the alternate binaural stimulus without central signs can be considered a peripheral sign. A Type 2 response on the stimultaneous binaural bithermal is more suggestive of a peripheral lesion, even though it measures more centrally active systems. It should be emphasized for the sake of discussion that acoustic neuromas are considered peripheral lesions.

A Type 3 or 4 response to the simultaneous binaural bithermal, with strong evidence for a directional preponderance, usually suggests a peripheral lesion. A Type 3 response alone without abnormalities in the alternate testing should make one suspicious of a central lesion.

If It is Peripheral, From Which Ear or Vestibular Nerve Is It Coming?

Again, the caloric testing indicating which side is a strong sign as to the ear. In addition, the presence of a fistula sign also indicates the ear and suggests an etiology. For a review of these procedures, see the following sample tracings (Figs. 21-21 through 21-32).

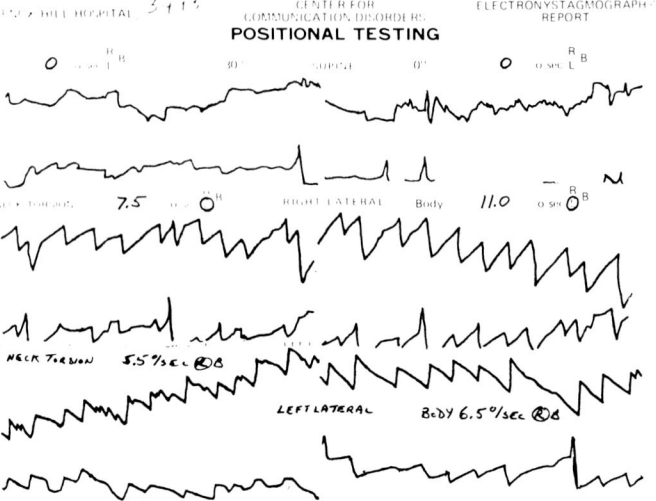

Fig. 21-24. The tracing of a patient with a direction-changing positional nystagmus. Note the neck torsion reducing nystagmus present from lying on that side. A left beating nystagmus with the right lateral position and the opposite with the left lateral position is also seen with the second phase of positional alcohol nystagmus.

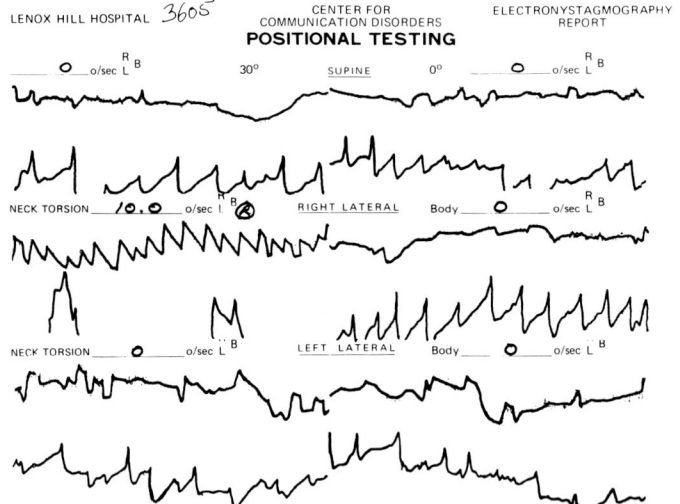

Fig. 21-25. Horizontal eye movement tracing reveals a right neck torsion nystagmus. This may indicate a neck-related lesion or, more likely, a modulation of the input of the potentials from each vestibular labyrinth. Note the eye blinks on some of the vertical tracings.

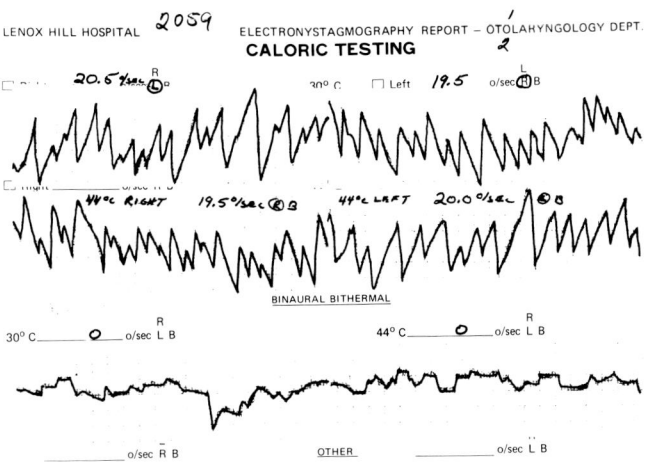

Fig. 21-26. The bithermal caloric testing in a patient with a normally functioning vestibular system. The top tracings reveal the cool responses to the right ear on the left of the page, and the responses to the left on the right side of the page. The middle line of tracings reveals the responses to the warm stimulus in each ear. The bottom line shows the responses to the simultaneous stimulation (SBB). On the bottom left is the cool response, revealing no nystagmus. The bottom right side reveals the absence of nystagmus to the simultaneous warm stimuli. The alternate binaural bithermal (ABB) are all between 5° and 25°/sec. The RVR is calculated at 1 percent and a DP at 2 percent. The absence of nystagmus to the SBB is a Type 1 which, coupled with the ABB, reveals a normally functioning vestibular system.

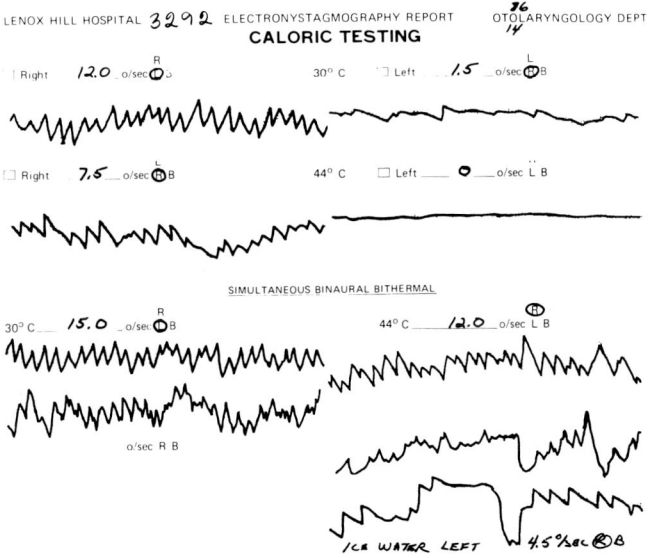

Fig. 21-27. The ABB of a patient with 86 percent RVR left. The SBB reveals a left beating cool and a right beating warm response revealing RVR left. Note the vertical tracing on the SBB with an upbeating cool and downbeating warm response. This suggests the head is not in the ideal position, with spillover of the stimuli to the vertically oriented semicircular canals. The ice water response reveals a consistently reduced response without evidence to suggest recruitment.

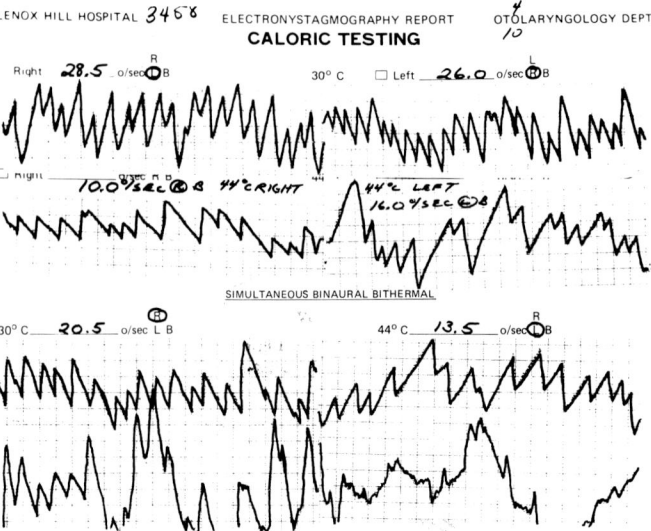

Fig. 21-28. The caloric testing in this patient reveals a normal response to the ABB with a 4 percent RVR and 10 percent DP. The SBB clearly shows an RVR right or a hyperactive left. Nevertheless, the SBB response is striking and clearly evidences vestibular pathology.

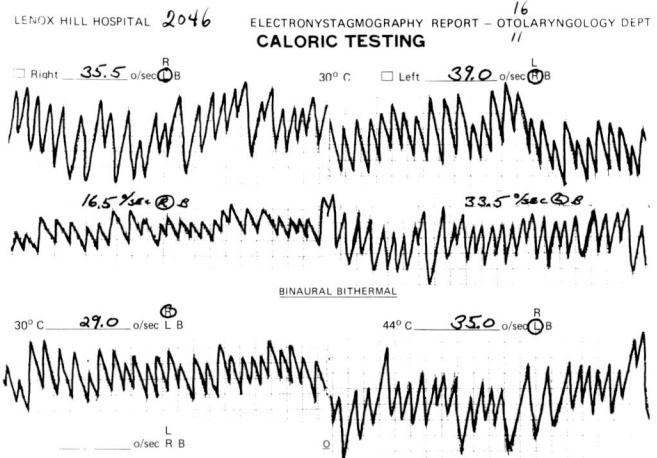

Fig. 21-29. Similar to Fig 28, but with more hyperactive responses. The SBB helps sort out the abnormality otherwise lost in the brisk response.

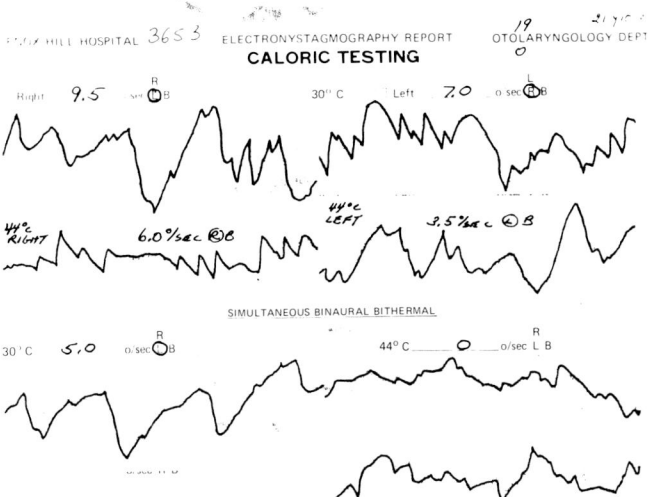

Fig. 21-30. Evidence of central dysrhythmia of all of the induced caloric responses. The SBB reveals a Type 4 response, which is a miscellaneous group in which both central and peripheral abnormalities can be found.

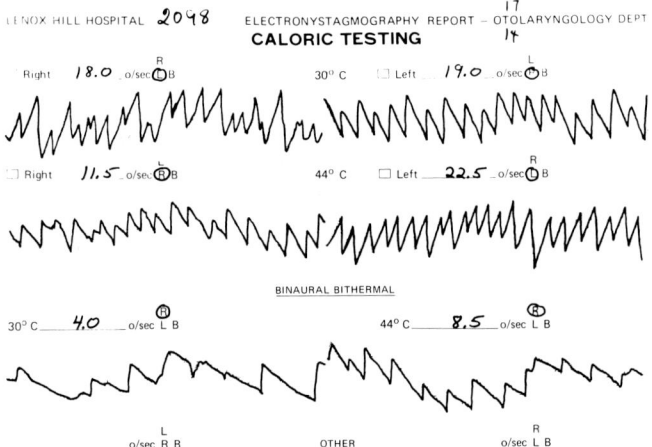

Fig. 21-31. The ABB shows normal responses with an RVR of 17 percent and DP of 14 percent. The SBB shows a Type 3 response. With the ABB findings, this could represent a central lesion.

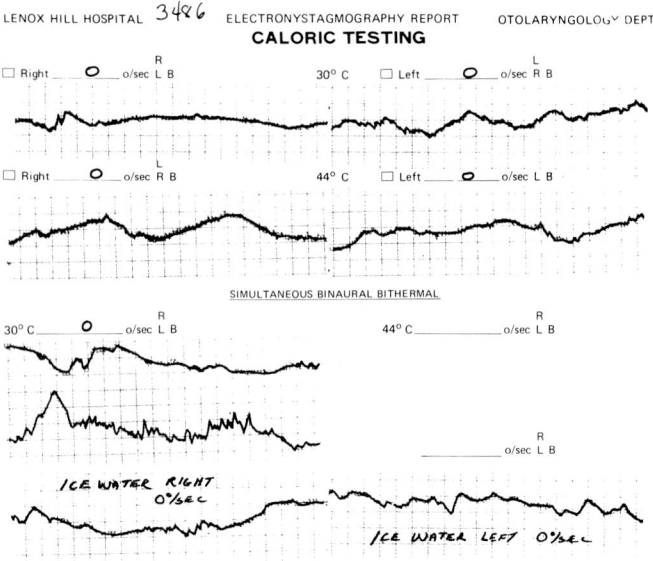

Fig. 21-32. The caloric responses are absent to ABB, SBB, and ice water in each ear. This tracing is consistent with an ototoxic etiology or brainstem suppression as might be seen with brainstem vascular compromise or an intense peripheral abnormality with maximum central inhibition.

REFERENCES

1. Fitzgerald G, Hallpike CS: Studies on the human vestibular function. I. Observations on the directional preponderance ("nystagmusbereitschaft") of caloric nystagmus resulting from central lesions. Brain 65:115-137, 1942
2. Brookler KH, Baker AH, Grams G: Closed loop water irrigation system. Otolaryngol Head Neck Surg 87:364-365, 1979
3. Brookler KH, Pulec JL: Computer analysis of electronystagmograph records. Trans Am Acad Ophthal Otolaryngol 74:563-575, 1970
4. Brookler KH: The simultaneous binaural bithermal: A caloric test utilizing electronystagmography. Laryngoscope 86:1241-1250, 1976

Mary S. MacDonald

22
The Principles and Practicality of Hearing Aid Dispensing

The goal of a hearing aid dispensing program within an otolaryngology practice is to provide not only convenience to the hearing impaired patient, but improved quality of hearing aid services as well. The purpose of this chapter is to provide to the physician a general overview of the process involved for the patient who is obtaining a hearing aid within the dispensing physician's office, as well as an overview of the equipment and personnel necessary for implementing a hearing aid dispensing program.

BACKGROUND

In 1977, following many years of activities by Congress, the hearing aid industry, and consumer groups, the Food and Drug Administration (FDA) issued regulations for professional and patient labeling and conditions for the sale of hearing aids. One provision of the FDA regulations mandated that patients undergo a medical evaluation of their hearing loss "by a physician, preferably a physician specializing in diseases of the ear" within 6 months prior to purchasing a hearing aid.[1] As a result of this provision, the hearing aid could no longer be considered an over-the-counter device. Although fully informed prospective adult hearing aid users do have the option of waiving the medical evaluation on the grounds of religious or personal beliefs, by signing a medical waiver statement, the vast majority of patients do choose to obtain the required medical clearance from an otolaryngologist. In an effort to provide comprehensive hearing health care services to their hearing impaired patients, many otolaryngologists have therefore become involved in hearing aid dispensing by adding dispensing audiologists to their clinical staff. Physicians who employ hearing aid dispensers are often referred to as, not surprisingly, "dispensing physicians."[2]

The decision as to whether to set up a hearing aid dispensing program within an otolaryngology office has become an important element in the provision of hearing health care services. Hearing aid dispensing may not be feasible for some otolaryngologists; careful consideration should be given in making this decision. The following information is intended to outline some important factors to be considered prior to implementing a hearing aid dispensing program.

EQUIPMENT

A fairly large number of otolaryngologists currently employ audiologists to perform audiological evaluations. Many physicians' offices are therefore equipped with speech audiometers and acoustically treated test booths. Assuming that this is the case, the physician interested in creating a hearing aid dispensing program within the office may need only to purchase a set of speakers and an amplifier (if necessary) that are compatible with the pre-existing audiometer. A well-calibrated audiometer and a good set of speakers are essential to obtaining accurate sound field information during the hearing aid selection process.

An instrument which is considered by many dispensing audiologists to be an invaluable piece of equipment is the electroacoustic analyzer. This instrument provides the dispenser with various measurements relative to the power output of the hearing aid being analyzed, the frequency response of the hearing aid, and the amount of distortion present within the hearing aid, in addition to various other electroacoustic measures. The electroacoustic analyzer is typically utilized to measure the electroacoustic characteristics of a new hearing aid, for quality control purposes, prior to dispensing the recommended hearing aid to the patient. The electroacoustic analyzer is also extremely useful for determining whether the origin of a hearing aid malfunction, as reported by the wearer, is actually within the hearing aid device itself, the earmold, or within the patient's ear. Hearing aid manufacturers are required by FDA regulation to provide various electroacoustic measurements and specifications with their hearing aids, which allows for easy comparison of data to determine whether or not the hearing aid in question is functioning within the manufacturer's specifications.

There are several assorted hand tools and related accessories which are necessary for the purpose of making minor repairs of and modifications to hearing aids and earmolds. While major hearing aid repairs are customarily handled by the manufacturer, minor in-house repairs are commonplace. For a detailed list of suggested tools and accessories, the reader is referred to Sorkowitz.[3]

PERSONNEL

There has been an ongoing professional debate in recent years, primarily among dispensing audiologists and hearing aid dealers, as to which group should be the primary provider of amplification and counseling to the hearing impaired patient. Characteristically, the training of nonaudiologist professionals is oriented to specialized aspects of the problem of hearing deficits rather than to total management of the hearing impaired individual. The otologist is generally fully occupied with the medical aspects of deafness and the hearing aid dealer's preparation rarely extends beyond fitting the hearing aid.[4] The audiologist, on the other hand, has received training in a broad range of areas, aimed at managing the total hearing impaired patient. Realizing that a hearing aid is only one part of an overall program of aural habilitation/rehabilitation, the Academy of Dispensing Audiologists says that "the audiologist is the best qualified professional practitioner to assume the responsibility for the non-medical habilitation/rehabilitation of the hearing impaired person."[5]

Prior to 1978, the American Speech-Language-Hearing Association (ASHA)—the national professional organization of audiologists and speech pathologists—in effect prohibited its audiologist members from engaging in the commercial dispensing and sale of hearing aids. In 1978, however, following a United States Supreme Court ruling, ASHA removed from its code of ethics any restrictions on its member audiologists regarding direct involvement in the dispensing and sale of hearing aids.[6] Within the last 10 years, then, the role of the audiologist in the hearing aid delivery system has changed dramatically. Traditionally, the audiologist evaluated a patient's hearing, selected a hearing aid that would provide optimum benefit to the patient, and then referred the patient to a hearing aid dealer who would in turn sell the hearing aid that was recommended by the audiologist to the patient. It was the patient's responsibility to schedule an appointment to return to the audiologist, who then assessed the patient's hearing with the newly purchased hearing aid. Audiologists are now directly involved not only with the initial audiometric testing and hearing aid evaluation, but also with the actual delivery of the hearing aid, including the earmold fitting, patient counseling, the hearing aid orientation, aural habilitation/rehabilitation, and any necessary additional follow-up services. While ASHA has lifted any restrictions on audiologists dispensing hearing aids on the national level, the vast majority of states do have their own dealer licensing laws. The licensing of hearing aid dealers—or, in some cases, their registration by state agencies—is, in fact, a relatively new phenomenon, having evolved during the last 25 years.[7]

It is helpful, though not essential, to allocate to a member of the office staff the responsibility of performing the many clerical duties associated with a hearing aid dispensing program. The clerical duties of such an employee typically include the scheduling of patient appointments; handling incoming and outgoing mail, which generally involves maintaining a complete record of hearing aids ordered and received from the various manufacturers; patient billing; typing patient reports and letters; and, in addition, handling the tremendous amount of paperwork involved in the third-party payment for hearing health care services. The competent clerical worker is unquestionably an invaluable member of the hearing aid dispensing program.

OBTAINING A HEARING AID

Otological Examination

Within the framework of a dispensing physician's office, the first step for the patient interested in obtaining a hearing aid is the otological examination. According to the FDA, the purpose of the medical evaluation is to assure that all medically treatable conditions that may affect hearing are identified and treated before the hearing aid is purchased. It is typically during the otological evaluation that routine audiometric testing takes place. The audiometric testing should include bilateral air conduction and bone conduction testing, speech reception threshold testing, and speech discrimination testing at an optimal intensity level. A tympanogram and special audiometric testing may also be indicated. Following the completed otological evaluation, the physician must sign a written statement, stating that the patient's hearing loss has been medically evaluated and that the patient is a candidate for amplification. At this point, the patient is referred to the staff dispensing audiologist. The actual hearing aid fitting and dispensing—as well as the related habilitation/rehabilitation—is typically carried out by the audiologist and does not involve the physician directly.

Hearing Aid Evaluation

The hearing aid evaluation generally begins with the audiologist taking a thorough case history of the patient's hearing loss, including information relative to the time of onset of the hearing loss; possible causes of, or contributing factors to, the hearing loss, including familial history of hearing loss, instances of exposure to excessive levels of noise, use of ototoxic medications, and so on; and a description of specific situations in which the patient experiences communication difficulties due to the presence of the hearing loss. Prospective hearing aid users are typically naive with respect to the nature and implications of hearing loss, the options which are available in terms of amplification, and expectations of the benefit to be derived from amplification. It is therefore essential that the audiologist spend an adequate amount of time discussing with the patient the nature and degree of the hearing loss, the communicative difficulties which typically result from the described hearing loss, and also the prognosis in terms of expected benefit from the use of hearing aids. Through such discussion, the audiologist is usually able to make a fairly accurate assessment of the patient's attitudes regarding the hearing loss, as well as of the motivation to wear a hearing aid.

The determination of which ear should be fitted with the hearing aid, or whether binaural amplification is indicated, is typically made by the audiologist. This determination is arrived at following a careful examination of the patient's audiometric test results, as well as a consideration of the patient's lifestyle and daily communicative demands. In the case of bilateral hearing loss, the use of binaural amplification is strongly recommended whenever possible.

There are essentially 4 styles of hearing aids on the market today. In order of decreasing physical size, they are as follows: the body-worn hearing aid, the postauricular hearing aid, the all-in-the ear hearing aid, and the canal hearing aid. The body-worn hearing aid is generally reserved for those patients who possess a profound bilateral hearing loss, or who are unable to manipulate the controls on the smaller, ear-level hearing aids. The postauricular, or behind-the-ear, hearing aids in general are capable of accommodating a wide range of hearing impairments, from mild hearing losses to severe and profound hearing losses. Postauricular hearing aids, which are coupled to various types of earmolds, are generally considered to be very flexible in terms of achieving the desired sound quality. In-the-ear and canal hearing aids, on the other hand, accommodate a somewhat narrower range of hearing impairments and allow for less flexibility, although improvements in this area are occurring at a rapid pace. Cosmetically, the in-the-ear and canal styles of hearing aids are generally most appealing, as they are considered to be the least conspicuous. Poor visual acuity and reduced movement of the fingers, which often accompanies aging, often precludes the successful use of these smaller instruments. The determination of which style hearing aid will best suit the patient's needs, then, must depend upon the patient's degree of hearing loss, the patient's overall physical condition, including visual acuity and manual dexterity, and on the patient's cosmetic concerns. Since the average first-time hearing aid user is for the most part unfamiliar with the various hearing aid styles that are currently available, it is good practice to provide to the patient, prior to the hearing aid evaluation, a brochure detailing the various hearing aid types and a brief summary of the hearing aid selection and orientation process. It is also helpful to include in the patient's hearing aid brochure the current fees for the hearing aid evaluation and any follow-up visits, together with a range of prices for the actual hearing aid devices, and information pertaining to the hearing aid trial period policy.

While there are numerous techniques and theories in use for the purpose of hearing aid selection, the majority of audiologists currently use a comparative approach, whereby 3 or more hearing aids are evaluated in the calibrated sound field while constant stimuli conditions and patient head positions are maintained. Typically, the hearing aid with which the patient receives the most natural sound quality and the greatest amount of benefit in the sound field testing situation is the hearing aid which is recommended to the patient by the audiologist.[8] The dispenser then typically orders from the appropriate manufacturer that specific hearing aid model which will in turn be purchased by the patient. It is also necessary at this time to take an impression of the ear(s) on which the patient's hearing aid(s) will be worn. The hardened ear impression will serve as the form from which either the earmold or the actual hearing aid will be made, depending upon the chosen hearing aid style.

The hearing aid selection is often a rather lengthy process, and requires the audiologist to have at his or her disposal an adequate supply of stock hearing aids, preferably from several hearing aid manufacturers. Such stock hearing aids are generally loaned to the dispenser by the individual hearing aid manufacturers on a consignment basis for the sole purpose of conducting hearing aid evaluations. A small number of hearing aid manufacturers do, however, require the dispenser to actually purchase their aids for their stock, and do not participate in a consignment program.

Hearing Aid Orientation

The hearing aid orientation usually takes place approximately 2–4 weeks following the hearing aid evaluation, although there is no hard and fast rule for this. The hearing aid orientation consists of exactly what the name implies: the patient is in essence introduced to the hearing aid(s) for the first time, an experience about which many first-time hearing aid users appear apprehensive. It is at this time that the patient will listen with the personal, individualized hearing aid for the first time, which may necessitate some minor adjustments of the internal frequency response, gain, and output-limiting controls of the hearing aid, as applicable, by the audiologist. Additional sound field testing with the hearing aid may also be indicated in order to confirm the benefit received from the recommended hearing aid.

It is also at this time that the audiologist instructs the new hearing aid user in the proper use of the hearing aid, including manipulation of the external user-operated controls on the hearing aid, as well as battery insertion, care and maintenance of the earmold and/or hearing aid, and various trouble-shooting techniques. FDA regulations also require that the dispenser provide for and review with the hearing aid user a copy of the manufacturer's user instructional brochure. The hearing aid orientation is an opportune time to review with the patient the importance of realistic expectations of the capabilities of the hearing aid, as well as potentially problematic listening situations for the hearing aid user. It is important that the audiologist attempt to instill confidence in the patient and encourage the patient to wear the hearing aid without creating false hopes and unrealistic expectations.

The majority of hearing aid dispensing offices now offer a trial period, whereby the hearing aid user is permitted to wear the newly purchased hearing aid on a trial basis without obligation to keep the hearing aid. The trial period is typically 30 days in length, within which time the patient is permitted to cancel for any reason the purchase of the hearing aid and receive a refund of the majority of the money paid for the hearing aid. Typically 10–15 percent of the amount paid for the hearing aid is retained as a rental fee for the short-term use of the returned aid. Most hearing aid dispensers require that the patient pay in full for the new hearing aid at the time the patient receives the hearing aid, i.e., immediately following the hearing aid orientation visit. It is essential that, upon receiving the hearing aid, the patient read and sign a "contract" which identifies the make and model of the hearing aid, the serial number of the hearing aid, the length of time that the hearing aid is covered by the manufacturer's warranty, the total price of the hearing aid, and the dispenser's name and business address, and includes a complete description of the dispenser's policy relative to a nonobligatory trial period for the new hearing aid. The original signed and dated purchase agreement should be given to the patient for personal records, and a copy of the signed agreement should be retained by the dispenser and secured in the patient's chart (Fig. 22-1).

Follow-up Visits

It is customary to schedule an appointment for the novice hearing aid user to return to the dispenser's office for a check-up visit within the trial period in order to determine whether any adjustments need to be made on the hearing aid and to discuss any

PURCHASE AGREEMENT

DATE_____ 19____

Seller: ________________ Purchaser: ________________

Address: ________________

Purchaser hereby purchases the articles as listed below from seller. The terms and conditions of the sale are as follows:

Hearing Aid(s)		Hearing Aid(s)	$______
Make and Model No.(s)	______	Earmold(s)	$______
Serial No.(s)	______	TOTAL	$______
Instrument Warranty	______		

The hearing aid(s) described above are New____ Used____ Reconditioned____

THE BUYER HAS THE RIGHT TO CANCEL THIS PURCHASE FOR ANY REASON AT ANY TIME PRIOR TO MIDNIGHT OF THE THIRTIETH CALENDAR DAY AFTER RECEIPT OF THE HEARING AID(S). In the event of cancellation of such sale the purchaser will be refunded the total cost of the Hearing aid(s) less 12%. Within this 30 day period the purchaser has the right to a free adjustment of the hearing aid(s) or to cancel this purchase by returning the aids described herein. Such hearing aid(s) must be returned in the same condition as when purchased, ordinary wear and tear excluded.

The purchaser agrees to pay for the hearing aid(s) in full on the day of delivery of such instruments. Receipt of one copy of this agreement is hereby acknowledged by the purchaser.

Seller Lic. No. Purchaser

Fig. 22-1. Example of a purchase agreement.

concerns or difficulties which the patient may be experiencing with the new hearing aid. It would be appropriate at this time for the patient to notify the audiologist of any intention to return or exchange the hearing aid. It is not entirely uncommon for a hearing aid user who is satisfied with the newly purchased hearing aids to cancel the check-up visit with the audiologist, despite the efforts of the audiologist to advise the patient of the importance of the check-up visit. Since the hearing aid orientation may be the last time the audiologist sees the new hearing aid user, it is essential that the orientation be as informative and thorough as possible. The patient should also be encouraged to contact the office in the event that a problem with the hearing aid should arise. In order to encourage patients to return to the office periodically for hearing aid check-up appointments, many offices routinely send annual check-up reminder postcards to their hearing aid users. This appears to be an effective method of recalling patients.

HEARING AID COSTS

The total cost to the patient for obtaining a hearing aid typically consists of 4 basic fees: the fee for the initial otological evaluation, the fee for the mandatory audiometric testing, the fee for the hearing aid evaluation, and the cost of the actual hearing aid device and earmold, if applicable. The amount charged to the patient for the hearing aid itself is generally a composite of the manufacturer's current list price for the recommended hearing aid model and a fixed amount for fitting the hearing aid, which is predetermined by the physician and/or dispensing audiologist.

Who pays for the hearing aid? In most cases, the patient personally pays for the hearing aid and the hearing aid evaluation. Third-party payment for hearing aids and related services is not totally nonexistent, however. In a recent study by Chwat and Gurland, it was found that slightly more than 10 percent of the private health insurance companies in this country routinely provide hearing aid coverage in their basic insurance plans, although approximately one-third of the insurance companies surveyed provided hearing aid coverage in their more costly insurance plans.[9] Although federally-funded assistance programs do not typically cover hearing aid services, many state-funded assistance programs do cover the costs of the hearing aid, the hearing aid evaluation, and related services for qualifying adults. State-assisted hearing aid services for hearing impaired children are more prevalent; it has been reported that every state in this country provides some sort of assistance for hearing aid services to eligible children.[10]

REPAIR OF HEARING AIDS

Each hearing aid manufacturer provides a warranty on its new hearing aids, which covers the cost of all repairs on the hearing aid, generally for a period of 1 or 2 years. Minor hearing aid repairs and modifications, such as simple tubing replacements and tone hook replacements, are typically carried out in the office by the audiologist. More intricate repairs, which commonly involve the internal circuitry of the hearing aid, typically require that the aid be sent to the manufacturer for service. The length of time which elapses before the repaired hearing aid is returned to the dispenser's office varies from one manufacturer to the next, although 1–2 weeks seems to be the average length of time involved in an out-of-house repair. Since many hearing aid users become somewhat dependent upon their hearing aids in order to function effectively in everyday life, it is helpful, and usually sincerely appreciated by the patient, if the audiologist has a hearing aid which may be loaned to the patient for the period of time that the aid is being serviced. This, of course, requires that the audiologist have access to a stock of loaner hearing aids, preferably of various power outputs and frequency responses. For record-keeping purposes, as well as legal purposes, it is customary for the patient to be required to "sign out" a loaner hearing aid, with the understanding that the patient is responsible for the loaner aid while it is in that patient's possession (Fig. 22-2).

Following the expiration of the manufacturer's warranty, the patient will be charged for any repairs on the hearing aid. The price of the repair quoted to the patient is generally the manufacturer's invoice cost plus a fixed amount, which is usually predetermined by the physician or the audiologist, for handling the repair of the hearing aid. Upon servicing an out-of-warranty hearing aid, the manufacturer generally provides a 6-month or 12-month guarantee on the repair.

CONCLUSION

From a practical standpoint, a hearing aid dispensing program within an otolaryngologist's office is beneficial for a number of reasons. It is a convenient arrangement for the physician in that it allows for easy follow-up of hearing impaired patients who were referred to the in-house dispenser for hearing aid services. In addition, the physician is able to refer immediately to the audiologist those patients who are current hearing aid users and are experiencing difficulties with their present hearing aids. Likewise, from the dispensing audiologist's perspective, a dispensing program within the physician's office is advantageous because it allows for the prompt medical evaluation of those hearing aid users who exhibit conditions which interfere with successful hearing aid use and which require medical attention (impacted cerumen, drainage from the ear, or skin irritation of the ear, to name just a few conditions which require medical attention). Last, but certainly not least, the dispensing physician's office is beneficial to the hearing impaired patient. In terms of convenience, by having the physician and the hearing aid dispenser under one roof, the hearing impaired patient is able to consult with the physician and

LOANER AID POLICY

I agree to be held responsible for the cost ($) of this loaner hearing aid should it be lost, stolen or damaged beyond repair. I will also assume payment of repair charges if the loaner hearing aid is damaged while in my possession. I understand that I may use this loaner hearing aid at no charge for a period of ________, after which time I will be required to pay $1.00 per day rental fee for as long as the hearing aid is in my possession.

MODEL# ________ PATIENT ________

SERIAL# ________ WITNESS ________

DATE ________

Fig. 22-2. Example of an agreement to be signed by patients when signing out loaner hearing aids.

the dispenser while at one location and often, by scheduling consecutive appointments, the same day. Overall, then, it could be said that an in-house hearing aid dispensing program offers a comprehensive hearing health care program which readily lends itself to the team approach to total management of its hearing impaired patients. The end result should therefore be the provision of quality hearing health care services to the patient.

A hearing aid dispensing program may not be appropriate for every otolaryngology practice. The decision to dispense should obviously be based realistically on several considerations, including the availability of office space and the availability and effectiveness of existing alternate hearing aid dispensing systems in the area. Should physicians involved in an otolaryngology practice decide that hearing aid dispensing is not for them, it is important that they investigate and become familiar with the best referral system available, as well as with the current trends in amplification.[11]

REFERENCES

1. Bebout M: Life after regulation. Hear J 37:7-13, 1984
2. Mahon W: The M.D. in hearing aid dispensing. Hear J 38:13-17, 1985
3. Sorkowitz M: Business aspects of hearing aid dispensing. In Pollack M (Ed.): Amplification for the Hearing-impaired (ed. 2). New York: Grune & Stratton, pp. 393-421, 1980
4. Sanders D: Hearing aid orientation and counseling. In Pollack M (Ed.): Amplification for the Hearing-impaired (ed. 2). New York: Grune & Stratton, pp. 343-391, 1980
5. Mahon W: New ADA paper defines audiologist's role. Hear J 37:12-13, 1984
6. Radcliffe D, Mahon W: Who is today's dispenser? Hear J 36:7-13, 1983
7. Mahon W: 1984 guide to state hearing aid & audiology licensing. Hear J 37:29-36, 1984
8. Ross M: Hearing aid evaluation. In Katz J (Ed.): Handbook of Clinical Audiology (Ed. 2). Baltimore: Williams and Wilkins, pp. 524-541, 1978
9. Chwat S, Gurland G: National trends in third party reimbursement in speech-language pathology and audiology: Our professional crisis. ASHA 7:27-31, 1984
10. Mahon W: Third-party payments: Who pays the bill for hearing services? Hear J 37:7-10, 1984
11. Bailey H, Pappas J, Graham S: Profile: The ear & nose-throat clinic. Hear J 38:24-25, 1985

Thomas V. McCaffrey
Eugene B. Kern

23

Rhinomanometry

Rhinomanometry is the technique for determining nasal airway resistance by measuring pressure and airflow through the nose simultaneously.[1] Nasal resistance can then be calculated using the following formula.

Equation 1.
$R_N = P/\dot{V}$ where R_N = nasal resistance
P = transnasal pressure
$\dot{V}$ = nasal airflow

Clinical methods for performing rhinomanometry can be characterized according to the method used to measure transnasal pressure and the method used to measure transnasal airflow. If the measurement of nasal pressure is performed at the nares, the technique is known as anterior rhinomanometry. If the measurement of transnasal pressure is made at the mouth, the method is known as posterior rhinomanometry. In both cases, nasal pressure and flow are measured during quiet nasal breathing.

ANTERIOR RHINOMANOMETRY

Figure 23-1 shows the technique of anterior rhinomanometry. In this case, one nostril is occluded. Since no airflow occurs through an occluded nostril, the pressure at the occluded nostril will equal nasopharyngeal pressure (transnasal pressure). This is the driving pressure for nasal airflow through the nonobstructed nostril. Airflow through the nonobstructed nostril is measured using a pneumotachograph. A mask is applied to the face so that all airflow through the nose is directed through the pneumotachograph. Simultaneous measurement of nasal pressure and flow will then permit calculation of nasal resistance. Only unilateral nasal resistance can be measured with this method. If a measurement of total nasal resistance is required, it can be calculated by the parallel resistance formula:

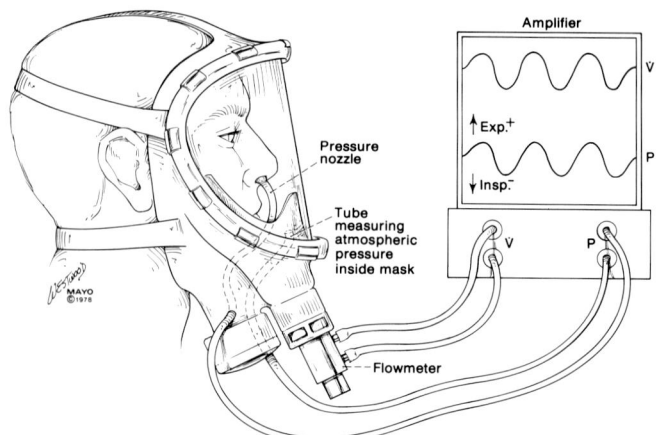

Fig. 23-1. Anterior rhinomanometry. Transnasal pressure is measured by an occluding pressure transducer in the nostril of the opposite nasal airway. This is a measure of the transnasal driving pressure. Flow through the measured nostril is determined with a pneumotachograph flowmeter.

$$R_{Tot} = \frac{R_L \times R_R}{R_L + R_R}$$

Equation 2.

where R_{Tot} = total nasal resistance
R_L = left-sided nasal resistance (Equation 1)
R_R = right-sided nasal resistance (Equation 1)

The method of anterior rhinomanometry also cannot be used in cases of total unilateral nasal obstruction or in cases of septal perforation, since nasal pressure does not reflect nasopharyngeal pressure accurately in these cases.

POSTERIOR RHINOMANOMETRY

To perform posterior rhinomanometry, nasopharyngeal pressure or nasal driving pressure is measured by placing a catheter in the mouth rather than in one of the nostrils (Fig. 23-2). In this way, it is possible to measure the nasal resistance through both nasal passages in parallel or to measure nasal resistance in cases of nasal septal perforation in which the nasal chambers communicate. Nasal airflow is measured as in anterior rhinomanometry by a face mask and pneumotachograph. If unilateral nasal resistance is to be measured with posterior rhinomanometry, one of the nostrils is obstructed. Although posterior rhinomanometry can be applied to situations not suitable for anterior rhinomanometry, such as septal perforations and total unilateral nasal obstruction, it is not often used clinically because of the difficulty in obtaining reliable nasopharyngeal pressures through the mouth. Palatal muscles need to be relaxed, and this may be difficult for some individuals during nasal breathing. Whether using anterior or posterior rhinomanometry, the pressure and flow recordings are displayed simultaneously on an XY recorder or oscilloscope. The resulting S-shaped curve depicts the resistance properties of

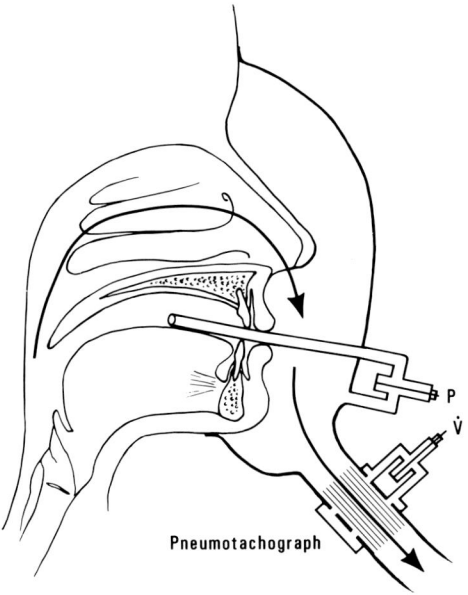

Fig. 23-2. Posterior rhinomanometry. Transnasal pressure is measured by a pressure catheter placed in the mouth. If the palate is relaxed, the pressure represents the transnasal driving pressure. Nasal airflow is measured with a pneumotachograph flowmeter.

the nose. These data can be used graphically, in which case increasing resistances are noted by clockwise rotation of the S-shaped curve; or nasal resistance ($\Delta P/\dot{V}$) can be calculated at a point on the curve. Since the relation of pressure to flow through the nose is curvilinear, the resistance calculated by Equation 1 will differ depending on the point on the curve that is used. Three methods are possible for selecting a point for the determination of resistance. These are shown in Figure 23-3.

CLINICAL EVALUATION OF NASAL OBSTRUCTION

Rhinomanometry provides only one aspect of the clinical evaluation of a patient with nasal obstruction. The measurement of nasal resistance must be interpreted along with the clinical history and physical examination. A study of a large number of patients with nasal obstruction has shown that, in general, the nasal resistance determined by

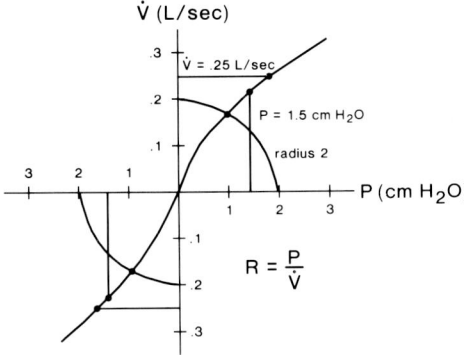

Fig. 23-3. Three possible ways to select a point on the pressure-flow curve for determining nasal resistance (R): A particular flow ($\dot{V}$), pressure (P), or radius can be used to define the point on the pressure-flow curve used to determine resistance. When a radius is used, the ratio of the pressure and flow axes must be 10:1.

rhinomanometry correlates with the subjective degree of nasal obstruction.[2] In addition, rhinomanometry provides objective information on the type and degree of nasal obstruction that could not be assessed by rhinoscopic examination alone.

In general, the two causes of nasal obstruction are mucosal hypertrophy or congestion and structural deformity of the nasal airway. By assessing nasal resistance before and after maximum nasal decongestion with topical phenylephrine, it is possible to determine the relative importance of mucosal versus structural nasal obstruction. For this reason, rhinomanometry in a clinical setting is usually performed in the following sequence:

1. Right-sided nasal resistance (no decongestion)
2. Left-sided nasal resistance (no decongestion)
3. One percent phenylephrine nasal spray—wait 10 minutes
4. Right-sided nasal resistance (after decongestion)
5. Left-sided nasal resistance (after decongestion)
6. Calculation of total nasal resistance from the measured unilateral resistances (Equation 2).

The nasal resistances measured are then compared to normal values (Fig. 23-4). A reversible or mucosal obstruction congestion could be expected to be reversed by decongestion, while obstruction from a structural abnormality would not come into the normal range after decongestion. The authors think that a nasal resistance greater than that of the 95th percentile of the normal population is definitely abnormal (Table 23-1). The threshold of subjective obstruction will, however, vary among individuals; some individuals with an apparently normal nasal resistance may experience obstructive symptoms at times.

INTERPRETATION OF NASAL RESISTANCE MEASUREMENTS

Nasal obstruction that is reversed by topical decongestion usually suggests a mucosal cause for the obstruction, such as nasal hyperreactivity as a result of allergy, vasomotor

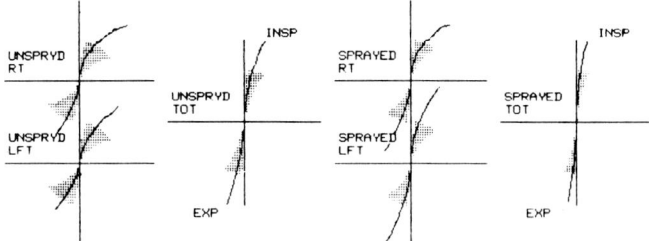

Fig. 23-4. Normal nasal resistance study. Nasal pressure flow curves calculated before and after decongestion with phenylephrine. The shaded areas represent the area bounded by the 5th and 95th percentile limits of normal nasal resistance. The total nasal resistance curve is derived mathematically from the unilateral nasal resistance measurements. Notice that after spray the variability is less, as shown by a smaller range of normal.

Table 23-1
Normal Nasal Resistance During Inspiration[a]

	Before Decongestion		After Decongestion 1% Phenylephrine	
	mean	range 5–95%	mean	range 5–95%
Radius 1	2.5	0.8–7.7	1.6	0.7–3.5
Radius 2	3.3	1.1–9.9	2.2	0.9–5.3

[a]At designated radii on pressure-flow curve before and after decongestion—based on 80 normal subjects from the authors' laboratory.

rhinitis, or exaggerated nasal cycle. In general, with mucosal hyperreactivity, the nose will have a greatly elevated resistance prior to decongestion and a normal resistance following decongestion with a topical vasoconstrictor (Fig. 23-5). A slightly elevated nasal resistance on one side, which returns to normal after decongestion and which does not produce an elevated total nasal resistance, can be considered to be an exaggerated nasal cycle (Fig. 23-6). The nose normally undergoes variations of nasal resistance with a pattern of alternating congestion and decongestion of the mucosa. In many individuals, the right nasal chamber is congested while the left is decongested, with an alternating period of 2–4 hours. This sequence of alternating congestion is termed the nasal cycle.[3] It is usually not of clinical significance, since total nasal resistance remains nearly constant. However, if a concomitant structural abnormality of the nasal airway exists, the cycle may produce a symptomatic obstruction during periods of congestion.

If nasal resistance remains elevated after topical decongestion, there is a structural abnormality of the nasal airway (Fig. 23-7). This could be a septal deformity, scarring, synechia, or irreversible mucosal abnormalities such as nasal polyps or hypertrophic turbinates. The precise etiology of the structural abnormality is usually apparent on rhinoscopic examination.

Rhinomanometry is particularly useful in the diagnosis of nasal obstruction that occurs as a result of dynamic changes in a nasal airway, since rhinoscopic examination may not detect these abnormalities. Nasal alar collapse (or nasal valve collapse) is a dynamic phenomenon in which the resiliant cartilaginous structures of the nasal ala

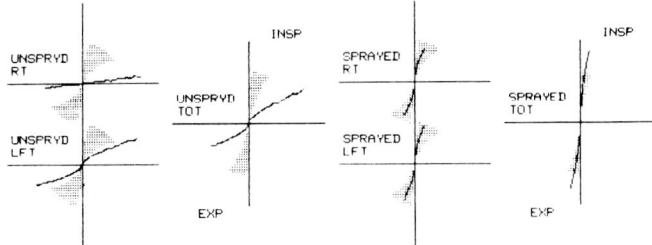

Fig. 23-5. Nasal mucosal obstruction. Prior to decongestion, there is a markedly elevated nasal resistance bilaterally (all curves outside the normal range). After decongestion, the nasal resistance is within normal limits. This demonstrates the reversibility of nasal mucosal obstruction.

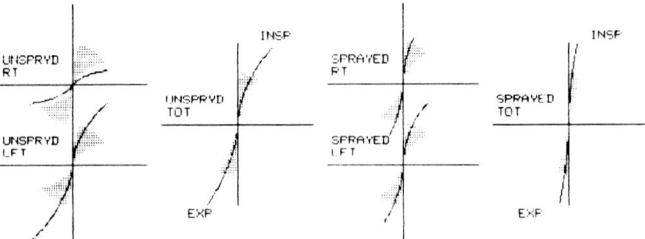

Fig. 23-6. Exaggerated nasal cycle. The nasal cycle is characterized by an alternating obstruction of the nasal airway. In the nondecongested nose, the right side is obstructed. However, total nasal resistance is normal. After decongestion, both nasal airways have a normal resistance.

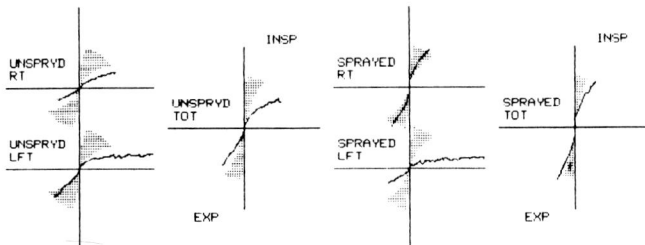

Fig. 23-7. Structural nasal obstruction. The obstruction of the left nasal airway is not reversed by decongestion and total nasal resistance remains elevated.

collapse during inspiration.[4] This phenomenon may be due to very localized obstruction in the area of the nasal valve or loss of structural cartilaginous support as a result of aging or nasal surgery (Fig. 23-8). If the negative pressure of the nasal airway is sufficient to overcome the elasticity of the cartilage, the airway collapses and nasal resistance increases. The typical finding on rhinomanometry in such collapse is an asymmetric nasal pressure flow curve. Since collapse occurs only during inspiration, inspiratory resistance is higher than expiratory resistance. In addition, collapse produces a flow limitation which can be detected as a plateau of the pressure-flow curve. Correction of alar collapse may require cartilage grafting to increase the rigidity of the nasal valve area.

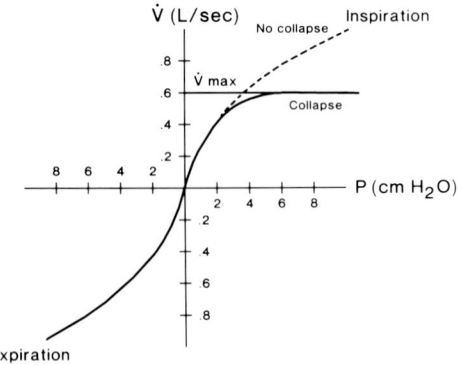

Fig. 23-8. Dynamic collapse of the nasal airway shown on a pressure-flow curve. Collapse of the nasal valve will produce a limitation of inspiratory airflow ($\dot{V}_{max}$). In spite of increased efforts, inspiratory flow cannot exceed this value when collapse occurs.

CONCLUSION

Rhinomanometry provides the following information which is useful in the diagnosis of nasal obstruction.

1. Nasal resistance is determined (normal versus elevated).
2. Reversible (mucosal) versus irreversible (structural) obstruction can be differentiated.
3. Dynamic changes of the nasal airway (such as alar collapse) can be detected.

The information derived from nasal resistance measurements can be used to determine which therapy would be most beneficial in a particular patient. In addition, following therapy, nasal resistance measurements are useful since they provide a comparison of pretreatment and post-treatment nasal resistance. The effectiveness of the treatment and the possible need to modify a therapeutic program can thus be assessed. A previous study has shown that success of nasal septal surgery can be predicted by preoperative nasal resistance measurements.[5]

REFERENCES

1. Clement PAR: Committee report on standardization of rhinomanometry. Rhinology 22:151–155, 1984
2. McCaffrey TV, Kern EB: Clinical evaluation of nasal obstruction. Arch Otolaryngol 105:542–545, 1979
3. Hasegawa M, Kern EB: The human nasal cycle. Mayo Clin Proc 53:28–34, 1977
4. Bridger GP, Proctor DF: Maximum nasal inspiratory flow and nasal resistance. Ann Otolaryngol 79:481–488, 1970
5. Mertz JS, McCaffrey TV, Kern EB: Objective evaluation of anterior septal surgical reconstruction. Otolaryngol Head Neck Surg 92:302–307, 1984

Frederick L. Sachs

24

The Clinical and Practical Aspects of Office Pulmonary Function Tests

The pulmonary function laboratory can provide the otolaryngologist with a great deal of information which may significantly aid in the diagnosis of a variety of conditions affecting the respiratory tract. In addition, the use of pulmonary function testing prior to proposed surgery can greatly reduce the incidence of postoperative complications. This chapter will attempt to provide the reader with a basic understanding of the use of the pulmonary laboratory.

SPIROMETRY

The spirometer provides the pulmonary physician with the means to assess lung capacities and lung volumes. Aberrations of lung function detected by assessment of these capacities and volumes can confirm the presence of disease states, suspected on the basis of history and physical examination. Figure 24-1 illustrates the commonly measured lung volumes and capacities. The tidal volume (VT) refers to the volume of air which is inhaled or exhaled during quiet breathing. Total lung capacity (TLC) refers to the amount of air contained in the lung at the end of a maximal inspiration. The vital capacity (VC) refers to the maximal volume of air that can be exhaled from the lungs from the height of inspiration. The residual volume (RV) refers to that volume of air remaining in the lung after a maximal exhalation. The functional residual capacity (FRC) is the volume of air remaining in the lung after an unforced exhalation. The expiratory reserve volume (ERV) is the volume of air that can be exhaled from the lung at the end of a quiet exhalation, i.e., FRC=ERV + RV. The inspiratory capacity (IC) refers to the volume of air that can be inhaled from the end of a normal expiration. The inspiratory reserve volume (IRV) is the additional volume of air which can be inhaled from the height of a normal inhalation. Dynamic lung volumes are obtained when the

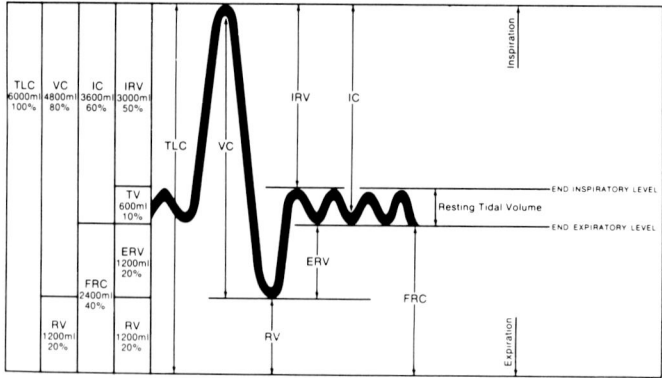

Fig. 24-1. The lung volumes and subdivisions expressed in milliliters as an approximate percentage of the total lung capacity. From Bickerman HA: Lung volumes, capacities, and thoracic volumes. In Chusid EL (Ed.): The Selective and Comprehensive Testing of Adult Pulmonary Function. Mt. Kisco, New York, Futura Publisher. p. 5, 1983. With permission.

patient is asked to perform a timed vital capacity. In this study, the patient performs the vital capacity maneuver as rapidly as possible. The value of the vital capacity performed in this manner is referred to as the FVC. By timing the forced vital capacity, it is possible to measure the volume of gas exhaled in the first second after exhalation (FEV_1), in the next second (FEV_2), and in the third second (FEV_3). By calculating the ratio FEV_1/FVC, it is possible to estimate whether or not flow is normal. The FEV_1/FVC value for a healthy individual is approximately 75 percent. Values below this indicate that there is obstruction to flow. The simplest spirometers available allow for measurement of the FVC and FEV_1. If one wishes to obtain FRC, RV, and TLC, more elaborate equipment is needed. Lung volumes are most commonly determined using gas dilution methods that employ helium or nitrogen. The details of the methods used to calculate these volumes are beyond the scope of this text.

THE FLOW VOLUME CURVE

The flow volume loop provides another method of evaluating pulmonary function. In this study, instantaneous flow (measured with a pneumotachygraph) is plotted against lung volume. Figure 24-2 illustrates a normal flow volume (FV) curve. It should be noted that when one measures function with a spirometer, flow is never directly measured. The spirometer provides data concerning volume exhaled in each unit of time, and from this information one estimates the adequacy of flow. In the flow volume study, however, the pneumotachygraph records instantaneous flow rates. The shape of the curve can be predicted by a knowledge of the physiologic derangement. Diseases that are associated with airway narrowing (such as asthma) will be characterized by a reduction in flow rates. The flow volume loop in these patients will reveal a concave shape as illustrated in Figure 24-2.

There are currently several companies that manufacture reliable and relatively inex-

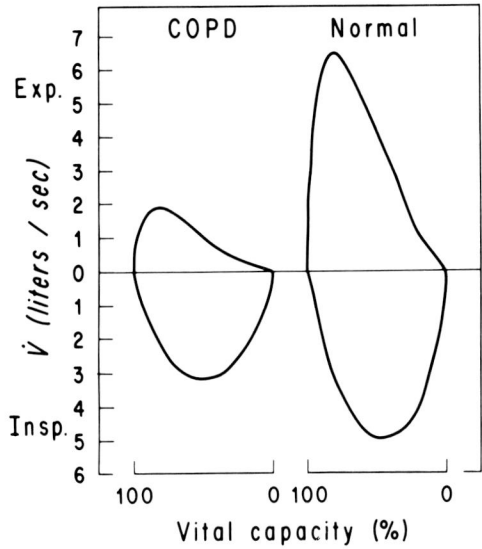

Fig. 24-2. Examples of typical FV loops. Left, in Chronic obstructive pulmonary disease (COPD). Right, normal. From Miller R, Hyatt RE: Evaluation of obstructing lesions of the trachea and larynx by flow-volume loops. Am Rev Respir Dis 108:478, 1973. With permission.

pensive devices to allow physicians to perform basic tests such as flow volume loops or simple spirometry in their offices. A normal spirometry or normal flow volume loop strongly suggests that there is no significant impairment in pulmonary function. Abnormal curves, however, may often be diagnostic of pulmonary pathology, indicating the presence of either limitation to flow or the presence of restrictive lung disease.

Diseases which are associated with limitation to airflow include asthma, a disease characterized by reversible obstruction to airflow, chronic bronchitis, and emphysema. In all of these disease states, the airway is narrowed and flow is reduced. The spirometer will detect this abnormality in the following manner: The vital capacity and the FEV_1 become reduced and the FEV_1/FVC ratio falls to below 75–80 percent. If functional residual capacity and residual volume are measured, it will be seen that these values are elevated. In many patients, total lung capacity will be elevated as well. The flow volume loop will also reflect the presence of obstruction to flow by demonstrating a reduction in flow rates and by producing its characteristic concave shape when displayed. Demonstrating that an individual patient has obstruction to airflow does not provide an exact diagnosis. However, more information can be provided with the use of bronchodilator medication. Patients with reversible airflow limitation will demonstrate an improvement of 15 percent or more in FEV_1. Lack of response to a bronchodilator does not make the diagnosis of reversible disease untenable, but the finding of a reversible component to airflow limitation is supporting evidence of reversible disease.

Restrictive lung diseases also produce changes in the simple spirometric tracing and flow volume loop. In restrictive lung diseases such as pulmonary fibrosis, the spirometer demonstrates a reduction in the FVC and FEV_1. The FEV_1/FVC ratio remains normal, however, and is actually often in the high normal range. If the TLC, RV, and FRC are measured, these are also below normal. The flow volume loop is also abnormal in patients with restrictive lung diseases. The volume axis reveals the reduction in vital capacity one would expect. The slope of the curve remains normal, however, since there is no limitation to flow. Restrictive lung diseases do not demonstrate any reversible component following the administration of bronchodilator.

Additional Uses of the Flow Volume Curve

The flow volume curve can also be used to confirm the presence of upper airway obstruction. In order to understand the curves produced by obstruction of the upper airway, it is necessary to be cognizant of the factors influencing airflow in the intrathoracic and extrathoracic airways.

During inhalation, the intrathoracic pleural pressure becomes more negative than during exhalation. The increasingly negative pleural pressure causes the intrathoracic airways to enlarge. In the extrathoracic airways, however, the increased negative pressure causes atmospheric pressure to exceed extrathoracic airway pressure. This phenomenon is associated with a slight narrowing of the extrathoracic airway lumen.

On exhalation, the opposite effects are found. During exhalation, pleural pressure becomes more positive and the intrathoracic airways become narrower due to dynamic compression. During exhalation, pressure in the extrathoracic airways becomes more positive than atmospheric pressure; this is reflected in a widening of the extrathoracic airway. These facts are illustrated in Figure 24-3.

Variably obstructing lesions of the extrathoracic airways are associated with abnormal flow volume curves. A lesion obstructing the extrathoracic airway will manifest itself by alerting the inspiratory portion of the curve because it is during inspiration that the extrathoracic airway is narrowest. Hence, a lesion that further narrows the extrathoracic lumen will distort the inspiratory curve. On exhalation, the extrathoracic lumen is normally slightly dilated and this tends to negate the effects of an obstructing extrathoracic lesion. Therefore, in patients with variable obstructing lesions of the extrathoracic airways, the inspiratory portion of the curve is flattened while the expiratory

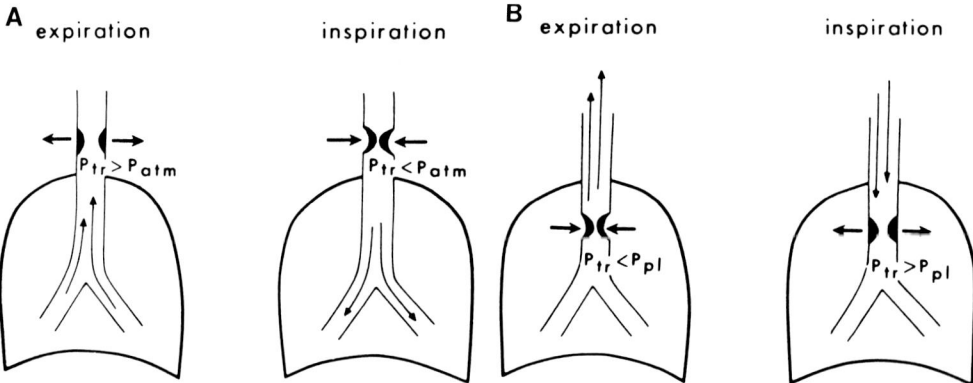

Fig. 24-3. (A) effect of the phase of respiration on an extrathoracic variable obstruction. Direction of airflow is indicated by the long, thin arrows. During forced expiration, the intratracheal pressure (P_{tr}) is greater than the pressure around the airway (P_{atm} = atmospheric pressure), resulting in a decrease of the obstruction. During forced inspiration, when the pressure around the airway exceeds the intratracheal pressure, the obstruction is increased. (B) Effect of the phase of respiration on an intrathoracic variable obstruction. During forced expiration, the pressure acting around the airway (P_{pl} = pleural pressure) may be greater than the intratracheal pressure, resulting in an increase in the obstruction. During forced inspiration, the intratracheal pressure is greater than the pleural pressure, thus decreasing the obstruction. From Kryger M, Biode F, Antic R, et al: Diagnosis of obstruction of the upper and central airways. Am J Med 61:87, 1976. With permission.

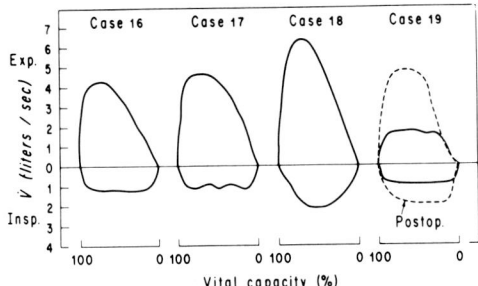

Fig. 24-4. Four examples of Group 2 (variable) lesions above the suprasternal notch. In cases 16, 17, and 18, vocal cord paralysis followed poliomyelitis, thyroidectomy, and polymyositis, respectively; in case 19, vocal cord paralysis was improved by arytenoidectomy. From Miller R, Hyatt RE: Evaluation of obstructing lesions of the trachea and larynx by flow-volume loops. Am Rev Respir Dis 108:478, 1973. With permission.

portion is relatively normal (Fig. 24-4). The clinical correlation with the physiological principles is striking. Children with epiglottitis have inspiratory stridor, reflecting the obstruction to the extrathoracic airway. Patients with oropharyngeal tumors often have subclinical compromise of the upper airway. This can be detected by the preoperative use of the flow volume loop and this information may enable the anesthetist and surgeon to prevent untoward intraoperative complications. Also of interest is the fact that individuals with intrathoracic obstructing lesions (such as large substernal goiters) may wheeze due to the effect of the goiter that compresses the airway lumen during expiration.

LUNG COMPLIANCE

The term compliance refers to distensibility. When one speaks of the compliance of the lung, one is therefore speaking of the distensibility of the lung parenchyma. A highly compliant lung is very distensible. Compliance is studied in the laboratory by measurements of the pressure required to produce a change in volume. In the very compliant lung, small changes in pressure can produce significant changes in lung volume. In the poorly compliant lung, large changes in pressure are required to produce volume changes. Elasticity is the term used to describe the physical characteristic of the lung by which it resists distortion. A highly compliant lung, which is easily distended by small pressure changes, has lost its elastic properties. On the other hand, a poorly compliant lung, which requires high pressures to evoke changes in volume, may be considered to be highly elastic. A highly elastic lung is a poorly compliant or "stiff" lung. The clinical correlate of these concepts is that the emphysematous lung which has lost its elastic properties becomes a highly distensible, highly compliant lung, whereas the lungs of patients with pulmonary fibrosis are highly elastic, poorly compliant, and require large pressure changes to produce significant volume changes. These facts are illustrated in Figure 24-5.

DIFFUSION

The diffusing capacity of the lung refers to the quantity of a specific gas that diffuses into the alveolar capillary from the alveolus during each unit time. The methods used to measure diffusion very among pulmonary physicians. In most laboratories, the single-breath test using carbon monoxide gas is the study commonly employed. Carbon monoxide has a great affinity for hemoglobin and the single-breath diffusion study provides

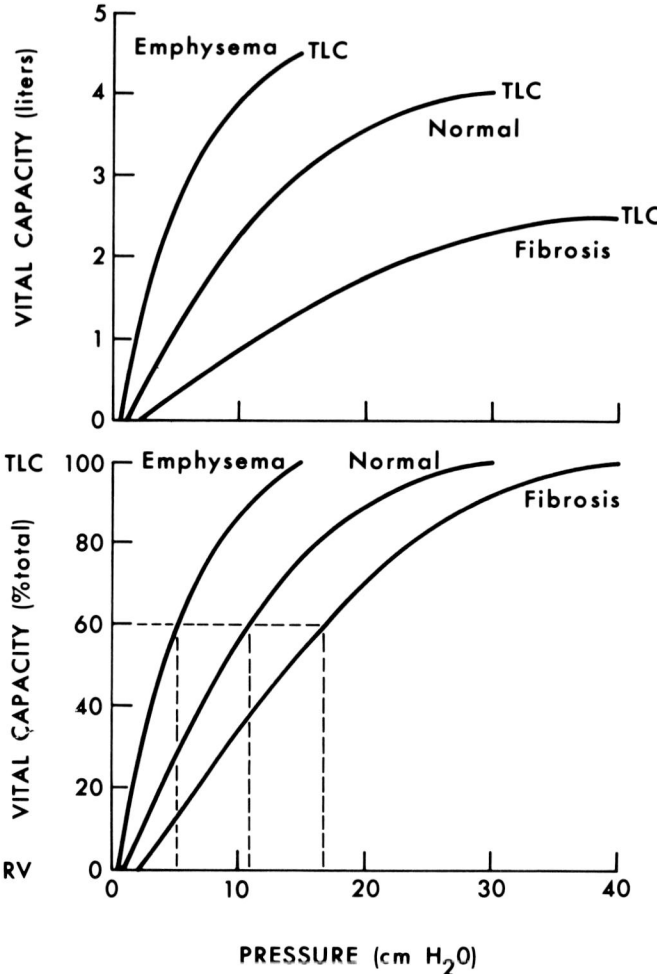

Fig. 24-5. Representative volume-pressure curves from adult subjects of the same age, sex, and body size showing changes caused by emphysema and pulmonary fibrosis, compared with normal lungs. *Upper panel* depicts volume-pressure relations in terms of measured (i.e., observed) vital capacity and demonstrates that emphysematous lungs are larger and fibrotic lungs smaller than normal. When expressed in terms of percentage of measured vital capacity (*lower panel*), at any given vital capacity (e.g., 60 percent, shown by dashed lines), elastic recoil pressure is less than normal in emphysema and greater than normal in fibrosis. From Murray JF: The Normal Lung—The Basis for Diagnosis and Treatment of Pulmonary Disease. Philadelphia: W.B. Saunders Company, p. 82, 1976. With permission.

information which can be used to estimate the size of the pulmonary vascular bed. For example, in patients with emphysema, there is a loss of pulmonary capillary volume and this is reflected in the low values recorded by single-breath diffusion methods. Many pulmonary physicians follow serial diffusion studies to estimate the loss of functioning capillary blood volume in interstitial diseases of the lung such as sarcoidosis or scleroderma.

BLOOD GASES

During breathing at tidal volumes, inspired air is distributed to both airways and alveoli. The volume of air in conducting airways does not participate in gas exchange and is referred to as the anatomical dead space. The volume of air in the alveoli which participates in gas exchange is called the alveolar volume. Alveolar ventilation is the amount of gas that moves into "functioning" terminal respiratory units during a given period. In every lung, there are terminal respiratory units that do not participate in gas exchange. For example, an alveolus which has no blood supply will not be involved in gas exchange. When added to the anatomical dead space, this volume is referred to as the physiologic dead space. In equation form, tidal volume (VT) = alveolar volume (VA) + dead space (VD). In order to calculate alveolar ventilation, the alveolar volume each breath (VA) is multiplied by the respiratory frequency (f).

Alveolar and arterial carbon dioxide tensions are equal and thus arterial PCO_2 is representative of alveolar carbon dioxide tension. The amount of carbon dioxide excreted by the lung is directly proportional to alveolar ventilation. The higher the level of alveolar ventilation, the greater the amount of carbon dioxide excreted, and the lower the level of alveolar carbon dioxide tension. High levels of alveolar ventilation is inversely proportional to alveolar carbon dioxide and therefore to arterial PCO_2. In practice, the arterial PCO_2 is used to measure the adequacy of alveolar ventilation. In patients with hypoventilation, the arterial PCO_2 will be elevated. In individuals with high levels of alveolar ventilation, such as patients with central hyperventilation due to a major central nervous system insult, arterial PCO_2 levels are below normal.

The sum of the partial pressures of gases contained in the lung is equal to the barometric pressure. Barometric pressure is relatively constant and, since water vapor pressure and the partial pressure of nitrogen do not vary to a great degree, the sum of the partial pressures of oxygen and carbon dioxide also remains constant. This relationship between alveolar oxygen tension and the tension of alveolar carbon dioxide dictates that as the level of alveolar oxygen rises, the level of alveolar carbon dioxide will fall. Through a series of equations beyond the scope of this text, one can calculate the value for alveolar oxygen tension (PAl_v) in the following manner:

Equation 1. $\qquad PAl_v = 148 - 1.2 \times PCO_2$

If the arterial oxygen tension is measured with a blood gas and the alveolar oxygen tension is calculated as above, it is possible to measure the alveolar-arterial gradient commonly called the A-a gradient. In a healthy lung, the gradient should be less than 10 mmHg. A-a gradients over 10 mmHg indicate the presence of intrinsic lung disease.

The most common cause of arterial hypoxemia is nonhomogeneous distribution of alveolar ventilation and blood flow. This is commonly referred to as ventilation perfusion abnormality (V/Q disturbance). Maldistribution of ventilation and perfusion oc-

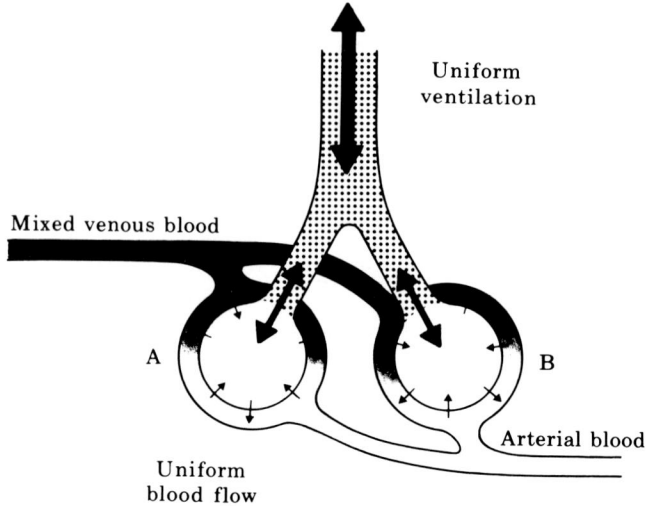

Fig. 24-6. Schematic representation of gas exchange in an idealized two-compartment model of the lung in which there is uniform distribution of ventilation and blood flow. Murray JF: The Normal Lung—The Basis for Diagnosis and Treatment of Pulmonary Disease. Philadelphia: W.B. Saunders Company, 1976; p. 173. With permission.

GAS EXCHANGE

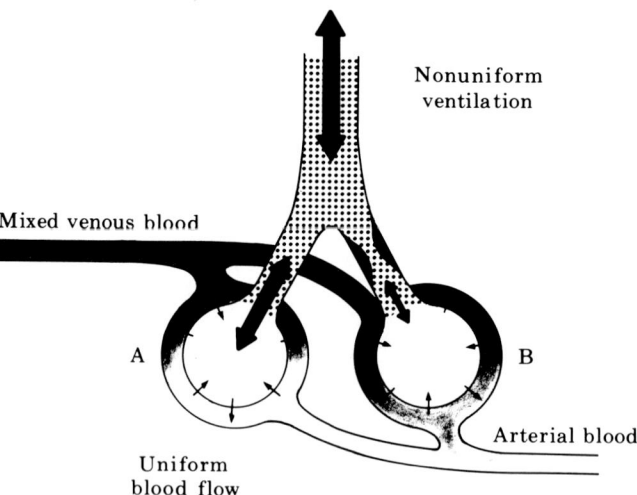

Fig. 24-7. Schematic representation of the effects of a ventilation-perfusion abnormality on gas exchange. Murray JF: The Normal Lung—The Basis for Diagnosis and Treatment of Pulmonary Disease. Philadelphia: W.B. Saunders Company, 1976; p. 179.

curs in patients with diseases such as asthma, chronic bronchitis, and emphysema. Figures 24-6 and 24-7 illustrate why ventilation and perfusion abnormalities produce hypoxemia. In alveolus A in Figure 24-6, the ventilation and perfusion are normal. The hemoglobin in red blood cells supplying alveolus A is fully saturated. In alveolus B, the situation is similar in that there is normal ventilation and perfusion, so that the hemoglobin in the red blood cells supplying alveolus B will also be fully saturated and the arterial blood will have a normal oxygen tension.

In Figure 24-7, however, the situation is somewhat different. In this lung, there is obstruction in the airway of alveolus A, which lowers the alveolar PCO_2 in alveolus A. This results in a reduction in the saturation of hemoglobin in the red cells of vessel A. Alveolus B has normal ventilation and perfusion so that the hemoglobin saturation in red blood cells supplying alveolus B will be normal. However, since the arterial blood is a sum of blood from vessels A and B, the arterial PCO_2 will be abnormally low.

It can be seen from the facts presented above that in patients with ventilation perfusion abnormalities, merely increasing the rate or depth of alveolar ventilation will not correct the hypoxemia. The impairment in ventilation will make it impossible to correct the low alveolar PCO_2 in alveolus A, and the low saturation of red cells from vessel A will remain. Since red cells from vessel B are already fully saturated, they cannot help to make up for the reduced saturation seen in red blood cells from vessel A.

If the inspired oxygen tension is raised, however, changes in arterial oxygen tension can be achieved. If the inspired oxygen tension is increased, this will lead to an increase in the alveolar oxygen tension in alveolus A. This increase in alveolar oxygen tension will result in an increase in the saturation of the hemoglobin contained in the red blood cells from vessel A. Relatively small increments in alveolar oxygen tension are associated with substantial improvements in saturation because of the shape of the oxyhemoglobin dissociation curve, as shown in Figure 24-8. At points along the steep portion of the curve, small increments in PCO_2 are associated with significant improvement in saturation. Thus, in patients with disturbances of ventilation/perfusion produced by diseases such as asthma, chronic bronchitis, and emphysema, hypoxemia can often be corrected by incremental increases in inspired oxygen tension.

It is necessary to use caution when raising the level of inspired oxygen in patients with chronic airflow obstruction accompanied by longstanding carbon dioxide retention. The rationale for this is related to the mechanisms by which the body controls ventilation. Ventilation is regulated in normal healthy individuals by chemoreceptors which monitor levels of carbon dioxide, oxygen, and pH in the arterial blood. Of these receptors, the most important is the response to carbon dioxide. Receptors involved in the ventilatory response to carbon dioxide are located on the ventral surface of the medulla. These receptors are bathed in cerebrospinal fluid (CSF), which is separated from the blood by the blood-brain barrier. Hydrogen and bicarbonate ions do not easily cross this barrier, but carbon dioxide does. Thus, when the arterial PCO_2 rises, carbon dioxide diffuses into the CSF and liberates hydrogen ions. The increase in hydrogen ion concentration causes an increase in ventilatory drive. In chronic states, however, renal compensation for increased PCO_2 leads to an increase in bicarbonate concentration. This increase in bicarbonate levels serves to restore the pH of the CSF and reduces the increase in ventilation produced by the elevation of PCO_2. There are peripheral chemoreceptors for carbon dioxide in the carotid and aortic bodies, but their contribution to ventilatory stimulation is small.

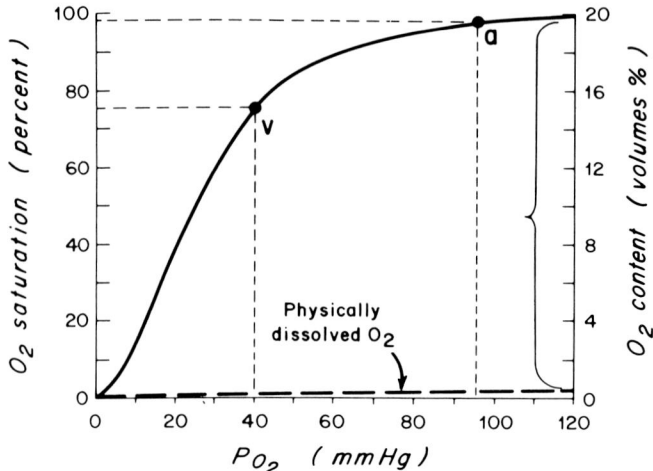

Fig. 24-8. Oxyhemoglobin dissociation curve. Oxygen saturation is given by the vertical axis on the left and oxygen content by the vertical axis on the right. Note the S shape of the curve and the location of arterial point *a* on the flat part of the dissociation curve and the venous point *v* on the steep portion of the curve. The hemoglobin content of this blood is 15 g/100 ml, and the amount of oxygen carried in physical solution is much less than that bound to hemoglobin, as indicated by the bracket on the oxygen content axis. From Kazemi H: Oxygen and carbon dioxide transport, disorders of the respiratory system. In: The Science and Practice of Clinical Medicine. New York: Grune & Stratton, (vol. 2). p. 42. With permission.

Hypoxemia effects ventilation through its effects on the peripheral receptors located in the carotid and aortic bodies. Reducing the arterial oxygen tension leads to an increase in ventilation.

Peripheral chemoreceptors are affected by pH, per se, but pH does not exert a major effect on ventilatory drive.

In patients with longstanding chronic airflow obstruction, ventilation perfusion mismatching often produces hypoxemia with accompanying carbon dioxide retention. Because of the chronicity of the carbon dioxide retention, these patients have developed renal compensation that raises the level of their serum bicarbonate, restores their arterial pH towards normal, and reduces the sensitivity of their central receptors to carbon dioxide. In these individuals, ventilation is driven largely by the level of arterial hypoxemia. Administration of too high an inspired oxygen tension may thus improve the arterial hypoxemia to a level at which the stimulus to breathe is markedly reduced and respiration may cease.

James J. Pappas
Sharon S. Graham

25

Development and Management of an Outpatient Surgical Facility in the Office of an Otolaryngological Group Practice

With the current economic and political climate for surgeons practicing in our country today, the advantages of outpatient surgery are becoming obvious, both as a means of containing spiraling medical costs, and as a means of improving the quality, efficiency, and delivery of health care services. In the past, many patients occupying hospital beds were receiving a more expensive level of care than was truly necessary. The 1976 Orkand report,[1] a government-sponsored study of outpatient procedures, concluded that outpatient surgery could significantly reduce costs, while at the same time delivery high-quality surgical care. Authors of this report felt that up to 40 percent of all surgical procedures performed in hospitals could be performed safely in outpatient settings. Yet, in 1980, a report published by O'Donovan[2] estimated that only 5–7 percent of surgical procedures performed in the United States were being done on an outpatient basis. O'Donovan estimated that if 40 percent of the services were done on an outpatient basis, the annual savings to the American health care system would exceed two billion dollars.

For many otolaryngological operative procedures, outpatient surgery represents an efficient and effective health care alternative.[3] Many otolaryngological procedures are carried out on patients who are in generally good health, and usually no blood replacement is required. The operating time is usually short, and postoperative ambulation may be allowed within a few hours.

The success of an outpatient surgical facility for an otolaryngological practice depends upon long-term and careful planning prior to the opening of such a facility. With such careful planning, an efficient operating room can be designed that will prove beneficial both to the patient and to the otolaryngologist.

Several essential steps are involved in planning an office surgical facility. Specific, detailed construction plans with blueprints must be drawn up in accordance with state health department regulations, as well as with the regulations of any other accrediting agency, such as the Joint Commission for Accreditation of Hospitals (JCAH) or the

American Association for Ambulatory Health Care (AAAHC). Along with such construction plans, arrangements must be made for funding the construction and purchase of equipment. Also, prior to any initiation of construction, provision must be made for anesthesia coverage, as well as for nursing coverage. Prospective fee schedules must be considered for the facility charges; this necessitates careful cost accounting of what charges will be incurred by the facility in carrying out any specific procedure, with a decision made regarding what charges will be made in excess of those costs (for a profit margin), while keeping charges within certain established guidelines, such as the Blue Cross allowable fee schedules. All of these factors—construction, funding, anesthesia, nursing, and fee schedules, must be planned in specific detail before the first major step in initiation of an outpatient facility is taken. This step is application for the certificate of need from the local health systems agency.

In most states, it is necessary to acquire this certificate prior to being licensed by the state health department and before any third-party carrier will consider payment to the facility. Certificate of need guidelines vary from state to state. Two major considerations on which the certificate of need is based are the capital expenditure law, which, in 1984 in many states, involves any capital expenditure in excess of $600,000, and the initiation of a new health service within a community. A certificate of need thus may be necessary if a new facility comes under either of these 2 criteria.

Formal application for a certificate of need usually includes submission of a detailed application form, which describes the services to be provided, the relationship of these services to the community's federal and state health systems plan, the relationship of the services to other similar services offered in the area, and specific details on construction and funding. Following this application, a formal presentation is made to the local health systems agency. Rulings on such applications for certificates of need have become highly political decisions in many areas of the country, based on the political pressure by area hospitals and other agencies against expansion of competitive operating room facilities in the community.

Once the certificate of need has been obtained from the health systems agency, the next step is application for a license from the state health department. This application is also typically a very detailed submission of all major policies and procedures for the facility. Often, in order to qualify for licensure, a constitution, bylaws, and articles of incorporation (including the name, purpose, board of governors, officers, administrators, and medical staff), and minutes of meetings must be submitted with the application. Also required may be submission of names of the governing body and steps by which the governing body plans to administer the facility, including a peer review committee, with plans for regularly scheduled meetings.

Rules of administration, which must be submitted prior to approval for a state license, may govern such requirements as specific recordkeeping, visitor policies, storage of patient valuables, disaster plans, emergency telephone numbers, and procedures to meet all established fire codes. Other procedure descriptions that may be required include personnel policies, communicable disease reports, nursing staff and procedure requirements, medication reports, exact requirements for medical record notation, and laboratory, radiology, and pharmacy procedures.

Also necessary is proof of provision for specialized surgical services similar to that required for a hospital, including proper operating room tables, lights, anesthetic equipment, cardiac monitor and defibrillator, conductive flooring, ungrounded electrical system, back-up emergency generator, stretchers, conductive footwear, central sterilization, inhalation therapy, periodic testing of emergency power supply and other equipment, and provision for housekeeping and laundry services.

Once specific, detailed documentation has been drawn up in writing for all of these types of administration, the state health department will review these written documents and conduct an on-site inspection of the facility. Once a license by the state health department has been issued, facilities are subject to future inspections and must meet any changes in regulations in order to keep the license.

Once the state license has been obtained, it is possible to begin pursuit of third-party approval for payment. This involves application for Medicaid provider numbers and other such provider numbers from state and federal agencies for payment of facility fees, since the facility itself may have a number separate and different from that of the operating surgeon. It is then wise to contact Blue Cross and Blue Shield, advising them of the existence of the new facility, and then to meet with them to discuss established fees for outpatient operating rooms, recovery rooms, and laboratory and radiographic studies. Having established facility fees, with consideration of the usual and customary fees in the local community, it is then wise to prepare a letter and a package of materials outlining the assigned facility fees, for use in notifying other third-party carriers.

In order to receive third-party payment from a number of organizations, it is becoming increasingly necessary to hold accreditation or certification from a national accrediting organization, such as the Joint Commission for Accreditation of Hospitals (JCAH). An alternate certifying organization is the American Association of Ambulatory Health Care (AAAHC), an association that certifies only outpatient or ambulatory facilities. With the increased regulation of outpatient facilities due to their growth in the last several years, it is most probable that in the future, accreditation will be necessary in order to receive third-party payment. Currently, in order to receive Medicare payment, as well as payment from other governmental agencies such as CHAMPUS, it is necessary to hold accreditation from JCAH or AAAHC.

In order to make application for JCAH accreditation, an outpatient facility must have been in business for at least one year. A lengthy and detailed application form must be submitted in order for the JCAH to consider the facility for accreditation. This application includes detailed and specific information regarding the: quality assurance program of the facility; quality of care procedures; medical records; rights of patients; governing bodies; administration; facilities and environment; educational activities; surgical and anesthesia services; emergency services; pharmaceutical services; pathology and medical laboratory services; radiology services; teaching and publication activities; and research activities. Only after submission of this detailed application and verification by JCAH officials that the application shows that the facility meets the initial criteria, is an initial inspection scheduled by a team of JCAH inspectors. This team includes a minimum of one physician and one medical administrator. The on-site inspection involves a very detailed investigation of all aspects of facility operation. Initial accreditation may be made on a temporary basis, if the facility meets most criteria, but not all. Any change in professional liability status should be carefully investigated. While the medical-legal climate differs from one community to another, it is mandatory to know if there are any changes in liability status and how these changes may affect the liability insurance premium. In some instances, having the outpatient facility in the same area and on the same floor as the physicians' private offices and examining rooms results in no change in liability status.

All outpatient facilities should have an agreement in writing with the nearest local hospital, ensuring admission of any patient from the outpatient facility should a medical problem arise. It may be necessary to submit a copy of this letter to the state health department in order to secure the state license. If the facility is not adjacent to a hospital, there should also be a written agreement regarding ambulance transportation.

The office surgical facility should be self-contained and completely equipped. The floor plan for the authors' office, including the outpatient surgery center, is shown in Figure 25-1. This plan was designed for the author's 5-physician group practice. The surgery center consists of an operating room, 15 × 20 feet or 300 square feet; a 4-bed recovery room, 21 × 24 feet or 504 square feet; a doctors' dressing room; a nurses' dressing room; a 2-sink scrub area; a nonsterile work area; and a clean work room for the autoclave and sterile supplies. Glass cabinets that can be stocked for the operating room are accessible from the clean work area. There is a separate storage area, away from the surgical facility, for bulk supplies. Ideally, there should be separate areas for preoperative and postoperative patients. Initially, the use of this facility was greatly underestimated, and thus it has been necessary to use the same recovery area for both preoperative and postoperative patients.

A major piece of equipment necessary for the authors' operating room is a back-up generator in case of power failure. Some health departments require conductive flooring to drain off static electricity, and an isolated power panel to prevent electrical shock in the event of an electrical short in any equipment. Planning should include sources for oxygen and nitrogen, apparatus to deliver these gases, a source for compressed air, and a central suction system. Operating room light sources, as well as the operating room table, should be chosen to meet specific individual needs. Another major item is the anesthesia unit. Also necessary are electric cauteries and an operating-room-quality sterilizer.

Operating facilities should have a full complement of emergency equipment. This includes a cardiac monitor and defibrillator, a tracheotomy tray, and a full emergency kit, including drugs. There should be an office alarm system, which can be used to alert the physician and nursing staff during any crisis in the operating room or recovery room.

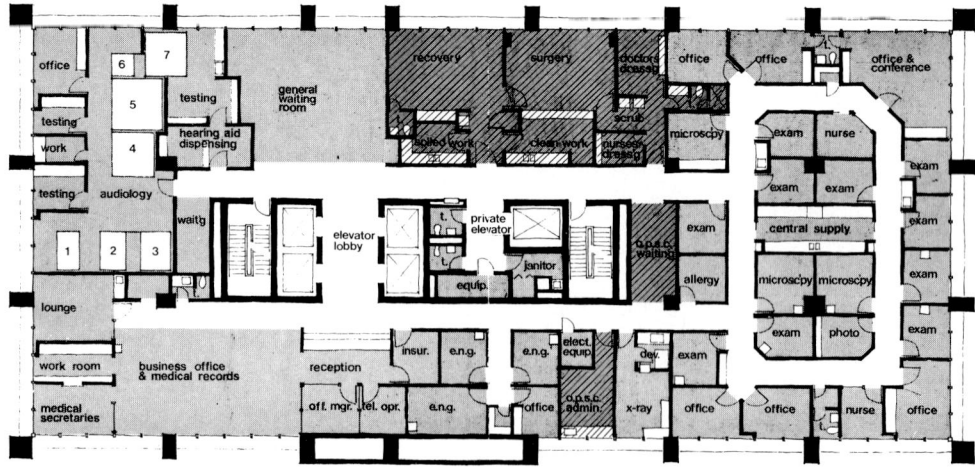

Fig. 25-1. Clinic floor plan, including the outpatient surgery center.

Also necessary is a prescribed fire escape plan and any equipment necessary to ensure safe removal of patients in the event of fire or other disaster. In the recovery room, movable carts, such as Stryker carts, are necessary, along with portable sources of oxygen and suction.

Once an office surgical facility has been designed and equipped, it is necessary to consider criteria for case selection. Cases should be those requiring short-term postoperative care. Patients should be in generally good health; elderly patients must be carefully evaluated prior to outpatient surgery. Work-up on an outpatient basis should include the same laboratory and radiographic studies as if the cases were to be done in the hospital. Patients should be carefully counseled at the time they are posted and receive both written and oral instructions regarding preoperative medications and NPO status.

Currently, a wide variety of otolaryngological and cosmetic facial surgery procedures are done in the authors' outpatient facility, as seen in Table 25-1. This facility did not begin performing this wide variety of procedures. Procedures were begun very cautiously; only those conservative procedures which the physicians felt completely secure about performing on an outpatient basis were performed. Gradually, as experience accumulated, the range of procedures was expanded, while the criteria for patient selection were maintained. The most commonly performed surgical procedures at this facility include

Table 25-1
Outpatient Otolaryngological Procedures

Ear	Head and neck
myringotomy with tube	basal cell excision
tympanoplasty	open reduction of trimalar fracture
stapedectomy	removal of arch bars
tympanomastoidectomy	open reduction of zygomatic fracture
meatoplasty	
Nose and sinus	Gillies procedure
septoplasty	flap revision
NA window	Plastic
Caldwell-Luc	rhinoplasty
closed reduction-fracture	blepharoplasty
polypectomy	facelift
Oral cavity and oronasopharynx	scar revision
adenoidectomy	otoplasty
tonsillectomy	brow lift
clip frenulum	mentoplasty
thyroglossal duct cyst	neck lift
ranula excision	dermabrasion
submaxillary gland excision	lip wedge excision
sublingual gland stone	face peel
Miscellaneous	eye wedge resection
Larynx and tracheobronchi	
laryngoscopy	
teflon injection, vocal cord	
section recurrent laryngeal nerve	
bronchoscopy	
bronchoscopy with esophagoscopy	
panendoscopy	

myringotomy, tonsillectomy and adenoidectomy, septoplasty, tympanoplasty, stapedectomy, and laryngoscopy. For some procedures, patients are asked to stay overnight in a motel in or near the building, if they live further than 30 minutes away by car. These patients return to the office on the morning following surgery for a brief examination and then are discharged to return to their homes.

In 9 years of experience with this outpatient facility, after over 10,000 cases, there have been no deaths. The facility has experienced 6 true emergencies, including one cardiac arrest following local injection of xylocaine with epinephrine 1:100,000 for a rhinoplasty. This patient was admitted to the hospital following resuscitation. Other complications experienced have included laryngospasms and bronchospasms. All of these emergencies were handled within the facility's operating room and/or recovery room, and there have been no serious consequences as a result of any of these emergencies. In 10,000 procedures, the admission rate to the hospital has been 0.5 percent.

Currently, 80 percent of all the cases done in the authors' outpatient surgical facility are performed under general anesthesia. Anesthesia is provided by a private group of anesthesiologists who assign coverage to the facility. This private anesthesia group bills the patients directly for services.

Recruitment of the nursing staff involves consideration of the case load, as well as of the need for ordering and stocking supplies and for cleaning not performed by janitorial services. All nurses should be trained in cardiopulmonary resuscitation. Coverage should include a scrub nurse, circulating nurse, and appropriate number of recovery room nurses for the case load, as well as someone responsible for cleaning instruments and rooms and for restocking supplies. There is an enormous amount of nursing administration necessary in order to run an outpatient facility effectively and efficiently. This includes not only the ordering of supplies, assignment of nursing services, and care of major equipment, but also detailed paperwork which is mandatory for meeting the requirements of the certifying agencies.

Scheduling of cases in the outpatient facility should be planned in a manner which makes the most effective use of the facility's time, staff, and beds. Short cases should be done first, as they generally have the shortest recovery times, thus freeing recovery beds for later patients requiring longer recovery. A general rule is that the recovery time for general anesthesia is twice that of the surgery time, and for local anesthesia, recovery time is equal to the surgery time.

In order to assure availability of adequate supplies, an agreement should be made with local dealers who are able to provide daily delivery service. When the case load of the facility reaches 40 cases each month, it may be possible to receive a volume discount on supplies. Sufficient operating room supplies should be stored to run a facility for 2–3 weeks, if possible. Cabinets in the operating room itself should hold enough supplies for 2–3 days without necessitating restocking. Disposable supplies are often preferable to nondisposable items for a number of reasons, including time saved by eliminating cleaning, manufacturer's provision of a sterility guarantee, and third-party cost reimbursement for disposable supplies.

Effective management of an office facility includes careful cost control. Detailed cost accounting analysis is necessary for such control and is required annually by Blue Cross and Blue Shield, which, in Arkansas, does not permit a profit factor of more than 10 percent. Such a monthly cost accounting analysis includes pro-rating the floor space, utilities, and maintenance, salaries of appropriate nursing and business personnel, supplies, equipment, and depreciation. This pro-rated monthly cost is then multiplied by 12 months and divided by the number of cases done each year; such a computation gives an estimate of the yearly facility cost for each case. Having this cost for each case, net proceeds can be deduced by looking at total facility charges and supply charges, less bad debts, which gives an overall estimate of profit.

SUMMARY

Numerous otolaryngological surgical procedures can be safely performed in an outpatient facility, under either general or local anesthesia. There are many advantages to outpatient surgery in otolaryngology, including the opportunity to improve the quality of health care delivered while reducing associated costs.

The authors have been performing outpatient surgery since 1975, and have demonstrated that there is a cost savings to patients when such surgery is compared to inpatient care. Some patients have no insurance; also, most insurance companies will not pay for elective cosmetic surgery. In these situations, outpatient surgery offers a significant savings to patients. With the advent of diagnostic related guidelines, preferred physician organizations, health maintenance organizations, etc, outpatient surgery has been firmly established as an efficient, effective, economical, and convenient way to perform certain indicated types of surgical procedures.

Outpatient surgery allows hospital operating rooms and beds to be kept available for emergency and extensive surgery cases. Convenience both to the patient and to the surgeon should not be underestimated. Basically, any operative procedure that allows the patient to be discharged safely on the day of surgery can be efficiently accomplished within an outpatient surgery facility. The authors' experience with over 10,000 procedures has demonstrated that outpatient surgery is safe for a wide variety of otolaryngological procedures.

REFERENCES

1. Orkand Corporation: Report to the Bureau of Health Planning and Resources Development of the Health Administration. Department of Health, Education and Welfare, Contract HEW-HRA 230-75-0071, 42–46, 1976
2. O'Donovan TR: Ambulatory surgery update. Same Day Surgery 6:44–45, 1980
3. Bailey HAT, Pappas JJ, Gay EC: O.P.S.C: Improving delivery of otolaryngological surgical care. Laryngoscope 88:1612–1616, 1978

Howard A. Tobin

26
Designing the Facility

With the rapid change in concepts and applications of office surgery, it must be recognized that any discussion of this nature will be subject to ongoing change. The author has had over 10 years of experience in designing and operating 2 office-based outpatient surgical facilities. The first was designed as an integral, functioning part of a medical office, while the second, which was recently completed, consists of a wholly independent outpatient surgical center that, while physically located within an office complex, exists as a fully licensed, independent entity. Since another chapter in this book discusses this more elaborate type of facility, aspects of office surgery that are applicable to the more limited type of facility will be emphasized here.

Recognizing that office surgery provides many advantages to both the surgeon and the patient, the question of economics cannot entirely be ignored. Although it is much more efficient to operate in one's own office, it still becomes a fairly expensive endeavor. Cost accounting becomes important in outpatient surgical facilities, creating an additional chore which is always burdensome, but even more so when the facility is first starting. As the movement toward outpatient surgery progresses, however, the practitioner who plans to build an operating room in the office must be fully aware of some important trends.

Third-party reimbursement is essential in this day of cost consciousness. Although insurance companies are becoming increasingly attuned to covering outpatient surgery, there is no assurance that this trend will continue to cover private operating rooms within the surgeon's office. It is therefore important to be aware of local, state, and federal legislation related to the construction and operation of freestanding ambulatory surgical facilities. Obtaining a certificate of need and building to comply with state health department and Medicare requirements might add considerably to the cost of the project, but could make the difference between operating in the red or in the black. The American Medical Association has prepared a monograph which gives some guidance in these areas.[1]

In Texas, one has 2 choices in regard to Medicare compliance. One can seek Medicare certification based on physical requirements alone, without participating in the

Medicare program, or one can fully participate. In the former situation, Medicare officials merely advise that the facility could physically comply with the regulations. The physician is not, in this case, required to participate in Medicare procedures, or to accept Medicare payment. This option allows the operator to comply with Medicare if it is so desired. Since Medicare appears to be the benchmark for coverage by other private insurance companies, it would seem to be advisable to comply with these basic physical requirements if at all possible.

Unfortunately, at the time of this writing, changes are so rapid as to preclude giving any accurate guidelines. Furthermore, it is important to realize that federal legislation (particularly in regard to Medicare) can be administered differently by the various states.

Finally, it is important to recognize that hospitals are keenly aware of the competition coming from private outpatient surgical facilities. Physicians are likely to see much more competitive pricing of outpatient surgery by hospitals, so the cost advantage in favor of the private practitioner is not as great as it was only a short time ago.

SELECTION OF CASES

Before entering into a discussion of the design and operation of an outpatient surgical facility, it is worthwhile to consider the types of surgery that will be carried out in the facility. Depending on the facilities developed, and the staff and equipment available, a large percentage of otolaryngology-head and neck surgery procedures can be performed in an office outpatient surgical facility. However, many facilities will have physical limitations that will preclude some of the more major operations. Whenever possible, it is best to determine, beforehand, the scope of surgical practice to be carried out, so that proper planning can be made. Of course, in many cases, there will be pre-existing limitations which may require the practitioner to suit the practice to the facility rather than the ideal situation, in which the facility is geared toward the desired practice.

It goes without saying that, whenever possible, it is wise to overplan and overbuild. It is rare that an individual builds a facility that that individual later feels is too big. Unfortunately, the opposite is often the case. The author has frequently talked to surgeons who were building a new facility and heard them say, "I don't need such and such, since I'm only going to do minor cases under local anesthesia." Unfortunately, these same surgeons usually find that after they have begun working in their offices and become comfortable with office surgery, they wish to expand the scope of their office surgery, only to find that they are now too limited by the physical plant to practice as they would desire.

This chapter is primarily concerned with the physical aspects of the design of the office operating suite. Before beginning this discussion, it must be stressed that the ultimate success or failure of an office surgery program depends on the skill, experience, and training of the entire staff. It should go without saying that an office operating room must not be used as an excuse to allow a surgeon to carry out procedures that that surgeon is not trained or qualified to do. Furthermore, the surgeon must realize that in the office operating room, the physician is, indeed, "the Captain of the Ship," and is responsible for many things that are taken care of by others in the hospital.

Adequate equipment and supplies for the planned procedure must be available. The surgeon must have instrumentation equal in quality and assortment to that which would be required in the hospital. Sutures, dressings, and medications must be available as required. A patient should never be expected to accept second best because that patient is undergoing office surgery. Furthermore, the surgeon must be equipped to handle any unforeseen situations that might reasonably be expected. This includes the ability to carry out advanced life support without outside assistance. Plans must be made ahead of time to allow for the transfer of patients to a hospital, if required. Transfer agreements with the hospital must be established in advance. There should be a roster of consultants who would be available for specific problems outside the range of the surgeon's expertise.

A thorough preoperative evaluation should be carried out which is adequate to ensure that the patient is in good enough general health to undergo the operation. This may be done by the operating surgeon or by another designated physician. A laboratory evaluation suitable for the requirements of the patient and procedure should be obtained, although this will frequently be less extensive than that required under cookbook regulations of hospitals. Patients must receive adequate counseling so that they will know what they should and should not do before and after the operation.

DESIGNING THE FACILITY

At this point, it would be appropriate to emphasize the value of visiting exiting facilities before embarking on one's own building venture. Textbooks like this will be of help, but there is no substitute for actually spending time at a functioning office outpatient surgical facility. Such a visit will provide an opportunity to evaluate the weaknesses and strengths of various designs. Physicians who have spent the time and effort to build their own surgical centers are proud of what they have accomplished and would welcome visitors for a day or so. During the visit, one should talk to the staff as well as the surgeon and inquire as to adequacy of space and equipment, traffic flow, and convenience. One should not hesitate to ask what problems were not adequately addressed and what would be done differently if the facility were built again.

Of course, one must take into consideration the type of practice for which the building was designed. A facility designed for general otolaryngology would be far different than one designed primarily for cosmetic surgery.

This discussion is based on the design of the operating facility that was part of The Facial Plastic Clinic & Surgical Center built in 1975 and its replacement facility, The

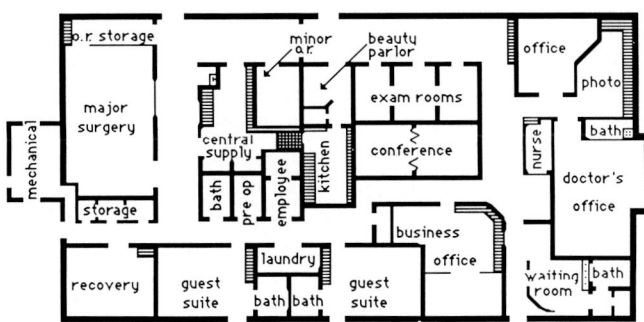

Fig. 26-1. Floor plan of new Facial Plastic & Cosmetic Surgical Center, Completed in 1985.

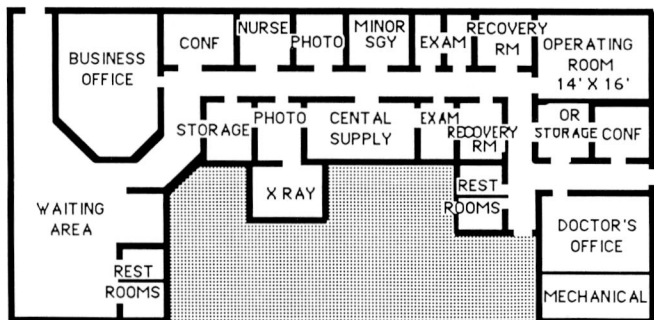

Fig. 26-2. Floor plan of original Facial Plastic & Surgical Center.

Facial Plastic & Cosmetic Surgical Center, constructed in 1984. Although the new facility consists of a totally isolated surgical center, it still exists as a part of a total office complex (Figure 26-1). Physical separation is accomplished through specially constructed fire walls, as stipulated by state code. Such physical separation is not required for accreditation, but very likely will be required for state licensure and Medicare certification. It should be stressed that the new facility has, in no way, expanded the scope of the author's office surgical practice. The changes were largely made for convenience, efficiency, aesthetics, compliance with anticipated regulatory change, and ego gratification.

Figure 26-2 shows the layout of the original clinic, which occupied about 3600 square feet. The operating room (OR), recovery rooms, and OR storage were at the end of a long corridor extending the length of the clinic, but were not isolated from the other areas of the office. Since only one surgeon used the clinic, this created no significant problems, but, in a group practice, more physical separation might be desirable. This could easily have been accomplished by placing a doorway in the corridor just to the left of the two recovery rooms.

OPERATING ROOM SIZE

The operating room size of 14 × 16 feet (Figure 26-3) proved to be quite adequate. The scrub sink was placed in the operating room—a great convenience, but contrary to state code for licensure. Barring legal requirements, it is helpful to have running water in the operating room, although the large scrub sink did prove to impinge on space that would have been otherwise useful. It is amazing how much equipment ends up in the operating room. The new facility has much more storage space than does the old, adjacent to the operating room, which has proven to be a great advantage.

DOORS, WALLS, AND CEILINGS

The doorways should be made wide enough for easy passage, giving consideration to the possible use of stretchers or wheelchairs. Although many patients are ambulatory by

Designing the Facility

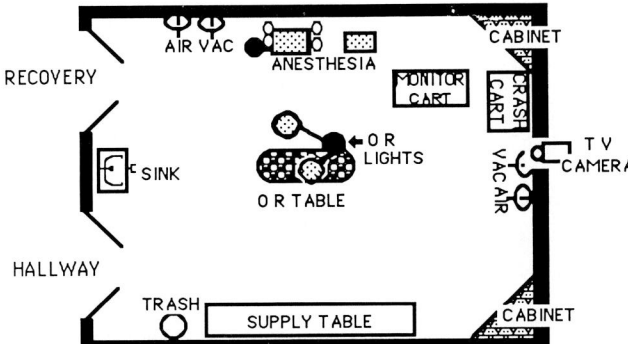

Fig. 26-3. Operating room of original Facial Plastic Clinic & Surgical Center. Note corner cabinets and sink. These have been removed in new operating room, but, otherwise, design has remained essentially the same.

the end of the operation, it is still frequently necessary to transport patients to the recovery area by stretcher. In the previous facility, it was occasionally necessary to carry them—obviously not an ideal situation.

Walls and floors should be durable. A high grade of vinyl wall covering was found to work quite well. In considering floor covering, economics will play a great role, since there is a great range in price and quality. If possible, a high-grade solid floor covering, preferably with some cushioning, is recommended. Scuff resistance is important, as is a no-wax finish.

A standard suspended ceiling with acoustic tile was initially utilized (again, not adequate for a licensed facility) and served quite well, though one should seriously consider the nonporous ceiling tiles, which are easier to clean and probably somewhat more sanitary. They are the type normally found in food-handling establishments. In the new facility, there is a solid ceiling, which is preferable from the standpoint of aesthetics, but somewhat more expensive than a suspended ceiling.

LIGHTS

If ceiling-mounted OR lights are to be installed, adequate structural support will have to be provided. This, of course, is quite variable, depending on the lights chosen. In the first facility, Burton dual flood lights suspended from the ceiling were used, and this was adequate, although the newer multiquartz or multihalogen lighting systems made by Burton (as well as other manufacturers) might be preferable if the surgeon depends heavily on the conventional type of OR lighting. As is true of many surgeons today, the author depends primarily on a head light, and so the type of ceiling light is relatively unimportant. Caution is advised if one is considering the single-source halogen lights, even when used in pairs. The author's facility originally installed these, but had to remove them because of the heavy shadows. The facility has standard Amsco hospital-type OR lights on tracks in the new operating room, having relegated the Burton lights to the minor surgery room.

STORAGE

In the initial operating room, cabinets were built in both corners on one side of the operating room and along the top of the opposite wall above the doorways (not shown in the diagram). An alternative, which the author believes to be preferable, is a solid wall of cabinets and drawers with a countertop at one end of the room. It is the author's opinion that one cannot have too much storage space, and this is probably the major shortcoming in most office surgical facilities. There is now a large storage room next to the operating, room which results in less clutter within the OR.

MEDICAL GASES

An adequate central source of suction is far preferable to individual suction units; it is much quieter and far more convenient. If portable units are to be utilized, one of high capacity should be chosen. The small portable suction units such as the Gomco (which is so familiar in hospital wards) are usually inadequate. With the advent of liposuction surgery, much more powerful units are now on the market that will serve nicely. In fact, during the move between the old and new facilities, the author's group was temporarily without central suction. The Wells Johnson liposuction aspirator served quite well.

Central oxygen was not installed in the first facility, but the author does feel that this would be advantageous, as well as economical, over a long period of time, and it is present in the new surgical center. The facility did have central compressed air, which was used to power the ventilator on the anesthesia machine, although oxygen is now used for this purpose.

ENVIRONMENTAL CONTROL

Special consideration is due to the heating and cooling requirements in the operating room—something that was neglected in the first OR! The temperatures desirable in the operating room are different than for the rest of the clinic, in that generally more air conditioning and less heating is required during surgery. A zone system, with the OR constituting a discrete zone, should work well. The author's group compensated by installing a standard ceiling fan in the OR, and this certainly saved the day, although the author doubts it would be allowed in a licensed facility.

ALTERNATE POWER

Adequate electrical power should be installed on several circuits, so that a failed breaker would not interrupt all of the electricity in the operating room. Grounded plugs, of course, are essential. An alternate source of power is highly desirable. A relatively small generator should suffice, with automatic activation of key circuits in case of power failure. The author's system provided current to the operating lights, a few of the hall lights, and to selected floor and wall plugs in the recovery area as well as the operating room and minor surgery. Since most of the modern office surgery tables are electric, it would be wise to put a floor plug where the plans call for table installation.

RECOVERY

Space dedicated to the recovery area can be conservative. The first facility utilized 2 small recovery rooms, each measuring about 8 × 8 feet. This provided enough room for a patient recliner chair, a chair for an attendant, a small table, and a rolling cart for monitoring equipment. Two of these recovery rooms have proven adequate, although a third, at times, would have been desirable. Occasionally conference rooms were used for recovery of patients. There is now a 3-bed recovery room with curtains separating each area. It has proven more convenient to have all postoperative patients in one area. There is a small preoperative room that can be used as a private recovery room if desired.

A nurse call system is installed so that the patient may be left under the temporary care of a family member who can summon the staff if needed. There is also video monitoring in the recovery room, which allows the staff to keep an eye on the patients, even if the staff is not physically present in the recovery room.

A bathroom should be located close to the operating room. It would be very helpful to have a wide door with uncluttered area around the commode, since patients will frequently need help after surgery. Support railings should be installed on the walls adjacent to the commode, and a "call for help" alarm switch within easy reach is certainly recommended.

Virtually all of the other areas utilized in the original facility were shared with the clinic area. Of special importance was the central supply area which was about 6 × 14 feet and well supplied with counters and cabinets, as well as having 2 sinks and a dishwasher. Although this proved adequate, the staff always felt limited in storage space. Again, the author stresses that it is almost impossible to include too much storage space.

PATIENT ACCESS

Patient access and egress is an important consideration. The original facility required patients to negotiate 3 steps at the back door. Obviously, a ramp would have been preferable. Remember that patients will usually require assistance when leaving and it would be very helpful to be able to negotiate the way easily with a wheelchair.

EQUIPMENT

In the discussion of the design of the office operating suite, reference has already been made to some items of equipment. This section will elaborate on some of those items, as well as mentioning items not already considered. Of course, no effort will be made to consider all of the equipment needed, rather, areas that are of particular importance or which the novice might be likely to overlook will be highlighted.

OPERATING ROOM TABLE

In the past, there was a very limited selection of OR tables for office use. Fortunately, this is no longer the case. Each surgeon should be able to find a table which will be suitable itself to the type of surgery that is to be carried out. The author's group originally did our surgery on a standard exam table with a back that elevated up to about 45°. It was somewhat tedious, but it worked! This is mentioned only to emphasize that some of the more major items of equipment do not have to be purchased right away.

The facility now uses one of the electric contour chair models, which has proven very adequate and reliable. With the advent of liposuction surgery, and with many otolaryngologists now doing body liposuction, it should be noted that the contour chairs are inadequate for this type of work. (The staff now finds itself again using the old exam table!) If an electric table is contemplated, it would be helpful to plan a floor plug adjacent to the site of the table.

AUTOCLAVE

Although the facility now has a full-size, hospital-type autoclave, the staff managed very nicely for years with a small tabletop steam autoclave supplemented by a small tabletop gas autoclave. This latter unit utilized ampules of ethylene oxide. It has proven indispensible for sterilizing many items that would not tolerate steam. Through the use of heavy plastic bags, these units control the escape of the ethylene oxide and are quite safe and effective. One source of this type of equipment is H. W. Anderson Products, Inc.; 11616 Industriplex Boulevard; Baton Rouge, LA 70809.

SUPPLIES AND INSTRUMENTS

Surgeons who plan an office operating room will have already had experience operating in the hospital, and so will have a pretty good idea of the instruments they will be using in their practice. They probably will not be aware of the cost of these instruments. Some discretion must be used in purchasing instruments, but a carpenter is only as good as the tools used. One positive aspect is that instruments will last much longer in a private operating room if they are given the care that they deserve. It is extremely rare for the author's group to replace an instrument.

With experience, one will find that it is possible to set up for cases with far fewer instruments than one is accustomed to using in the hospital, since the set-up will be specifically designed for the individual surgeon. Trays should consist of only those instruments that are likely to be used. Items only used on occasion can be kept sterile and opened when needed.

It is simply astounding how many sources for purchase of supplies can be accumulated. Sometimes, it may prove wiser to select a few general sources to avoid some of the bookkeeping problems that result from multiple accounts. The monthly deluge of bills can be truly overwhelming. However, direct purchasing can, at times, result in significant savings. This, of course, is another advantage of having adequate storage space—it allows shopping in quantity for bargains.

EMERGENCY EQUIPMENT

A major consideration in an office operating room should be the management of emergencies. The fact that emergencies so rarely occur makes it all the more difficult to prepare for them. Adequate equipment must be available. The author's operating room contains, in addition to cardiac and blood pressure monitors, a defibrillator and a readily available ambu bag. As mentioned, there are outlets for oxygen from the central manifold (which, in turn, has automatic switching from 2 banks of cylinders). A Banyon emergency kit (available from Banyon International Corporation) is utilized, which contains a laryngoscope, endotracheal tubes, blood pressure cuff, IV fluid, emergency cut-down tray, and all the usual necessary emergency medications. This kit, with slight modification to suit particular needs, is kept available for emergency use. Medications or supplies are never removed for routine needs, and the kit is restocked whenever used. Periodically, the dated supplies are exchanged for fresh drugs.

Of course, just having the proper equipment is not enough. The office staff should be instructed as to individual responsibilities in an emergency situation. Periodic drills should be used to emphasize each person's role. Everyone should have some designated responsibility—even if it is just to stand by for further instructions.

COMMUNICATION

Unlike the hospital, the operating room will function as a part of the total clinic. Most likely, personnel will be shared. Communication between the OR and the rest of the clinic is important. The author's facility has a telephone in the operating room with a speakerphone attachment to allow hands-off conversation. This is especially useful for obtaining lab reports such as those on frozen sections. In addition, there is an outlet for an electrocardiograph (EKG) machine that is linked to a computer analysis system, which can be used in case of emergency.

Paging is also available over a loudspeaker system so that needed personnel can be summoned, even when their exact location is uncertain. This also allows music throughout the building.

A nurse call system is installed in the recovery room so that patients can summon assistance. Since family is often allowed to stay with patients in the recovery room after the patients have awakened, it is important that family know how to summon help if needed. There is also a nurse call alarm installed in the patient bathroom in the surgical area, which has a distinct buzzer so that one can differentiate this from the routine recovery room call. Finally, a panic alarm can be triggered from the operating room to alert the entire office staff to a potential emergency.

Careful attention to planning communications in the office can result in the surgical unit functioning in a maximally orderly manner, and can save a great deal of wasted time and effort.

PROCEDURES AND ANESTHESIA

Patients undergoing surgery in the office receive preoperative counseling both verbally and through written instructions. The preoperative work-up is individualized on the basis of the patient's age, medical history, and physical exam. Whenever it is deemed advisable, the staff recommends a medical work-up by the patient's family doctor or an internist. Chest x-rays, electrocardiograms with computer analysis, hematocrit, and urinalysis can all be done in the clinic; these constitute the usual preoperative laboratory work-up. Other tests are run by outside laboratories of the patient's choice.

Patients are premedicated, before entering the operating room, with 200 mg of Dramamine (Searle) and 100 mg of Seconol (Lilly), which is given with a small sip of water. This provides adequate relaxation and has almost entirely eliminated the problem of postoperative nausea in these patients. The patient is then escorted to the preoperative room, where the IV is started.

The author's facility has had extensive experience with the use of low-dose Ketalar (Parke-Davis) and Valium (Roche) as an adjunct to local anesthesia,[2] and this is the facility's preferred technique when surgery is carried out under local anesthesia. In these cases, the anesthesia is administered and supervised by the surgeon. Most of the facility's surgery, however, is carried out under general anesthesia, and in these cases, the anesthetic is administered by certified nurse-anesthetists under the direct supervision of the surgeon.

Frequently, surgeons question the liability incurred with the use of nurse-anesthetists as opposed to M.D. anesthesiologists. The author is not aware of any data that would provide an answer to this question, except to state that the carrier that insures the author and his clinic makes no distinction based on the selection of M.D. or nurse anesthesia providers. In some cases, prevailing practice in the community may provide an answer to that question, but usually the choice will be individual, based on availability and the skill and experience of the individuals involved.

Otolaryngologists/head and neck surgeons are in the unique position of having training in the management of airway problems. A large percentage of the calamities involving general anesthesia are directly related to problems with the airway. It behooves all those who operate in their own facilities to maintain their airway management skills regardless of what aspect of the specialty is practiced. These skills, plus an up-to-date knowledge of and experience in advanced cardiopulmonary resuscitation (CPR) should be adequate to initiate treatment for any emergency that might arise.

It goes without saying that the equipment present in the office OR must be completely adequate for the type of anesthesia used. If general anesthesia is used, then, obviously, adequate anesthesia equipment must be provided. Whenever possible, a second back-up unit should be available, since equipment failures will occur, and usually at the most inopportune time. Drugs and gases in suitable amounts and varieties should be on hand for both routine procedures and emergencies. Dated drugs must be watched and replaced as needed.

After surgery, patients are brought to the recovery room by stretcher. As previously mentioned, in the author's past office, the patients were usually walked to the recovery area or brought by wheelchair. It is certainly feasible to do this, but the author's staff has thoroughly enjoyed the wide corridors and doorways in the new facility, which allow transport of the patients while they are lying down. Actually, the stretchers that we use are intensive care unit (ICU) beds. The staff prefers these because of their slightly larger size and softer mattresses. They are much more comfortable than standard stretchers. They are brought into the OR after surgery and the patient is moved over. Patients then stay on these beds until they are ready to leave the recovery room. In most cases, the patients are awake enough after surgery to slide over by themselves. If not, we use a short roller to help move them.

In many cases, the patients are awake enough when they reach the recovery room to allow their families to sit with them. Video monitoring and a call system allow the staff

Designing the Facility

to remain in close supervision without actually sitting by the patient. When patients are fully recovered, as determined by the operating surgeon, they are assisted to their car or to one of the private guest suites.

The inclusion of private living suites within the clinic adds a new dimension to an outpatient surgical center. Much greater flexibility can be added to the services offered. Located in west Texas, as the author's facility is, many of the facility's patients come from great distances. In the past, these people were required to stay in nearby motels for a day or two before and after surgery. Now they can stay in the clinic itself. The suites consist of a hospital-type bed and an additional daybed. Each room contains a small kitchenette with refrigerator and microwave oven. A telephone and television are furnished. In the bathroom is a combination shower-steam bath with handicap railings for security. Each suite has an entrance into the clinic as well as a private entrance to an outside courtyard. At night, the clinic entrance is locked, but the outside access remains open.

The suites are not intended to serve as hospital rooms. Patients are required to have someone stay with them if they are postoperative. Patients are not discharged to the suites if it is felt that hospitalization is indicated. Nevertheless, it obviously much more convenient and comfortable for patients to go to their suites than it would be for them to go home or to a nearby hotel. It is also much more convenient for the surgeon, since the patients can easily be checked the evening of surgery and the following morning. Staying within the clinic also offers the patients a strong sense of security.

ACCREDITATION

In reading this chapter, it has surely become obvious that the most striking feature of office surgery is the change that is constantly occurring. For those who see operating in the office as a means of avoiding red tape and regulation, some reconsideration is unfortunately in order. As surgeons increase their efforts to obtain third-party payment for surgery performed in the office, and especially as they seek payment for the facility as well as their own services, government agencies and insurance companies are taking a new look at these facilities and beginning to impose criteria that must be met if the facility is to qualify for coverage.

At the present time, it is still quite feasible to build an operating room within an office without complying with any regulatory criteria. However, it is quite possible that, in the near future, regulations may be imposed that will impose a certain standard on office operating rooms. At this point, licensure may be prohibitory for most physicians. An alternative is for the operator of the facility to seek accreditation.

Accreditation is available to owners of outpatient surgical facilities or office operating rooms through the Accreditation Association for Ambulatory Health Care, Inc. (AAAHC) Incorporated in 1979 as an offshoot of the Joint Commission on Accreditation of Hospitals, the purpose of the AAAHC is "to organize and operate a peer-based assizement, education, and accreditation program for ambulatory health care organizations as a means of assisting them to provide the highest achievable level of care for recipients in the most efficient and economically sound manner."[3]

Sponsoring organizations of the AAAHC include The American Academy of Facial Plastic and Reconstructive Surgery, Free Standing Ambulatory Surgical Association, Society for Office Based Surgery, and the Outpatient Ophthalmic Surgery Society, among others. This assures that the AAAHC will remain responsive to the needs of those involved in outpatient surgery.

Organizations seeking accreditation begin by writing to AAAHC requesting their Handbook,[3] which will describe the standards that must be met. If the facility feels that it can meet the standards, an accreditation survey will be scheduled. Surveyors are physicians, dentists, nurses, and administrators who are chosen and trained by the AAAHC. Surveyors are all volunteers who are actively involved with ambulatory care, thus assuring that they are in touch with the problems faced by the facility. Each survey is tailored to the type of facility being visited. The results of the survey are reviewed with the organization and then forwarded to AAAHC, after which a decision is made regarding accreditation. The organization can receive approval for 1 year or 3 years, or approval can be deferred or denied based on deficiencies discovered during the evaluation. If an organization is unsure regarding whether it could comply with the requirements of AAAHC, it can request a consultative evaluation. This type of survey allows the organization to seek assistance in preparing for accreditation. Problems are identified and recommendations are made for improvement, but no decision is made regarding accreditation.

At the present time, accreditation often makes it much easier to obtain reimbursement from insurance companies. In the case of CHAMPUS, for example, accreditation by AAAHC ensures coverage if the organization is otherwise in compliance with CHAMPUS regulations. It appears likely that in the future, accreditation will be important both for licensure and Medicare reimbursement. Of equal importance is the fact that, by achieving accreditation, the organization or facility assures itself and its patients that it is committed to the highest possible standards of care. With office operating rooms being outside of the usual bounds of peer review, this takes on increasing importance.

REFERENCES

1. Establishing Freestanding Ambulatory Surgery Centers. Chicago: American Medical Association, 1982
2. Tobin HA: Low-dose ketamine and diazepam. Arch Otolaryngol 108:439–440, 1982
3. Accreditation Handbook for Ambulatory Health Care—1985 ed. Skokie, IL: Accreditation Association for Ambulatory Health Care, Inc.,

John V. Barto
Carol H. Stewart

27
The Computer for Business

In addition to the many professional requirements of a newly established medical practice, the implementation of sound procedures to control the business aspect of the office is essential. The basic responsibility of the bookkeeping or administrative staff is to maintain a good cash flow. This includes billing the patients properly, the control and collection of patient balances, verifying the payment of expenses and performing all remaining clerical functions, too numerous to mention. This chapter will address the use of the computer to assist in the control and organization of the business office.

The major advantage of a computer is its capacity to store and remember large amounts of information and to recall and present this information quickly. Another advantage is the computer's ability to update (effect) multiple files simultaneously, i.e., the billing, history, recall, and service analysis files. In addition to reducing space requirements, the computer could, as the practice grows, reduce the need to employ additional staff. Also, the stored patient demographic data, accounts receivable balances, and other information will be copied daily onto disks or magnetic tape for storage in another location to ensure office continuity in case of fire or other disaster. A well-thought-out administrative computer installation will enable the staff to maintain daily accounting control.

There are two predominant ways in which a computer system can be integrated into the business office. First, the office may use a leased work station and printer. This remote system is connected to a main computer data bank located off-site at a service bureau. This arrangement, while requiring a relatively low investment, usually limits administrative flexibility and managerial control. The other method locates the computer hardware in the office. Hence, it is always available for more effective use. An in-house computer presents the opportunity to continually add new applications or enhance existing ones. The installation of an in-house computer would require a greater initial investment, but would eventually present a payback not available with a leased remote system.

The placement of a computer into an established office with firmly rooted procedures may require a different approach than the installation for a new practice. Most important in the established office, the computer applications must parallel current basic methods. This installation could potentially replace a manual system which maintains thousands of billing cards and the hand entries needed to control the proper account balances.

The decision to install an in-house computer system involves many considerations. Assistance should be sought, and most often will come from an accountant in addition to a computer specialist. The accountant will help establish the method of accounts receivable control most suitable for a particular practice and will also offer advice regarding the proper way to control cash, bank deposits, billing, and accounts payable. The computer specialist will assist in determining the proper type of computer, the required storage capacity, the number of work stations, and expansion necessary for practice growth and the addition of other applications. Together, these two consultants should establish the proper methods, procedures, and controls to efficiently and effectively manage the office. The objective, once these items are established, is for the office to run smoothly with a minimum of supervision and follow-up.

It is not necessarily a requirement that the physician know in detail all the ramifications of a successful computer installation. But being knowledgeable, in general, of what is involved will develop confidence. In addition, the physician will be able to introduce personal requirements of the system, e.g., a monthly analysis of the services performed, diagnoses, billings, and collections. Having the physician involved in the design or selection of the layout of the patient bill and monthly patient statement is essential. This will guarantee, for example, that all information necessary for insurance purposes is included. Also, the patient statement cycle should be considered, with input from the accountant and office staff. A properly thought-out system will produce the data needed by the accountant to verify the proper treatment of all billing, cash, and credit adjustment entries. A check and balance of the operation will maintain the doctor's confidence in the office personnel.

Prior to making a decision regarding the purchase and installation of a computer, and in order to limit future misunderstandings, a number of questions should be satisfactorily answered by the computer consultant and the software and hardware vendor. Some of these should be included in a contract with the software (programming) vendor and others with the hardware (computer) manufacturer. A typical listing of considerations might include:

1. Equipment maintenance—on-site? How quickly? Cost of different types?
2. Similar models in the area to use in case of an emergency
3. Special electrical requirements
4. How much additional work would the conversion or start-up require of the office staff? How much interruption?
5. Are the programs flexible? Can they be modified or altered to accommodate procedural changes? Can they be enhanced locally?
6. Can the computer and programs operate in a multi-task environment? Simultaneous jobs from different work stations?
7. Are the internal data files expandable to allow for additional professional staff?
8. Does the program allow for the integration and addition of a new module, i.e., accounts payable?

The Computer for Business

9. Can the programs and data files be easily copied for storage in another location?
10. How many patients and visits will the system accommodate on-line at one time?
11. Who will be responsible for form design?
12. Exactly what does training and installation consist of? How many hours and where?
13. Should you perform the major functions, such as billing, using both the old method and the computer for a period of time?
14. Will the installation of a new computer require staff reorganization?
15. What type of warranty is offered on the operation of the programs?
16. On-line printer speed; this is based on the amount of printing required
17. Does the patient billing form allow ample space to print the multiple diagnoses and the more detailed procedure descriptions now required by insurance companies? To be sure, a billing sample should be reviewed by the claims department of one of the major carriers.

If possible, it would be very beneficial to visit an office that is currently in operation with the system under consideration. Include a member of your staff to observe what is necessary for inputing data, retrieving historical information, and other daily operations. Be sure to ask if the system is menu driven and actually go through the steps needed to seek and perform a repetitive function. Notice the noise level of the printer, so that the best location for its operation can be determined. This will avoid any unnecessary annoyance to your patients. Review the way in which diagnoses and procedural information are communicated to the billing clerk. Determine what is involved in the preparation of the patient billing. Find out if there is a line of patients at the front desk under normal conditions. It would also be beneficial if you could observe the operation of the bookkeeper to better understand the responsibilities of business control.

For the most part, it is not necessary to employ a computer specialist on the staff. Most employees will, with little difficulty, learn and operate the repetitive daily or weekly operations. However, if there is an employee with a particular interest and a high level of comprehension concerning the logic of the system's operation, it would be helpful to make available instruction either from one of the vendors or a local continuing education course. This could save on consultant fees and eliminate confusion.

As soon as the discussion of a potential computer purchase reaches the staff, some anxiety and fear could develop. This could not only affect the current operation but could greatly hamper the future computer installation. Therefore, try to include as many staff as possible in the initial discussion. Staff who have given suggestions, or other input, into the decisionmaking process will feel like part of the entire installation and become very instrumental in its success.

Discipline within the computer operation is also very important to its continued success. Daily, the total dollar value of all input and data files should be compared to a manual balance total to ensure proper function and input. Input edits should be listed and stored for future use and data file copies should be made without fail. Be sure that new employees are trained before being allowed to operate the equipment. This will develop confidence, in addition to minimizing an inadvertent destruction of data.

There are many jobs a computer can efficiently perform for the office. The following is a listing of many such reports and operations. One must remember that not all are necessary and some will work better than others, depending upon the requirements. Some offices will have a particular need for some of the applications and some will have no need at all. Also, it would be to your benefit to have a good understanding prior to the first conversations with a software vendor.

The applications are classified into 2 groupings. The primary grouping lists those items necessary for office cash control. The secondary grouping lists those items not necessary for an initial installation, but which could be considered beneficial at a later time.

PRIMARY APPLICATIONS AND REPORTS

Daily Patient Billing

At some point, patient visit data must be entered into the computer. If this can be accomplished at the secretary's desk at the time of the visit, the encounter form will not have to be handled twice, i.e., to create a manual billing document and then later to enter the data into the computer. In addition, a computer-created billing does not require any calculation and will be presented in an organized fashion.

Accounts Receivable Report

This report summarizes and lists all patients who have not completely paid their bills. It can show the telephone number, address of the guarantor, and the date and amount of the last payment. Its total should indicate the amount in arrears that is overdue by 30 days, 60 days, etc.

Delinquency Report

The purpose of this list, which is much the same as the accounts receivable report, is to segregate those patients who owe amounts overdue by more than 60 days, and hence need special attention.

Service Analysis

An itemization of the number of diagnoses and procedures performed is presented for analysis monthly. It can show totals by location and different staff doctors. This information can easily be given to your accountant in this form for tax purposes.

Patient Statements

These reminders are sent to all patients monthly to encourage payment of outstanding bills. They can show payments recorded this month and additional procedures that have been included. Statements can be selected so as not to be sent to various city, state, or federal agencies.

Cash and Adjustment Lists

These listings present a hard copy of all cash received and adjustments applied to open accounts. The cash total should balance to the sum of the cash received in the mail and the cash received at the time of visits. This total should then agree with the amount deposited in the bank. It is good practice to have one office person record and total the mail payments. A second person should apply the cash to open accounts and deposit the money. Periodically, all accounts receivable adjustments, i.e., insurance only, professional courtesy, employee visits, should be reviewed for authenticity.

Patient History

This itemization will present a review of all diagnoses, procedures, payments, and account adjustments for each patient. It will indicate the date, the visit number, the doctor, and the location of the encounter.

SECONDARY APPLICATIONS

Recall Listings

This weekly or monthly reminder can list those patients due for another visit. It can show name, address, telephone number, and a code for the visit purpose. Also, mailing labels could be prepared for post-reminders.

Office Scheduling

Some offices may be able to use the computer to schedule office visits. When an appointment is made, the name and date could be keyed into the computer. Daily, a listing of scheduled appointments would be run to prepare the patient's chart for the visit.

Referring Physician Reports

Doctors may wish to accumulate data by referring physician. This can be done by keying into the machine a code for each referring physician and later printing a summarization.

Accounts Payable

This computer module will summarize all office vendor payments by an expense account number, will print checks, list a check register, and store the data to assist the monthly check reconciliation. Listings can be presented monthly indicating exactly what the checks were for and to whom they were made out. A monthly office profit and loss statement could be prepared by combining this module with the monthly service analysis. These statements could be presented to the accountant for analysis and audit.

Office Payroll

The many requirements of the office payroll could be prepared on a computer. Data for federal and state reports could be prepared. Payroll checks and a payroll register would also be listed. The office payroll might best be prepared and maintained by a bank or another service bureau. It would be good to look into each method.

Before investing in a system for an otolaryngological office, one should determine exactly what the system and program can do. The program should include additional features that are necessary to operate a successful otolaryngological office.

A well-thought-out program might include these features:

1. Detailed specification listing of complicated otolaryngological procedures as required by most insurance companies. Do *not* just list ENG or site lesion audiological testing.
2. Ability to separate and credit payments to separate doctors if practicing in a group with productivity incentive.
3. Ability to apply payments to the earliest charge or to divide the payments to separate doctors if there are 2 visits on the same date and the patient consulted 2 physicians.
4. At the same time, the program must be flexible enough to be able to apply payments as requested by a patient and not necessarily follow item 3 above.
5. Conformity to the various Health Maintenance Organization (HMO) requirements. Each HMO has different fee schedules, different formats for reimbursement, and different time limits for filing claims. HMOs require proper submission of claims and within specific time frames before payment. Be sure the program can assist in the initial billing and be able to follow up at a later date if no payment is received. Also, with HMOs one must be able to produce a printout listing each claim and show the percentage of reimbursement at the end of the year. This will enable the office to recoup any risk-pool money due if the HMO should show a profit.
6. Ability to apply professional courtesy adjustments while maintaining the normal charges on the original bill. The first copy—the insurance copy—would not show the professional courtesy adjustment. The second copy—the patient's copy—would show the courtesy adjustment.
7. In the case of HMO billing or the courtesy adjustment, the full amount of the bill due should be posted to the Accounts Receivable in the program, yet the program should flag the account to accept insurance only. When the insurance payment is received, the program will cancel the remaining balance.
8. Ability to allow the office manager to enter into the program immediately to correct errors (e.g., to change an incorrect payment code entered in error). A printout will automatically be produced at the end of every business day showing all changes made for that day. This will allow you to review all corrections daily.
9. Ability to provide a profile on new physicians, along with the percentage of collectibles on patients they treated and billed. This information is used in administering their salary.

In closing, it must be said that even the best and most expensive systems will be worthless if the program cannot be adapted to your office's particular needs. The program should work in accordance with your office style, not the other way around.

By investing in a custom-designed program, your office will not lose the personal touch that is important in successfully treating your patients.

Index

Page numbers in *italics* indicate illustrations.
Page numbers followed by *t* indicate tables.

ABR. *See* Auditory brainstem response
Abrasion, corneal, complicating blepharoplasty, 146
Accounts payable, computer for, 319
Accounts receivable report, computer for, 318
Accreditation for outpatient surgical facility, 313–314
Acne scars
  chemical peel for, 80
  collagen injections for, 122
Acoustic neurinoma, 16
Advancement flap, 98
Age, ABR outcome and, 239
Aid, hearing, 267–275. *See also* Hearing aid(s)
Air-blowing test in preoperative evaluation for voice restoration, 185–186
Airflow obstruction, chronic, ventilation in, 253–294
Airway
  extrathoracic, obstruction of, flow volume curve in, 288–289
  upper, obstruction of, flow volume curve in, 288
Allergen immunotherapy, 222–226. *See also* Immunotherapy
Allergen screening
  with multiple-allergen discs, 221
  with RAST, 221, 222*t*
Allergic drug reactions complicating fiberoptic esophagoscopy, 59
Allergic response to collagen, 123–124
Allergic rhinitis
  diagnosis of, 216–217
    laboratory in, 217–222
    radioallergosorbent test in, 218–222. *See also* Radioallergosorbent test (RAST)
  immunotherapy for, 222–226. *See also* Immunotherapy for allergic rhinitis
Allergic rhinosinusitis, 12
Allergy
  immunotherapy for, 212–213
  modified RAST and, 215–226. *See also* Radioallergosorbent test (RAST), modified
  skin testing for, 207–214
    equipment for, 207
    patient selection and preparation for, 208
    preparation of trays for, 207–208
    responses to
      abnormal, 211–213
      normal, 210–211
    serial dilution titration technique of, 208–210
Alveolar-arterial (A-a) gradient, 291
Alveolar ventilation, carbon dioxide tensions and, 291
Anesthesia
  for blepharoplasty, 138–139
  for carbon dioxide laser, 194–195
  local, for head and neck examination, 1
  for outpatient surgical facility, 311–313
Angina, Ludwig's, 14
Anterior rhinomanometry, 277–278
Antihelical fold, lack of, 4–5
Arrhythmias, cardiac, complicating chemical peel, 86

Arterial oxygen tension, changes in, 291–293
Arteriol-venous fistulas complicating hair transplantation, 115
Aspiration pneumonia complicating fiberoptic esophagoscopy, 59
Asthma, flow volume curve in, 287
Auditory brainstem response (ABR), 229–244
  administration of test for, 242–243
  amplifier in, 236
  clinical applications of, 243–244
  equipment for, 235–238
    investment in, reasons for, 230
    selection of, 237–238
  hearing aids and, 244
  history of, 229–230
  infant, 235
  interpretation of, 231–235
  monitoring techniques for, 244
  outcome of, factors influencing, 238–243
  preamplifier in, 236
  preparation for, 240–242
  sensitivity of, 243–244
  signal averager in, 237
  stimulation system in, 236
  terminology for, 229
Augmentation malarplasty, buccal fat extraction with, 170–171
Augmentation mentoplasty, cervico-facial lipo-suction with, *162, 163, 164*
Auscultation of neck masses, 7
Autoclave for outpatient surgical facility, 310

Backer's formula for facial peel, 81
Baldness
  hair transplantation for, 103–117. *See also* Hair, transplantation of
  male-pattern, classification of, 105t
Barrett's epithelium, fiberoptic esophagoscopy for, 57
Basal cell carcinoma of skin, cryosurgery for, 203
Bell's palsy, 16
Billing, daily patient, computer for, 318
Bilobed flap, 99
Blaise-Raphael voice prosthesis, insertion of, *186, 187,* 188–190
Bleeding
  complicating blepharoplasty, 145–146
  complicating hair transplantation, 114–115
  esophageal, complicating fiberoptic esophagoscopy, 59

Blepharochalasis, 135
Blepharoplasty, 135–147
  anatomy for, 136
  anesthesia for, 138–139
  complications of, 145–147
  for eyebrow ptosis and eyelid ptosis, 137
  lower eyelid tone and, 137–138
  lower lid, 142–144
  photographic projections for, 25t
  postoperative care in, 144–145
  preoperative evaluation for, 136
  surgical techniques for, 139–144
  upper lid, 139–142
Blindness complicating blepharoplasty, 146
Blood gases in pulmonary function testing, 291–294
Broken line geometric closure in scar revision, 97
Bronchitis, chronic, flow volume curve in, 287
Bronchoscopy, fiberoptic, 41–45
  care of equipment for, 42
  clinical examination and laboratory evaluation before, 42–43
  complications of, 45
  indications for, 42
  procedure for, 43–45
  types of, 41–42
  use of, 41
Brymill unit for cryosurgery, 201
Buccal fat pad, lipo-suction for, 167–171
Burns, reconstructive hair transplantation after, 114
Business, computer, 315–320. *See also* Computer for business

Cameras, video, for videolaryngoscopy, 65–66
CAMERAS pneumonic, 20
Cannula for cervical-facial lipo-suction, 151–152
Carbon dioxide laser, 191–198
  anesthesia for, 194–195
  basic concepts of, 191–192
  complications of, 196–197
  informed consent for, 195
  instrumentation for, 195–196
  laser unit for, selection of, 192
  patient selection for, 193–194
  room organization for, 193
Carbon dioxide tensions, alveolar ventilation and, 291

Index

Carcinoma
  basal cell, of skin, cryosurgery for, 203
  in-situ, of larynx, cryosurgery for, 202
  squamous cell, of skin, cryosurgery for, 203
Cardiac arrhythmias complicating chemical peel, 86
Cartilage splitting otoplasty, 130–132
Cash and adjustment lists, computer for, 318–319
Cervical-facial changes, nature of, 151
Cervical-facial lipo-suction, 149–183. *See also* Lipo-suction, cervical-facial
Chemical peel, 79–87
  complications of, 86
  indications for, 79–80
  patient selection for, 80
  postoperative instructions after, 85
  procedure for, 81–84
Choanal polyp, 12
Cholesteatoma, 8
Coaxial illumination for head and neck examination, 1
Cochlear hearing loss, auditory brainstem response in, 234
Collagen injection, 119–124
  adverse reaction to, 123–124
  implantation techniques for, 120–122
  materials for, 119
  patient selection for, 119–120
Communication for outpatient surgical facility, 311
Computer for business, 315–320
  introduction to, 316–318
  in-house vs. remote, 315
  primary applications and reports of, 318–319
  program for, 320
  secondary applications of, 319–320
Conductive hearing loss
  auditory brainstem response in, 233
  testing for, 9
Consent
  informed, for carbon dioxide laser, 195
  photographic, 26
Contractures, scar, z-plasty for, 95–96
Corneal abrasion complicating blepharoplasty, 146
Cranial nerves, examination of, 15–17
Cryobiology, 199–200
Cryosurgery, 199–205
  apparatus for, 201, *202, 203*
  for benign oral pathology, 202
  clinical applications of, 200
  for head malignancy, 204
  for laryngeal pathology, 202
  for nasal pathology, 201
  for neck malignancy, 204
  for skin malignancy, 203–204
  therapeutic applications of, 201–204
Cyst(s)
  dermoid, nasal, 11
  thyroglossal duct, 7

Dacryocystitis, 13
Delinquency reports, computer for, 318
Demerol for fiberoptic esophagoscopy, 54
Dental occlusion in head and neck examination, 4
Dermabrasion, 87–91
  complications of, 90–91
  indications for, 87
  periorbital, 89
  postoperative course of, 89
  postoperative instructions after, 89–90
  precautions for, 88
  preoperative preparation for, 88–89
  procedure for, 87–88
Dermatochalasis, 136
Dermoid cyst, nasal, 11
Diabetes mellitus, external otitis in, 8
Diagnosis, physical, of head and neck, 1–17
  external examination in, 2–8
    anatomy in, 3
    inspection, 2–5
    lymphatic drainage pattern in, 6–7
    morphology in, 4
    neck masses in, 7
    palpation in, 508
    salivary glands in, 6
    sinuses in, 5
    skin in, 4
    submandibular glands in, 5–6
    symmetry in, 4
    thyroid gland in, 7–8
  internal examination in, 8–17
    of cranial nerves, 15–17
    of ear, 8–11
    epistaxis in, 13
    of larynx, 15
    of nose, 11–12
    of oral cavity, 14
    of sinuses, 12–13
Diffusion in pulmonary function testing, 289, 291

Dimpling, skin, complicating cervical-facial lipo-suction, 180–181
Dizziness, evaluation of, 10
Dressing(s)
  for cervico-facial fat extraction with augmentation mentoplasty, 164
  for dermabrasion, 89
  for jowl fat pad extraction, 161
  for submental fat pad extraction, 157, 159
Drugs, allergic reactions to, complicating fiberoptic esophagoscopy, 59

Ear(s)
  examination of, 8–11
  foreign body removal from, 74–75
  lop deformities of, otoplasty for, 125–133. See also Otoplasty
Ectropion, postoperative, complicating blepharoplasty, 147
Edema
  after facial peel, 83
  complicating hair transplantation, 115
Electronystagmography (ENG), 247–266
  equipment for, 247–249
  interpretation of, 258–266
    abnormal evaluation in, 259
    for central or peripheral abnormality, 259
    for peripheral lesion, 261
  nonroutine testing in, 256–257
  preparation of tracing in, 257–258
  technical staff for, 249
  testing routine for, 249–256
Emergency equipment for outpatient surgical facility, 310–311
Emphysema, flow volume curve in, 287
Endoscopy of eustachian tube, 37
Endotracheal tube, ignition of, complicating carbon dioxide laser, 197
ENG. See Electronystagmography
Enophthalmos complicating blepharoplasty, 146
Environmental control for outpatient surgical facility, 308
Epiphora complicating blepharoplasty, 146
Epistaxis, evaluation of, 13
Eipthelium, Barrett's, fiberoptic esophagoscopy for, 57
Esophagitis, fiberoptic esophagoscopy for, 57
Esophagoscopy, fiberoptic, 49–60
  advantages of, 49–50
  for benign esophageal conditions, 55–57
  complications of, 59
  contraindications to, 54t
  examination procedure for, 53–55
  indications for, 53
  for malignant esophageal conditions, 57, 58t
  prophylaxis for, 60t
  requirements for, 50–53
  therapeutic options with, 58–59
Esophagus
  bleeding from, complicating fiberoptic esophagoscopy, 59
  conditions of
    benign, fiberoptic esophagoscopy for, 55–57
    malignant, fiberoptic esophagoscopy for, 57, 58t
  perforation of, complicating fiberoptic esophagoscopy, 59
  strictures of
    dilatation of, fiberoptic esophagoscopy in, 58–59
    fiberoptic esophagoscopy for, 57
  varices of, fiberoptic esophagoscopy for, 57
Ethmoid sinusitis, 12–13
Eustachian tube, endoscopy of, 37
Exostosis of external auditory canal, 8
Eyebrow ptosis, blepharoplasty for, 137
Eyelid(s)
  lower
    blepharoplasty for, 142–144
    tone of, evaluation of, for blepharoplasty, 137–138
  plastic surgery of, 135–147. See also Blepharoplasty
  ptosis of, blepharoplasty for, 137
  upper, blepharoplasty for, 139–142

Face superficial anatomy of, 150
Face peel, procedure for, 81–82
Facial flap(s), 97–102
  advancement, 98
  bilobed, 99
  glabellar, 100–101, 102
  island, 101–102
  local, replacement of skin loss with, 97–98
  midline forehead, 101
  nasolabial, 98–99
  in O-Z closure, 100
  rhomboid, 99–100
  rotation, 98
Facial paralysis, 16–17

Index

Familial hemorrhagic telangiectasia, surgery for, 201
Fatty tissue
  removal of, from face and neck, 149–183. *See also* Lipo-suction, cervical-facial
  structure of, 150
Fiberoptic bronchoscopy, 41–45. *See also* Bronchoscopy, fiberoptic
Fiberoptic esophagoscopy, 49–60. *See also* Esophagoscopy, fiberoptic
Fiberoptic nasopharyngolaryngoscopy, 31–40. *See also* Nasopharyngolaryngoscopy, fiberoptic
Fiberoptic nasopharyngoscope for head and neck examination, 2
Fiberoscope(s)
  care of, 38
  flexible, for videolaryngoscopy, 64
Fiberscopic videolaryngoscopy (transnasal), 67–68, 68–69
  and telescopic videolaryngoscopy, comparison of, 65t
Film, color, in medical photography, 21
Fish-scaling technique of otoplasty, 125–130
Fistula, arteriol-venous, complicating hair transplantation, 115
Fistula test, 11
Flaps, facial, 97–102. *See also* Facial flap(s)
Flash response in allergy skin testing, 211, *212*
Flexible fiberscopes for videolaryngoscopy, 64
Flow volume curve in pulmonary function testing, 286–289
Food impactions, esophageal, removal of, fiberoptic esophagoscopy in, 58
Forehead flap, midline, 101
Foreign body(ies)
  esophageal, removal of, fiberoptic esophagoscopy in, 58
  removal of
    from ear, 74–75
    instruments for, 76, 77
    from nose, 73–74
    from throat, 75
Frontal sinusitis, 13

Gases
  blood, in pulmonary function testing, 291–294
  medical, for outpatient surgical facility, 308
Gastrointestinal endoscopy areas, establishment of, guidelines for, 50–53

Gender, ABR outcome and, 239
Glabellar flap, 100–101, *102*
Gland(s)
  salivary, palpation of, 5–6
  submandibular, palpation of, 5–6
Glomus jugulare tumor, 17
Grafts, mini, for hair transplantation, 112–113
Granulation tissue complicating hair transplantation, 115

Hair
  growth of, failure of, complicating hair transplantation, 115
  transplantation of, 103–117
    complications of, 114–115
    donor site for, 107–109
    mini grafts in, 112–113
    patient selection for, 104–106
    photographic projections for, 25t
    postoperative procedures for, 112
    preoperative tasks in, 107
    recipient site for, 110–112
    reconstructive, after burns of, 114
    scalp reduction and, 113–114
Head
  malignancy of, cryosurgery for, 204
  and neck, physical diagnosis of, 147. *See also* Diagnosis, physical, of head and neck
Hearing aid(s)
  auditory brainstem response and, 244
  costs of, 273
  dispensing, 267–275
    background on, 267–268
    equipment for, 268
    follow-up visits in, 272–273
    hearing aid evaluation in, 270–271
    hearing aid orientation in, 271–272
    otological examination, 269–270
    personnel for, 268–269
  repair of, 273–274
Hearing loss
  conductive
    auditory brainstem response in, 233
    testing for, 9
  sensorineural, testing for, 9
Hematoma
  complicating cervical-facial lipo-suction, 182
  orbital, complicating blepharoplasty, 146
Hemorrhage. *See* Bleeding
Hemorrhagic telangiectasia, familial, cryosurgery for, 201

Hernia, hiatal, fiberoptic esophagoscopy for, 56–57
Herpes simplex, oral, cryosurgery for, 202
Herpetic infection
  complicating chemical peel, 86
  complicating dermabrasion, 91
Hiatal hernia, fiberoptic esophagoscopy for, 56–57
Hourglass reaction in allergy skin testing, 212, *213*
Hyperpigmentation
  chemical peel for, 80
  complicating chemical peel, 86
  dermabrasion for, 87, 90
Hypopigmentation
  complicating chemical peel, 86
  complicating dermabrasion, 90

Illumination, coaxial, for head and neck examination, 1
Immunotherapy, 212–213
  for allergic rhinitis
    effectiveness of, 223
    length of, 226
    preparation of individual patient treatment set vials for, 225
    preparation of serially-diluted stock solutions for, 224–225
    prognosis for, 226
    RAST-based, 223–224
    results of, 225–226
Implantation techniques for collagen injection, 120–122
Infants, auditory brainstem response in, 235
Infection(s)
  complicating fiberoptic esophagoscopy, 59
  complicating hair transplantation, 115
  herpetic
    complicating chemical peel, 86
    complicating dermabrasion, 91
Injection, collagen, 119–124. *See also* Collagen injection, 119–124
Inspection in head and neck examination, 2–5
Instruments
  for foreign body removal, *76, 77*
  for outpatient surgical facility, 310
Intensity, ABR outcome and, 238
Island flap, 101–102

Jowl fat pad, lipo-suction for, *158*, 159–161

Keratosis
  chemical peel for, 80
  dermabrasion for, 87
Keratosis obturans, 8

Laryngectomy, total, voice restoration after, 185–190. *See also* Voice restoration
Laryngoscope
  for head and neck examination, 2
  for videolaryngoscopy, 64–65
Larynx
  examination of, 15
  pathology of, cryosurgery for, 202
Laser, carbon dioxide, 191–198. *See also* Carbon dioxide laser
Leukoplakia, 14
  intraoral, cryosurgery for, 202
Lichen planus, 14
Light source(s)
  for fiberoptic nasopharyngolaryngoscopy, 33, *34*
  for outpatient surgical facility, 307
  for videolaryngoscopy, 66
Lipo-suction, cervical-facial, 149–183
  cannula for, 151–152
  complications of, 180–182
  concepts of, 151–152
  equipment for, 152–153, *154*
  fatty tissue structure for, 150
  preoperative consultation for, 153–156
  preoperative preparation for, *154*, 156
  superficial anatomy for, 150
  techniques of, 157–180
    with augmentation mentoplasty, *162, 163*–164
    for buccal fat pad, 167–171
    for jowl fat pad, *158*, 159–161
    for melolabial mound extraction, 165–167
    with rhytidectomy, 172–180, *181*
    for sad pad, 171–172
    for submental fat pad, *155, 156*, 157–159
    for total neck extraction, *160*, 161–162
Lop ear deformities, otoplasty for, 125–133. *See also* Otoplasty
Ludwig's angina, 14
Lung(s)
  compliance of, in pulmonary function testing, 289, *290*
  diffusing capacity of, 289, 291
  diseases of, restrictive, flow volume curve in, 287

Lymphatic drainage in head and neck examination, 6–7

Machida ENT-4L (or 3L) flexible nasopharyngolaryngoscope, 31–33, 64
Magnification in medical photograpy, 22–23
Malarplasty, augmentation, buccal fat extraction with, 176–181
Malignancy
  esophageal, fiberoptic esophagoscopy for, 57, 58t
  head, cryosurgery for, 204
  neck, cryosurgery for, 204
  oral, cryosurgery for, 204
  skin, cyrosurgery for, 203–204
Medical gases for outpatient surgical facility, 308
Medical photography, 18–28. *See also* Photography office
Melolabial mound extraction, lipo-suction for, 165–167
Mentoplasty, augmentation, cervico-facial lipo-suction with, *162*, 163–164
Milia
  complicating chemical peel, 86
  complicating dermabrasion, 90
Mini grafts for hair transplantation, 112–113
Mirrors for head and neck examination, 1
Mucocele of sphenoid sinus, 13

Nasal airway resistance, determining, rhinomanometry in, 277–283. *See also* Rhinomanometry
Nasal polyp, 12
Nasal resistance measurements, interpretation of, 280–282
Nasolabial flap, 98–99
Nasopharyngolaryngoscope, flexible, Machida ENT-4L (or 3L), 31–33, 64
Naso-pharyngo Laryngoscope, flexible,/Wolf, 32
Nasopharyngolaryngoscopy, fiberoptic, 31–40
  advantages of, 38–39
  anatomic structures seen during, 36
  care of fiberscope in, 38
  clinical applications of, 37–38
  disadvantages of, 39
  documentation in, 39
  equipment for, 31–33
  for head and neck examination, 2

preparation for, 33–34
technique of, 34–37
Neck
  fat extraction from, lipo-suction for, *160*, 161–162
  and head, physical diagnosis of, 1–17. *See also* Diagnosis, physical, of head and neck
  malignancy of, cryosurgery for, 204
  masses of, palpation of, 7
  superficial anatomy of, 150
Neonates, auditory brainstem response in, 235
Nerve(s)
  cranial, examination of, 15–17
  injury to, complicating cervical lipo-suction, 182
Neurinoma, acoustic, 16
Nose
  examination of, 11–12
  foreign body removal from, 73–74
  obstruction of, clinical evaluation of, rhinomanometry in, 279–280
  pathology of, cryosurgery for, 201
Numbness complicating hair transplantation, 115
Nystagmus, 10–11
  electronystagmography for, 247–266. *See also* Electronystagmography

Occlusion, dental, in head and neck examination, 4
Office payroll, computer for, 319
Office scheduling, computer for, 319
Olympus ENF-P flexible rhinolaryngofiberscopic, 31–33, 64
Olympus fiberoptic bronchoscopes, 42
Operating room, size of, for outpatient surgical facility, 306
Operating room table for outpatient surgical facility, 309–310
Oral cavity
  examination of, 14
  malignancy of, cryosurgery for, 204
  pathology of, benign, cryosurgery for, 202
Otitis, external, 8
Otolaryngological group practice, development and management of outpatient surgical facility in office of, 295–301. *See also* Surgical facility, outpatient
Otologic examination, 10

Otoplasty, 125–133
  cartilage splitting, 130–132
  fish-scaling technique for, 125–130
  photographic projections for, 25t
Oversedation complicating fiberoptic esophagoscopy, 59
Oxygen tension, arterial, changes in, 291–293
O-Z closure, 100

Palpation in head and neck examination, 5–8
Papillomatosis, laryngeal, cryosurgery for, 202
Paralysis, facial, 16–17
Patient billing, daily, computer for, 318
Patient history, computer for, 319
Patient statements, computer for, 318
Payroll, office, computer for, 319
Peel, chemical, 79–87. See also Chemical peel
Pendulum nystagmus, 10–11
Perforation, esophageal, complicating fiberoptic esophagoscopy, 59
Photography, office, 19–28
  accessories in, 24–26
  adjustments in, 21–22
  basic steps in, 27
  color film in, 21
  conclusion on, 27–28
  developing skills in, 20
  equipment in, 23
  magnification in, 22–23
  reasons for, 19–20
  reproduction in, 23–24
  standards in, 26
  views for, 24, 25t
Physician reports, referring, computer for, 319
Plastic surgery, facial, photographic projections for, 25t
Plateau response in allergy skin testing, 211–212
Pneumonia, aspiration, complicating fiberoptic esophagoscopy, 59
Polarity, ABR outcome and, 238
Polyp(s)
  choanal, 12
  nasal, 12
Positional vertigo, 11
Posterior rhinomanometry, 278–279
Power, alternate, for outpatient surgical facility, 308
Prosthesis, voice, Blaise-Raphael, insertion of, 186, 187, 188–190
Pseudomonas aeruginosa, 8

Psychologic evaluation for chemical peel, 80
Ptosis, eyebrow and eyelid, blepharoplasty for, 137
Pulmonary function tests, office
  blood gases as, 291–294
  clinical and practical aspects of, 285–294
  diffusion as, 289, 291
  flow volume curve as, 286–289
  lung compliance as, 289, 290
  spirometry as, 285–286

Radioallergosorbent test (RAST)
  immunotherapy based on, 223–224
  results of, 225–226
  modified, in allergy diagnosis and management, 215–226
  advantages of, 220
  allergen screening with, 221, 22t
  background of, 215
  inappropriate and appropriate uses of, 222
  performance of, 218
  principles of, 219t
  scoring system for, 219–220
Radiography in head and neck examination, 6
RAST. See Radioallergosorbent test
Recall listings, computer for, 319
Recovery area for outpatient surgical facility, 309
Referring physician reports, computer for, 319
Repetition rate, ABR outcome and, 239
Restrictive lung diseases, flow volume curve in, 287
Retrocochlear disorders, auditory brainstem response in, 234–235
Rhinitis
  allergic, 216–226. See also Allergic rhinitis
  vasomotor, cryosurgery for, 201
Rhinolaryngofiberscope, flexible, Olympus ENF-P, 31–33, 64
Rhinomanometry, 277–283
  anterior, 277–278
  in clinical evaluation of nasal obstruction, 279–280
  interpretation of nasal resistance measurements in, 280–282
  posterior, 278–279
Rhinoplasty, photographic projections for, 25t
Rhinosinusitis, allergic, 12
Rhomboid flap, 99–100
Rhytidectomy, cerico-facial lipo-suction with, 172–180, 181

Index

Rinne test in otologic examination, 10
Rotation flap, 98

Sad pad, lipo-suction for, 171–172
Salivary glands, palpation of, 5–6
Scalp, plastic surgery on, photographic projections for, 25t
Scalp reduction, hair transplantation and, 113–114
Scar(s)
  acne
    chemical peel for, 80
    collagen injections for, 122
  complicating chemical peel, 86
  complicating dermabrasion, 91
  complicating hair transplantation, 115
  facial, photographic projections for, 25t
  post-traumatic, collagen injections for, 123
  revision of, 93–97
    avoidance of, 93–95
    broken line geometric closure in, 97
    w-plasty in, 96
    z-plasty in, 95–96
Scheduling, office, computer for, 319
Sedation
  for chemical peel, 81
  for dermabrasion, 88
Sensorineural hearing loss, testing for, 9
Serial dilution titration technique of allergy skin testing, 208–214. *See also* Allergy, skin testing for
Seroma complicating cervical-facial lipo-suction, 182
Service analysis, computer for, 318
Sialography in head and neck examination, 6–7
Singer-Blom procedure for voice restoration, 185–187
Sinus(es)
  examination of, 12–13
  palpation of, 5
  sphenoid, 13
Sinusitis
  frontal, 13
  ethmoid, 12–13
Skin
  complications of cervical-facial lipo-suction involving, 180–181
  in head and neck examination, 4
  loss of, replacement of, with local flaps, 97–98
  malignancy of, cryosurgery for, 203–204
  pigmentation of, chemical peel and, 80
  testing of, allergy, 207–214. *See also* Allergy, skin testing for
  texture of, chemical peel and, 80
Sphenoid sinus, 13
Spirometry, 285–286
Spontenaeous nystagmus, 10
Squamous cell carcinoma of skin, cryosurgery for, 203
Storage for outpatient surgical facility, 308
Strictures, esophageal, fiberoptic esophagoscopy for, 57
Submandibular gland, palpation of, 5–6
Submental fat-pad, lipo-suction for, *155, 156,* 157–159
Surgical facility, outpatient
  accreditation of, 313–314
  alternate power in, 308
  anesthesia in, 312
  autoclave for, 310
  ceilings of, 307
  communication in, 311
  cost control in, 300–301
  designing of, 305–306
  development and management of, 295–301
    accreditation application in, 297
    case selection in, 299, 304–305
    certificate of need application in, 296
    equipment in, 298–299
    floor plan in, 298
    state license application in, 296–297
    third-party payment application in, 297
  doorways in, 306–307
  emergency equipment for, 310–311
  environmental control in, 308
  equipment for, 309–311
  floors of, 307
  lights for, 307
  medical gases in, 308
  operating room size in, 306
  operating room table in, 309–310
  patient access to, 309
  procedures for, 311–313
  procedures performed in, 299–300
  recovery area in, 309
  scheduling in, 300
  staffing, 300
  storage in, 308
  supplies and instruments for, 310
  walls of, 307

Swelling
  after face peel, 83
  complicating hair transplantation, 115

Tape
  removal of, after face peel, 83–84
  skin reactions to, complicating cervical-facial lipo-suction, 181
Telangiectasis, hemorrhagic, familial, cryosurgery for, 201
Telescopes, rigid right-angled, for videolaryngoscopy, 64–65
Telescopic videolaryngoscopy, 68, 69
  and fiberscopic videolaryngoscopy, comparison of, 65t
Tension, scarring and, 94–95
Throat, foreign, body removal from, 75
Thyroglossal duct cysts, 7
Thyroid gland, palpation of, 7–8
Transoral videolaryngoscopy, 68
Topography mapping in facial paralysis, 16
Transnasal videolaryngoscopy, 67–68
Transplant, hair, 103–117. See also Hair, transplantation of
Tufting complicating hair transplantation, 115
Tuning fork, use of, 9–10
Tympanic membrane, examination of, 8–9
Tympanosclerosis, 9

Upper airway obstruction, flow volume curve in, 288

Valium for fiberoptic esophagoscopy for, 54–55
Varices, esophageal, fiberoptic esophagoscopy, 57
Ventilation
  alveolar, carbon dixoide tensions and, 291
  regulation of, 293–294
Ventilation perfusion abnormality, 291–293
Vertigo, positional, evaluation of, 10
Vestibular testing, electronystagmography for, 247–266. See also Electronystagmography
Vestibulitis, 11

Video adaptors for videolaryngoscopy, 66
Video cameras for videolaryngoscopy, 65–66
Video recorder for videolaryngoscopy, 67
Videolaryngoscopy, 63–70
  equipment for, 64–67
  fiberscopic, 67–68, 68–69
    and telescopic, comparison of, 65t
  indications for, 69–70
  laryngoscopes for, 64–65
  light source for, 66
  recorder for, 67
  results of, 68
  technique for, 67–68
  telescopic, 68, 69
  video adaptors for, 66
  video cameras for, 65–66
Vigilon dressing for dermabrasion, 89
Vocal cords, examination of, 15
Voice restoration, 185–190
  Blaise-Raphael prosthesis for, 186, 187, 188–190
  Singer-Bloom procedure for, 185–187

Webbing complicating blepharoplasty, 147
Weber test in otologic examination, 10
Whealing in allergy skin testing, 210–211
  abnormal, 211–212
Wolf flexible Naso-pharyngo laryngoscope, 32
W-plasty in scar revision, 96
Wrinkles
  collagen injections for, 122–123
  complicating blepharoplasty, 146–147
  complicating cervical-facial lipo-suction, 180–181
  fine
    chemical peel for, 80
    dermabrasion for, 87

Xerophthalmia complicating blepharoplasty, 146

Z-plasty in scar revision, 95–96
Zyderm collagen implant, 119–124. See also Collagen injection